ATLAS OF
NORMAL HISTOLOGY

MARIANO S. H. di FIORE
Former Associate Professor of Histology and Embryology,
Faculty of Medical Sciences, University of Buenos Aires;
Former Professor and Head of Histology of the National Institute of Higher Learning;
Former Head of the Laboratory of the Juan A. Fernandez Hospital

SIXTH EDITION

Edited by

VICTOR P. EROSCHENKO, PH.D.
Professor of Anatomy
Department of Biological Sciences
and
WAMI Medical Program,
University of Idaho, Moscow, Idaho

122 ORIGINAL COLOR PLATES

231 FIGURES

Lea & Febiger　　　Philadelphia ● London

Lea & Febiger
600 Washington Square
Philadelphia, PA   19106-4198
U.S.A.
(215) 922-1330

ATLAS DE HISTOLOGIA NORMAL
Libreria "El Ateneo" Editorial
Buenos Aires, Argentina

FIRST EDITION, 1957 *Reprinted 1958, 1959, 1960, 1961, 1962*
SECOND EDITION, 1963 *Reprinted 1964, 1965*
THIRD EDITION, 1967 *Reprinted 1968, 1969, 1970, 1971, 1972, 1973*
FOURTH EDITION, 1974 *Reprinted 1975, 1976, 1977, 1978, 1979, 1980, 1981*
FIFTH EDITION, 1981 *Reprinted 1981, 1982, 1983, 1985, 1987*

Library of Congress Cataloging in Publication Data

Fiore, Mariano S. H. di.
  [Atlas de histologia normal. English]
  Atlas of normal histology / Mariano S.H. di Fiore.—
6th ed. / rev. and edited by Victor P. Eroschenko.
    p.   cm.
  Rev. translation of: Atlas de histología normal.
  Includes index.
  ISBN 0-8121-1126-5
  1. Histology—Atlases. I. Eroschenko, Victor P. II.
Title.
QM557.F5513 1988
611'.018'0222–dc19   88-21526
                         CIP

Printed in the United States of America

Print No.: 10   9   8   7   6   5   4   3   2

PREFACE

Dr. di Fiore's *Atlas of Human Histology* remains a highly popular reference source with students of histology. Since its first publication over 30 years ago, the *Atlas* has become a valuable teaching aid, not only to these students, but also to their instructors.

In revising the *Atlas* for the sixth edition, I attempted to retain and improve all the features that made it popular. The title has been changed to *Atlas of Normal Histology*. This change reflects more accurately its contents because of the numerous histologic illustrations that represent animal tissues or organs. In addition, the text contents have been edited and updated. Also, certain headings and labels have been altered in the text and the illustrations to conform with those found in contemporary textbooks of histology. Six old illustrations have been replaced with new and original drawings. These plates were prepared in my laboratory from histology slides by a medical illustrator, Ms. Amy Ruth Werner of Washington State University, Pullman, Washington.

The contents and emphasis in contemporary histology courses continue to change; however, certain basic concepts and typical histologic structures must still be learned for students to comprehend the total complexity of the living organism. This *Atlas* enhances that learning by depicting a composite of structural variations on a single illustration that would not normally be seen on a single slide. When I studied histology, I found that these composite illustrations greatly increased my confidence in understanding the "complete picture" of a particular specimen. In observing the students in my own histology classes, I find that many continue to use this book in essentially the same manner and for the same purpose. It is hoped that, with the revisions incorporated in the new edition, the *Atlas* will continue to serve students of histology and biology as a valuable supplement.

In my continuous efforts to revise and edit this *Atlas*, I welcome all comments from students and instructors who have used or are presently using the new edition. All constructive suggestions will be greatly appreciated and incorporated in the book wherever possible.

Finally, I wish to thank my former histology instructor, Dr. Robert Hunter of the School of Medicine, University of California at Davis, for recommending me to Lea & Febiger; and to acknowledge the efforts of Mr. George H. Mundorff, Mr. Thomas J. Colaiezzi, and Mr. John F. Spahr of that company in assisting me during the revision of this *Atlas*.

Victor P. Eroschenko, Ph.D.
Moscow, Idaho

PREFACE TO THE FIFTH EDITION

Dr. di Fiore's *Atlas of Human Histology* is presented as an admirable reference for the student of histology. It is not intended to supplant a textbook of histology but to be used as a supplement.

The *Atlas* consists of color plates prepared from histologic slides of tissues and organs that show reasonably typical structure. Most are stained with routine stains, others with special stains to demonstrate specific features. Principal features of each tissue and organ are clearly labeled, and are supplemented by an accompanying text. Details of structure must be acquired from textbooks of histology.

Electron micrographs have not been included in the *Atlas*. It is felt that textbooks now contain so complete a number of these, often at the expense of routinely prepared slides, that the *Atlas* serves a better purpose by presenting only the latter.

The color plates throughout all editions of the *Atlas* are from water color drawings prepared by Professor Celia M. Ishii de Sato under Dr. di Fiore's supervision. Slides for plates in the first and second editions and several new ones for the third edition were from Dr. di Fiore's laboratory. All additional ones for the third, fourth and fifth editions were contributed mainly by the Anatomy Departments of the University of Cincinnati and the University of Alabama in Birmingham, and were sent to Dr. di Fiore for processing.

The earlier editions of Dr. di Fiore's *Atlas* met with unusual success. The third, fourth and fifth editions have been revised by Dr. Ida G. Schmidt, Department of Anatomy, University of Alabama Medical Center, Birmingham. Excellent suggestions have come from many students and faculty who have used the book. Dr. Schmidt has utilized many of these in revising much of the text and improving the illustrations. For the fifth edition, the *Atlas* has been enhanced by 18 new figures in addition to the original ones and those added to the third and fourth editions. Terminology and text have been brought up to date, using *Nomina Anatomica*, fourth edition, 1977, as a guide for the former; most of this terminology has already been incorporated into current textbooks of histology. Figures and text have been revised or improved wherever necessary. The fifth edition, therefore, should be even more useful to its audience than heretofore.

We are pleased to acknowledge the efforts of Dr. Schmidt in her revisions of this *Atlas* making it more useful to students of histology. We are indeed grateful for her contributions over many years.

The sixth edition has been revised by Dr. Victor P. Eroschenko, Professor of Anatomy, Department of Biological Sciences and WAMI Medical Program, University of Idaho, Moscow, Idaho.

Lea & Febiger
Philadelphia, Pennsylvania

CONTENTS

Preface 3

Preface to the Fifth Edition 4

Index of Plates 9

Abbreviations on Plates............................. 13

TISSUES

Epithelial Tissue

Simple Squamous Epithelium 14

Simple Columnar Epithelium 16

Stratified Squamous Epithelium..................... 18

Pseudostratified Columnar Ciliated Epithelium and
    Transitional Epithelium 20

Simple Branched Tubular Gland (Diagram) 22

Compound Tubuloalveolar Gland (Diagram)....... 24

Compound Alveolar Gland (Diagram).............. 26

Connective Tissue

Loose (Irregular) Connective Tissue: Spread 28

Loose (Irregular) Connective Tissue 30

Dense Regular Connective Tissue.................... 32

Dense Irregular and Loose Connective Tissue....... 34

Cartilage 36

    Hyaline 36

    Fibrous.. 38

Bone, Mature 40

    Compact (Dried).................................. 40

    Cancellous....................................... 42

Bone, Developing.................................... 42

    Intramembranous Ossification 42

    Endochondral Ossification 44

    Formation of Bone Osteons....................... 48

    Secondary (Epiphyseal) Ossification Centers...... 50

Blood

Peripheral Blood.................................... 52

Bone Marrow 56

Muscle Tissue

Smooth and Skeletal Muscle Fibers 60

Skeletal, Smooth, and Cardiac Muscle.............. 62

Nerve Terminations in Skeletal Muscle 64

Nervous Tissue and Nervous System

Nervous Tissue: Gray Matter 66

Fibrous Astrocytes and Oligodendrocytes
    of the Brain..................................... 70

Nerve Fibers and Nerves........................... 72

Dorsal Root Ganglion 76

Spinal Cord: Cervical Region....................... 78

Spinal Cord: Mid-Thoracic Region 80

Cerebellum.. 82

Cerebral Cortex 84

ORGANS

Cardiovascular System

Blood and Lymphatic Vessels 86
Neurovascular Bundle 88
Heart: Left Atrium and Ventricle 90
Heart: Pulmonary Trunk, Pulmonary Valve,
    Right Ventricle; Purkinje Fibers 92

Lymphatic System

Lymph Node 94
Lymph Node and Palatine Tonsil 98
Thymus 100
Spleen 102

Integument

Skin 104
Sweat Gland (Diagram) 106
Scalp, Sebaceous Gland, and Hair Follicle 108
Glomus in Dermis of Thick Skin and
    Pacinian Corpuscles 110

Digestive System

Lip 112
Tongue 114
Tooth, Dried 120
Tooth, Developing 122
Salivary Glands 124
    Parotid 124
    Submandibular 126
    Sublingual 128
Esophagus 130
Cardia 136
Stomach 138
    Fundus or Body 138
    Pyloric Region 144
Pyloric-Duodenal Junction 146
Small Intestine 148
    Duodenum 148
    Jejunum-Ileum and Glands 150
    Ileum and Villi 152
Large Intestine: Colon 154
    Appendix 158
    Rectum 160
    Anal Canal 162
Liver 164
    Lobules 164
    Mitochondria, Fat Droplets, Glycogen, and
    Reticular Fibers 168
Gallbladder 170
Pancreas 172

Respiratory System

Olfactory Mucosa 174
Epiglottis 176
Larynx 178
Trachea 180
Lung 182

Urinary System

Kidney 186
    Cortex and One Pyramid 186
    Deep Cortical Area and Outer Medulla 188
Ureter 192
Urinary Bladder 194

Endocrine System

Hypophysis (Pituitary Gland) 196
Thyroid Gland 200
Thyroid and Parathyroid Glands 202
Adrenal (Suprarenal) Gland 204

Male Reproductive System

Testis, Tubules, Rete Testis, Ductuli Efferentes 206
Testis: Seminiferous Tubules........................208
Ductuli Efferentes and Ductus Epididymis 210
Ductus Deferens....................................212

Prostate Gland.......................................214
Seminal Vesicle and Bulbourethral Gland 216
Penis and Cavernous Urethra.......................218

Female Reproductive System

Ovary 220
Ovary: Ovarian Cortex, Primary and Growing
   Follicles 222
Ovary: Corpora Lutea and Follicular Atresia 224
   Corpus Luteum 226
Uterine Tube......................................228
Uterus..230
   Proliferative Phase 230
   Secretory Phase 232
   Menstrual Phase..............................234

Placenta..236
Cervix..238
Vagina..240
Vagina: Exfoliate Cytology 242
Mammary Gland.......................................244
   Inactive 244
   Seventh Month of Pregnancy and
      During Lactation 246

Organs of Special Sense and Associated Structures

Eyelid 248
Lacrimal Gland and Cornea.......................250

Eye 252
   Sagittal Section 252
   Retina, Choroid, and Sclera.....................254
Inner Ear (Cochlea)................................256

Index...259

INDEX OF PLATES

TISSUES

Epithelial Tissue

PLATE

1. Fig. 1. Simple squamous epithelium: dissociated squamous epithelial cells.......... 15
   Fig. 2. Simple squamous epithelium: surface view of peritoneal mesothelium........ 15
   Fig. 3. Simple squamous epithelium: transverse section of peritoneal mesothelium......................... 15
2. Fig. 1. Simple columnar epithelium 17
   Fig. 2. Simple columnar epithelium: cells with striated borders and goblet cells 17

PLATE

3. Fig. 1. Stratified squamous epithelium (transverse section from esophagus) 19
   Fig. 2. Stratified squamous epithelium (tangential section from esophagus)........ 19
4. Fig. 1. Pseudostratified columnar ciliated epithelium 21
   Fig. 2. Transitional epithelium 21
5. Simple branched tubular gland (diagram)...... 23
6. Compound tubuloalveolar gland (diagram) 25
7. Compound alveolar gland (diagram)........... 27

Connective Tissue

PLATE

8. Fig. 1. Loose (irregular) connective tissue: spread 29
   Fig. 2. Cells of loose connective tissue in sections 29
9. Fig. 1. Loose (irregular) connective tissue 31
   Fig. 2. Dense irregular connective tissue (dense fibroelastic connective tissue)... 31
10. Fig. 1. Dense regular connective tissue: tendon (longitudinal section).............. 33
    Fig. 2. Dense regular connective tissue: tendon (transverse section)................ 33
11. Fig. 1. Dense irregular and loose connective tissue 35
    Fig. 2. Adipose tissue 35
    Fig. 3. Embryonic connective tissue 35
12. Fig. 1. Fetal cartilage: early development of hyaline cartilage...................... 37
    Fig. 1A. Fetal cartilage: sectional view 37
    Fig. 2. Mature hyaline cartilage 37
    Fig. 3. Newly formed hyaline cartilage of the trachea............................. 37

PLATE

13. Fig. 1. Fibrous cartilage: intervertebral disc.... 39
    Fig. 2. Elastic cartilage: epiglottis.............. 39
14. Fig. 1. Compact bone, dried: diaphysis of the tibia (transverse section) 41
    Fig. 2. Compact bone, dried: diaphysis of the tibia (longitudinal section) 41
15. Fig. 1. Cancellous bone: adult sternum (transverse section, decalcified) 43
    Fig. 2. Intramembranous ossification: mandible of a five-month fetus (transverse section, decalcified) 43
16. Endochondral ossification: developing metacarpal bone (panoramic view, longitudinal section) 45
17. Endochondral ossification (sectional view) 47
18. Formation of bone: development of osteons (Haversian systems) (decalcified, transverse section) 49
19. Formation of bone: secondary (epiphyseal) ossification centers (decalcified, longitudinal section) 51

Blood

PLATE

20. Peripheral blood smear 53
21. Fig. 1. Supravital stain: blood cells 55
    Fig. 2. Pappenheim's and Celani's stains: blood smears........................ 55

PLATE

22. Fig. 1. Bone marrow of a rabbit (section)...... 57
    Fig. 2. Bone marrow of a rabbit, India ink preparation (section) 57
23. Bone marrow: smear........................... 59

Muscle Tissue

PLATE

24. Fig. 1. Smooth muscle fibers 61
    Fig. 2. Skeletal (striated) muscle fibers
            (dissociated)........................... 61
25. Fig. 1. Skeletal muscles of the tongue........ 63
    Fig. 2. Smooth muscle layers of the intestine.. 63
    Fig. 3. Cardiac muscle (myocardium).......... 63

PLATE

    Fig. 4. Skeletal muscle (longitudinal section) .. 63
    Fig. 5. Cardiac muscle (longitudinal section) .. 63
26. Fig. 1. Nerve terminations in skeletal muscle:
            muscle spindle (transverse section) 65
    Fig. 2. Nerve terminations in skeletal muscle:
            motor end plates...................... 65

Nervous Tissue and Nervous System

PLATE

27. Fig. 1. Gray matter: anterior horn of the spi-
            nal cord (Nissl's method) 67
    Fig. 2. Gray matter: anterior horn of the spi-
            nal cord (Cajal's method) 67
28. Fig. 1. Gray matter: anterior horn of the spi-
            nal cord (Golgi's method).............. 69
    Fig. 2. Gray matter: anterior horn of the spi-
            nal cord (modified Weigert-Pal's
            method)................................ 69
29. Fig. 1. Microglia: fibrous astrocytes of the
            brain 71
    Fig. 2. Microglia: oligodendrocytes of the
            brain 71
    Fig. 3. Microglia of the brain 71
30. Fig. 1. Myelinated nerve fibers (dissociated) .. 73
    Fig. 2. Nerve (transverse section) 73
31. Fig. 1. Nerve (sciatic), panoramic view, longi-
            tudinal section (hematoxylin-eosin) 75
    Fig. 2. Nerve (sciatic), longitudinal section
            (hematoxylin-eosin) 75
    Fig. 3. Nerve (sciatic), transverse section (he-
            matoxylin-eosin) 75
    Fig. 4. Nerve (sciatic), longitudinal section
            (Protargol and aniline blue)........... 75

PLATE

    Fig. 5. Nerve (sciatic), transverse section (Pro-
            targol and aniline blue) 75
    Fig. 6. Nerve (sciatic), transverse section
            (Mallory-azan) 75
32. Fig. 1. Dorsal root ganglion: panoramic view
            (longitudinal section)................. 77
    Fig. 2. Section of a dorsal root ganglion....... 77
    Fig. 3. Section of a sympathetic trunk
            ganglion 77
33. Fig. 1. Spinal cord: cervical region (panoramic
            view), transverse section.............. 79
    Fig. 2. Spinal cord: anterior gray horn and
            adjacent anterior white matter 79
34. Fig. 1. Spinal cord: mid-thoracic region (trans-
            verse section, panoramic view) 81
    Fig. 2. Nerve cells of some typical regions of
            the spinal cord....................... 81
35. Fig. 1. Cerebellum: sectional view, transverse
            section 83
    Fig. 2. Cerebellum: cortex 83
36. Fig. 1. Cerebral cortex: section perpendicular
            to the cortical surface 85
    Fig. 2. Cerebral cortex: central area of cortex.. 85

ORGANS

Cardiovascular System

PLATE

37. Fig. 1. Blood and lymphatic vessels 87
    Fig. 2. Large vein: portal vein (transverse
            section) 87
38. Fig. 1. Neurovascular bundle (transverse
            section) 89
    Fig. 2. Large artery: aorta (transverse section). 89
39. Heart: Left atrium and ventricle (panoramic
    view, longitudinal section) 91

PLATE

40. Fig. 1. Heart: pulmonary trunk, pulmonary
            valve, right ventricle (panoramic view,
            longitudinal section) 93
    Fig. 2. Heart: Purkinje fibers (impulse-con-
            ducting fibers, hematoxylin-eosin) 93
    Fig. 3. Heart: Purkinje fibers (impulse-con-
            ducting fibers, Mallory-azan).......... 93

Lymphatic System

PLATE

41. Lymph node (panoramic view) 95
42. Fig. 1. Lymph node (sectional view) 97
    Fig. 2. Lymph node: reticular fibers of the
            stroma 97
43. Fig. 1. Lymph node: proliferation of
            lymphocytes 99
    Fig. 2. Palatine tonsil........................ 99

PLATE

44. Fig. 1. Thymus: panoramic view 101
    Fig. 2. Thymus: sectional view 101
45. Fig. 1. Spleen: panoramic view................ 103
    Fig. 2. Spleen: red and white pulp 103
    Fig. 3. Development of lymphocytes and re-
            lated cells 103

Integument

PLATE

46. Fig. 1. Integument: thin skin (Cajal's trichrome stain) 105
Fig. 2. Thick skin, palm: superficial layers 105
47. Integument: sweat gland (diagram) 107
48. Fig. 1. Integument: skin (scalp) 109
Fig. 2. Sebaceous gland and adjacent hair
follicle................................. 109

PLATE

Fig. 3. Bulb of hair follicle and adjacent sweat
gland................................... 109
49. Fig. 1. Integument: glomus in the dermis of
thick skin 111
Fig. 2. Pacinian corpuscles in the deep dermis
of thick skin........................... 111

Digestive System

PLATE

50. Lip (longitudinal section) 113
51. Tongue: apex (longitudinal section, panoramic
view)... 115
52. Fig. 1. Tongue: circumvallate papilla (vertical
section) 117
Fig. 2. Taste buds 117
53. Fig. 1. Posterior tongue near circumvallate
papilla (longitudinal section)........... 119
Fig. 2. Lingual tonsils (transverse section)..... 119
54. Fig. 1. Dried tooth: panoramic view, longitudinal section 121
Fig. 2. Dried tooth: layers of the crown 121
Fig. 3. Dried tooth: layers of the root 121
55. Fig. 1. Developing tooth: panoramic view..... 123
Fig. 2. Developing tooth: sectional view....... 123
56. Salivary gland: parotid 125
57. Salivary gland: submandibular................. 127
58. Salivary gland: sublingual..................... 129
59. Upper esophagus: wall (transverse section)..... 131
60. Upper esophagus: mucosa and submucosa
(transverse section) 133
61. Fig. 1. Upper esophagus: transverse section
(Mallory's trichrome stain) 135
Fig. 2. Lower esophagus: transverse section
(Van Gieson's trichrome stain) 135
62. Cardia (longitudinal section) 137
63. Stomach: fundus or body (transverse section)... 139
64. Stomach: mucosa of the fundus or body (transverse section) 141
65. Fig. 1. Stomach: fundus or body, superficial
region of the gastric mucosa 143
Fig. 2. Deep region of the mucosa 143
66. Stomach: mucosa of the pyloric region.......... 145
67. Pyloric-duodenal junction (longitudinal
section) 147

PLATE

68. Small intestine: duodenum (longitudinal
section) 149
69. Fig. 1. Small intestine: jejunum-ileum (transverse section) 151
Fig. 2. Intestinal glands with Paneth cells..... 151
Fig. 3. Intestinal glands with enteroendocrine
cells................................... 151
70. Fig. 1. Small intestine: ileum with aggregated
nodules (Peyer's patch), transverse
section 153
Fig. 2. Small intestine: villi 153
71. Large intestine: colon (panoramic view, transverse section) and mesentery 155
72. Large intestine: colon (wall, transverse section) 157
73. Appendix (panoramic view, transverse section) 159
74. Rectum: panoramic view, transverse section 161
75. Anal canal (longitudinal section)............... 163
76. Liver lobule (panoramic view, transverse
section) 165
77. Fig. 1. Liver lobule (sectional view, transverse
section) 167
Fig. 2. Liver: Kupffer cells (India ink
preparation)........................... 167
Fig. 3. Liver: bile canaliculi (osmic acid
preparation)........................... 167
78. Fig. 1. Mitochondria and fat droplets in liver
cells (Altmann's stain) 169
Fig. 2. Glycogen in liver cells (Best's carmine
stain).................................. 169
Fig. 3. Reticular fibers in a hepatic lobule (Del
Rio Hortega's stain) 169
79. Gallbladder 171
80. Fig. 1. Pancreas (sectional view)............... 173
Fig. 2. Pancreatic acini (special preparation)... 173
Fig. 3. Pancreatic islets (special preparation) .. 173

Respiratory System

PLATE

81. Fig. 1. Olfactory mucosa and superior concha,
Rhesus monkey (general view)......... 175
Fig. 2. Olfactory mucosa: Detail of a transition
area 175
82. Epiglottis (longitudinal section) 177
83. Larynx (frontal section) 177
84. Fig. 1. Trachea: panoramic view, transverse
section 181

PLATE

Fig. 2. Trachea: sectional view 181
Fig. 3. Trachea: sectional view (elastin stain) .. 181
85. Lung (panoramic view) 183
86. Fig. 1. Lung: intrapulmonary bronchus 185
Fig. 2. Lung: terminal bronchiole.............. 185
Fig. 3. Lung: respiratory bronchiole........... 185
Fig. 4. Lung: alveolar walls (interalveolar
septa) 185

Urinary System

PLATE

87. Kidney: cortex and one pyramid (panoramic view)............................... 187
88. Fig. 1. Kidney: deep cortical area and outer medulla 189
    Fig. 2. Kidney cortex: the juxtaglomerular apparatus 189
89. Fig. 1. Kidney medulla: papilla (transverse section) 191

PLATE

Fig. 2. Kidney medulla: papilla adjacent to a calyx (longitudinal section)............. 191
90. Fig. 1. Ureter: transverse section 193
    Fig. 2. Ureter wall: transverse section 193
91. Fig. 1. Urinary bladder, superior surface: wall (transverse section) 195
    Fig. 2. Urinary bladder: mucosa.............. 195

Endocrine System

PLATE

92. Fig. 1. Hypophysis (pituitary gland): panoramic view, sagittal section............. 197
    Fig. 2. Hypophysis (pituitary gland): sectional view 197
93. Fig. 1. Hypophysis: pars distalis (azan stain) 199
    Fig. 2. Hypophysis: cell groups (azan stain)... 199

PLATE

94. Fig. 1. Thyroid gland: general view 201
    Fig. 2. Thyroid gland: follicles (sectional view) 201
    Fig. 3. Thyroid gland: parafollicular cells...... 201
95. Fig. 1. Thyroid and parathyroid glands 203
    Fig. 2. Parathyroid gland..................... 203
96. Adrenal (suprarenal) gland 205

Male Reproductive System

PLATE

97. Fig. 1. Testis 207
    Fig. 2. Seminiferous tubules, straight tubules, rete testis and ductuli efferentes (efferent ducts) 207
98. Testis: seminiferous tubules (transverse section) 209
99. Fig. 1. Ductuli efferentes and transition to ductus epididymis 211
    Fig. 2. Ductus epididymis................... 211

PLATE

100. Fig. 1. Ductus deferens (transverse section)... 213
     Fig. 2. Ampulla of the ductus deferens (transverse section) 213
101. Fig. 1. Prostate gland with prostatic urethra .. 215
     Fig. 2. Prostate gland (sectional view)........ 215
102. Fig. 1. Seminal vesicle........................ 217
     Fig. 2. Bulbourethral gland................... 217
103. Fig. 1. Penis (transverse section) 219
     Fig. 2. Cavernous urethra (transverse section) 219

Female Reproductive System

PLATE

104. Ovary: panoramic view 221
105. Fig. 1. Ovary: ovarian cortex, primary and growing follicles 223
     Fig. 2. Ovary: wall of a mature follicle 223
106. Ovary: corpora lutea and follicular atresia (human ovary).. 225
107. Fig. 1. Corpus luteum: panoramic view 227
     Fig. 2. Corpus luteum: peripheral wall........ 227
108. Fig. 1. Uterine tube: ampulla (panoramic view, transverse section) 229
     Fig. 2. Uterine tube: mucosal folds (early proliferative phase) 229
     Fig. 3. Uterine tube: mucosal folds (early pregnancy) 229
109. Uterus: proliferative (follicular) phase........... 231
110. Uterus: secretory (luteal) phase 233
111. Uterus: menstrual phase 235
112. Fig. 1. Placenta: five months' pregnancy (panoramic view) 237
     Fig. 2. Placenta: chorionic villi (placenta at five months) 237

PLATE

Fig. 3. Placenta: chorionic villi (placenta at term)................................. 237
113. Cervix: longitudinal section 239
114. Fig. 1. Vagina: longitudinal section........... 241
     Fig. 2. Glycogen in human vaginal epithelium 241
115. Vagina: exfoliate cytology (vaginal smears) 243
     Fig. 1. Post-menstrual phase, 5th day of menstrual cycle........................... 243
     Fig. 2. Ovulatory phase, 14th day............. 243
     Fig. 3. Luteal phase, 21st day 243
     Fig. 4. Premenstrual phase, 28th day......... 243
     Fig. 5. Three months' pregnancy............. 243
     Fig. 6. Menopause, atrophic phase........... 243
     Fig. 7. Types of cells found in vaginal smears of a normal cycle..................... 243
116. Fig. 1. Mammary gland, inactive............. 245
     Fig. 2. Mammary gland during the first half of pregnancy......................... 245
117. Fig. 1. Mammary gland, seventh month of pregnancy........................... 247
     Fig. 2. Mammary gland during lactation 247

Organs of Special Sense and
Associated Structures

PLATE

118. Eyelid (sagittal section)..........................249

119. Fig. 1.   Lacrimal gland 251

Fig. 2.   Cornea (transverse section) 251

120. Eye (sagittal section) 253

121. Fig. 1.   Retina, choroid, and sclera: panoramic
view 255

PLATE

Fig. 2.   Layers of the retina and choroid in
detail.................................. 255

122. Fig. 1.   Inner ear: cochlea (vertical section)..... 257

Fig. 2.   Inner ear: cochlear duct (scala media).. 257

ABBREVIATIONS ON PLATES

h.s.—horizontal section
l.s.—longitudinal section
o.s.—oblique section
tg. s.—tangential section
t.s.—transverse section
v.s.—vertical section

Epithelial Tissue

PLATE 1 (Fig. 1)

SIMPLE SQUAMOUS EPITHELIUM:
DISSOCIATED SQUAMOUS EPITHELIAL CELLS

Illustrated is a "fresh" preparation of dissociated squamous epithelial cells obtained by scraping the superficial layers of the oral cavity. The cells are seen as either isolated (1, 6), or in sheets (2) in which the cells remain firmly attached to each other.

In surface view, the squamous cells exhibit irregular polygonal shape (1, 6) and distinct cell membranes (3). Their cytoplasm is finely granular (4) and the round or oval nuclei (5) have either a cental or an eccentric position (8) in the cell. In lateral view (7), the squamous cells are thin and spindle-shaped with thin, rod-like nuclei.

PLATE 1 (Fig. 2)

SIMPLE SQUAMOUS EPITHELIUM:
SURFACE VIEW OF PERITONEAL MESOTHELIUM

To visualize the surface of the simple epithelium, a small piece of mesentery was fixed and stained with silver nitrate and counterstained with hematoxylin. The cells of the simple epithelium (mesothelium) are flat, adhere tightly to each other, and form a sheet of a single cell layer in thickness. The irregular cell boundaries (1) appear highly visible as a result of silver deposition and form a characteristic mosaic pattern. The blue-gray cell nuclei (2) are usually centrally located within the yellow- to brown-stained cytoplasm (3).

Simple squamous epithelium is common in the body. It is often found lining the surfaces that allow passive transport of gases or fluids as well as lining the pleural, pericardial, and peritoneal cavities.

PLATE 1 (Fig. 3)

SIMPLE SQUAMOUS EPITHELIUM:
TRANSVERSE SECTION OF PERITONEAL MESOTHELIUM

Illustrated is a simple squamous epithelium, the mesothelium, seen in a transverse section as it covers the wall of the jejunum. The cells are spindle-shaped with prominent, oval nuclei (1). Cell boundaries are not seen distinctly but are indicated at cell junctions (2). A fine basement membrane is recognizable under the mesothelium (3). In surface view, the cells appear similar to those illustrated in Figure 2.

Mesothelium (1) and the underlying layer of connective tissue (4) form the serosa of the peritoneal cavity, the outermost layer of the jejunal wall. Serosa is attached to the muscularis externa, which consists of smooth muscle fibers (6). In the connective tissue layer are seen small blood vessels, lined by a simple squamous epithelium, the endothelium (5).

PLATE 1

EPITHELIAL TISSUE

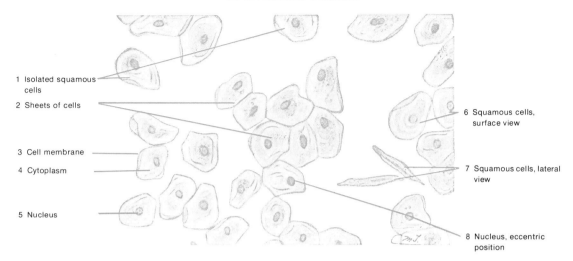

1 Isolated squamous cells

2 Sheets of cells

3 Cell membrane

4 Cytoplasm

5 Nucleus

6 Squamous cells, surface view

7 Squamous cells, lateral view

8 Nucleus, eccentric position

Fig. 1.   *Simple squamous epithelium. Dissociated squamous epithelial cells. Observed in the fresh state. 110×.*

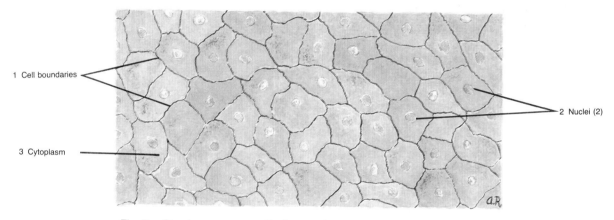

1 Cell boundaries

2 Nuclei (2)

3 Cytoplasm

Fig. 2.   *Simple squamous epithelium: surface view of peritoneal mesothelium.*
Stain: silver nitrate with hematoxylin.

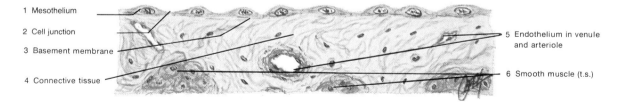

1 Mesothelium

2 Cell junction

3 Basement membrane

4 Connective tissue

5 Endothelium in venule and arteriole

6 Smooth muscle (t.s.)

Fig. 3.   *Simple squamous epithelium: transverse section of peritoneal mesothelium.*
Stain: hematoxylin-eosin: 500×.

PLATE 2 (Fig. 1)

SIMPLE COLUMNAR EPITHELIUM

A simple columnar epithelium which lines the surface of the stomach is illustrated.

The tall columnar cells (2) are arranged in a single row. The ovoid nuclei (7) with perpendicular orientation in the cells are located in the basal region. A thin, barely visible basement membrane (3) separates the epithelium from the underlying connective tissue layer (4, 10), the lamina propria of the gastric mucosa. Small blood vessels (5) lined with endothelium are seen in the connective tissue.

In some areas the epithelium has been sectioned transversely or obliquely. Where a plane of section passes close to the free surface of the epithelium, the sectioned apical regions of these cells resemble a mosaic of enucleated polygonal cells (1). Where a plane of section passes through basal regions of the epithelial cells, the nuclei are cut transversely and resemble a stratified epithelium (6).

The columnar, surface cells of the stomach secrete mucus. The light appearance of the cell cytoplasm is due to the routine preparation of the tissues. The mucigen droplets that filled these cell apices (9) were lost during section preparation. The more granular cytoplasm exhibits a basal location (8) and stains more acidophilic.

Examples of other columnar epithelia may be seen in the lining of the gallbladder (see Plate 79:14); in certain salivary gland ducts (see Plate 56:6, 14, IV; Plate 57: 1, 7, III); in bile ducts of the liver (see Plate 77, Fig. 1:7, 14); and in interlobular ducts of the pancreas (see Plate 80, Fig. 1:19, III).

A simple cuboidal epithelium is illustrated in the smallest ducts of the pancreas (see Plate 80, Fig. 1:1, 5, 20, II) and in the follicles of the thyroid gland (see Plate 94, Fig. 1:5 and Fig. 2:2).

PLATE 2 (Fig. 2)

SIMPLE COLUMNAR EPITHELIUM:
CELLS WITH STRIATED BORDERS AND GOBLET CELLS

Free ends of intestinal villi (1) illustrate simple columnar epithelium with two types of cells: columnar cells with striated border (2, 14) and goblet cells (8, 12). Striated border (13) is seen as a reddish outer membrane with faint vertical striations representing the microvilli on the apices of the columnar cells. In an area of contiguous cells, the striated border appears continuous. Cytoplasm of these cells is finely granular and the oval nuclei are located in the basal portions of the cells.

Goblet cells (8, 12) are interspersed among the columnar cells. During routine histological preparation, the mucus was lost and the goblet cell cytoplasm appears clear or only lightly stained (12). Normally, the mucigen droplets occupy the apical portion of the cell while the nucleus is in the basal cytoplasm (8).

The epithelium at the tip of the villus in the lower center of the figure has been sectioned at an oblique angle. The apices of the columnar cells appear as a mosaic (7) of enucleated cells, while the basal regions, where the plane of section passes through the nuclei, appear stratified (7).

The basement membrane (5) is slightly more visible than in Figure 1. In the connective tissue (the lamina propria) (10) are seen a lymphatic vessel, the central lacteal (3), a capillary (9) lined with endothelium, and smooth muscle fibers (4, 11) as either single fibers or small groups of fibers.

Other examples of cells with striated borders and goblet cells may be seen in a section of jejunum-ileum (see Plate 69, Fig. 2:1, 2 and, unlabeled, in Fig. 3).

PLATE 2

EPITHELIAL TISSUE

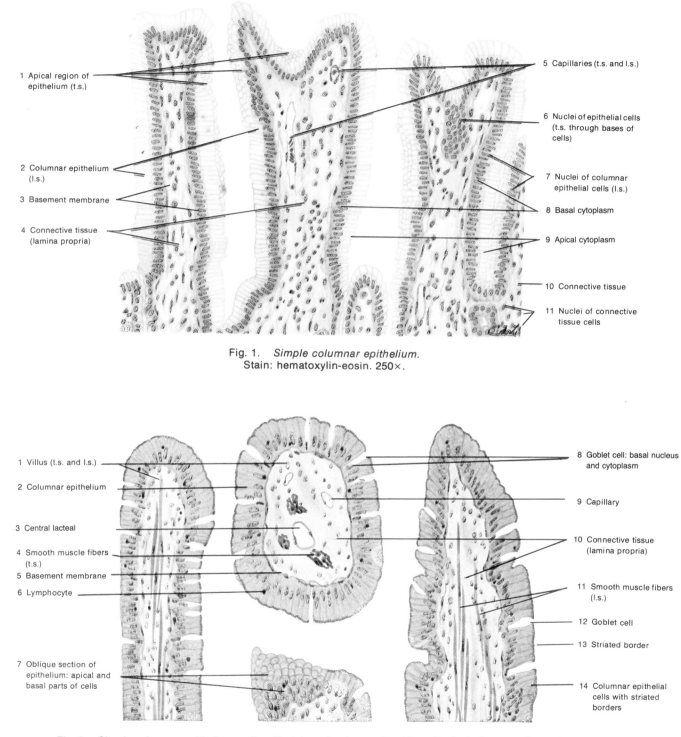

1 Apical region of epithelium (t.s.)

2 Columnar epithelium (l.s.)

3 Basement membrane

4 Connective tissue (lamina propria)

5 Capillaries (t.s. and l.s.)

6 Nuclei of epithelial cells (t.s. through bases of cells)

7 Nuclei of columnar epithelial cells (l.s.)

8 Basal cytoplasm

9 Apical cytoplasm

10 Connective tissue

11 Nuclei of connective tissue cells

Fig. 1. *Simple columnar epithelium.*
Stain: hematoxylin-eosin. 250×.

1 Villus (t.s. and l.s.)

2 Columnar epithelium

3 Central lacteal

4 Smooth muscle fibers (t.s.)

5 Basement membrane

6 Lymphocyte

7 Oblique section of epithelium: apical and basal parts of cells

8 Goblet cell: basal nucleus and cytoplasm

9 Capillary

10 Connective tissue (lamina propria)

11 Smooth muscle fibers (l.s.)

12 Goblet cell

13 Striated border

14 Columnar epithelial cells with striated borders

Fig. 2. *Simple columnar epithelium: cells with striated borders and goblet cells.* Stain: hematoxylin-eosin. 250 ×.

PLATE 3 (Fig. 1)

STRATIFIED SQUAMOUS EPITHELIUM
(TRANSVERSE SECTION FROM ESOPHAGUS)

The stratified squamous epithelium is composed of numerous layers of cells exhibiting a characteristic structure and arrangement. The thickness of this type of epithelium varies in different regions of the body and, as a result, the cell arrangement is altered.

Illustrated in this figure is an example of a moist type of epithelium (1) that lines the oral cavity and the esophagus. The cells in the basal layer are cuboidal or low columnar (5). The cytoplasm is finely granular and the oval nucleus, rich in chromatin, occupies most of the cell.

The cells in the intermediate layers are polyhedral (4) with round or oval nuclei and more visible cell membranes. Mitotic activity (7) can be frequently observed in the cells of the deeper layers and the basal cells.

Above the polyhedral cells in the intermediate layer are several rows of squamous cells (3). Cells and nuclei progressively flatten as the cells migrate toward the free surface.

A fine basement membrane (8), barely visible, separates the epithelium (1) from the underlying connective tissue (2), the lamina propria. Papillae of connective tissue (12) indent the lower surface of the epithelium, giving it a characteristic wavy appearance. The connective tissue contains collagen fibers (11), the connective tissue cells, the fibroblasts (10), and small blood vessels (6, 9, 13, 14).

Other examples of moist stratified squamous epithelium may be seen on Plates 52, 59, 60, 113, and 114.

When the stratified squamous epithelium is exposed to increased wear and tear, the outermost layer, the stratum corneum, becomes very thick and consists of non-nucleated cornified (keratinized) cells, as illustrated in the epidermis of the palm on Plate 46, Fig. 2.

An example of thin, stratified squamous epithelium without connective tissue papillae indentations is illustrated in the cornea of the eye, Plate 119, Fig. 2; the surface underlying the epithelium is smooth. This type of epithelium is only a few cell layers thick but shows the characteristic arrangement of basal columnar, polyhedral, and squamous cells, the most superficial cells on the cornea.

PLATE 3 (Fig. 2)

STRATIFIED SQUAMOUS EPITHELIUM
(TANGENTIAL SECTION FROM ESOPHAGUS)

A section made parallel to the surface of the epithelium at line a-a in Figure 1 passes through several epithelial downgrowths and their connective tissue papillae, both of which are seen in transverse sections.

In the connective tissue papillae (1, 5, 8) are seen collagen fibers, fibroblasts (3), and capillaries (2, 4). Basal cells of the epithelium (6) surround the papillae, while the polyhedral cells (7) of the intermediate layers occupy the remaining area.

PLATE 3

EPITHELIAL TISSUE

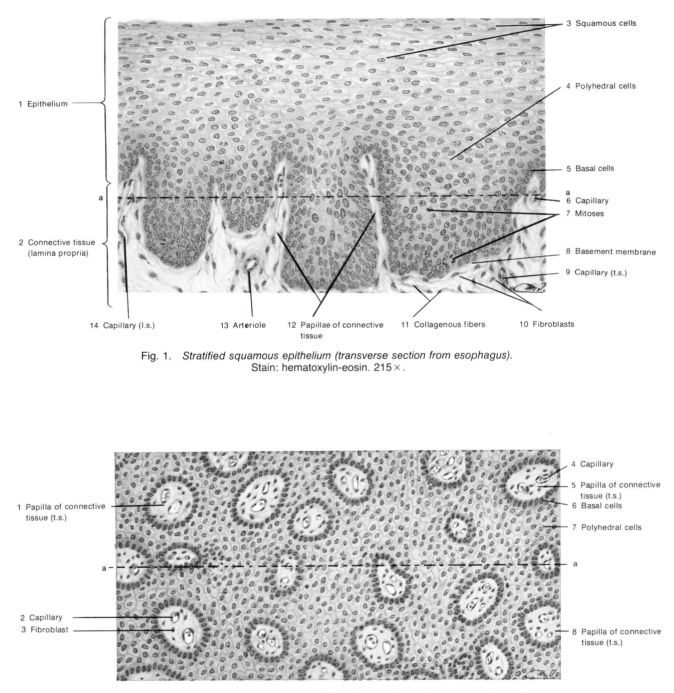

Fig. 1. *Stratified squamous epithelium (transverse section from esophagus).*
Stain: hematoxylin-eosin. 215×.

Fig. 2. *Stratified squamous epithelium (tangential section from esophagus).*
Stain: hematoxylin-eosin. 215×.

PLATE 4 (Fig. 1)

PSEUDOSTRATIFIED COLUMNAR CILIATED EPITHELIUM

The illustrated epithelium is from the upper respiratory passages of such organs as the trachea and bronchi. In this type of epithelium, the cells appear to be located in several layers because their nuclei are situated at different levels. Serial sections show that all cells are in contact with the basement membrane; however, since the cells are of different shapes and heights, not all reach the surface. For this reason, the epithelium is considered pseudostratified instead of stratified.

The more deeply placed nuclei belong to short basal cells (7) and intermediate cells. The more superficial, oval nuclei belong to the columnar ciliated cells (5). Interspersed among these cells are goblet cells (6). The small, round, heavily stained nuclei with no visible surrounding cytoplasm are those of lymphocytes (9) migrating from the connective tissue through the epithelium.

The short, motile cilia (3) are numerous and spaced close together at the cell apices. Each cilium arises from a basal body (4) which is identical to the centriole. The basal bodies are located beneath the surface membrane of the cell and adjacent to each other, and often give the appearance of a continuous membrane (4).

The basement membrane (8) is clearly visible, separating the surface epithelium (1) from the underlying connective tissue of the lamina propria (2, 11). It is thick and prominent, in contrast to the very thin basement membrane seen under other epithelia.

In the connective tissue (11) are seen the collagen fibers, cells (fibroblasts), scattered lymphocytes, and small blood vessels (10). Deeper in the connective tissue is found the glandular epithelium in the form of serous (12) and mucous alveoli (13).

Other examples of pseudostratified columnar ciliated epithelium are seen on Plate 83:14 and Plate 84, Fig. 1:13 and Fig. 2:5, 6.

PLATE 4 (Fig. 2)

TRANSITIONAL EPITHELIUM

Transitional epithelium (1) is found exclusively in the excretory passages of the urinary system. This epithelium is stratified and composed of several layers of generally similar cells (4, 5, 6) which are usually cuboidal with round nuclei. This similarity in cell morphology differentiates this epithelium from the stratified squamous epithelium (which it may resemble during different functional states), in which the cells of various layers exhibit different shapes.

This epithelium (1) has the ability to rearrange the number of cell layers, depending on whether it is in a distended or contracted state. When the epithelium is in a contracted state, the cells may be cuboidal or even columnar (4, 5, 6) and the epithelium exhibits numerous layers. When the epithelium is distended, the number of cell layers is normally reduced. The cells in the outer layers are then more elongated or flattened, but not to the degree seen in typically squamous epithelium. (Compare this transitional epithelium with stratified squamous epithelium of the cornea, Plate 119, Fig. 2).

Transitional epithelium (1) rests on a connective tissue (2, 8) base; between the epithelium and the connective tissue is a thin basement membrane. The base of the epithelium is not indented by connective tissue papillae and therefore presents an even contour. Small blood vessels (9, 10, 11) are present in the connective tissue. Deeper in the connective tissue are groups of smooth muscle fibers (12), which indicate a layer of smooth muscle.

Other examples of transitional epithelium are seen in both figures in Plates 90 and 91.

PLATE 4

EPITHELIAL TISSUE

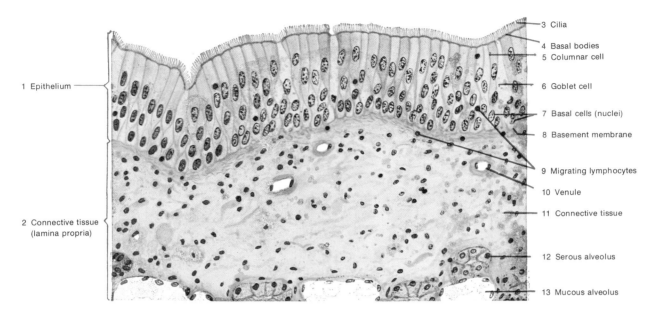

3 Cilia
4 Basal bodies
5 Columnar cell
6 Goblet cell
7 Basal cells (nuclei)
8 Basement membrane
9 Migrating lymphocytes
10 Venule
11 Connective tissue
12 Serous alveolus
13 Mucous alveolus

1 Epithelium

2 Connective tissue
(lamina propria)

Fig. 1.   *Pseudostratified columnar ciliated epithelium.*
Stain: hematoxylin-eosin. 330×.

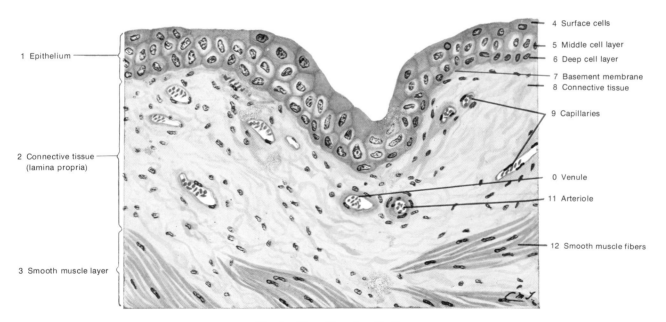

4 Surface cells
5 Middle cell layer
6 Deep cell layer
7 Basement membrane
8 Connective tissue
9 Capillaries
0 Venule
11 Arteriole
12 Smooth muscle fibers

1 Epithelium

2 Connective tissue
(lamina propria)

3 Smooth muscle layer

Fig. 2.   *Transitional epithelium.*
Stain: hematoxylin-eosin. 300×.

PLATE 5

SIMPLE BRANCHED TUBULAR GLAND (DIAGRAM)

In the center of the plate is a diagram of a simple branched tubular gland consisting of a long duct (2) and a branched terminal secretory portion of 4 tubules (3) arising from the basal portion of the duct. The diagram illustrates the general structure of a gland of this type; however, there are also variations in different glands.

The duct (2) is lined with simple low columnar epithelium with oval nuclei located basally in the cells; the duct opens onto an epithelial surface of similar cells (1). The low columnar epithelium in the duct decreases in height toward the secretory portion of the gland. The glandular epithelium (3) is low columnar to cuboidal and the nuclei are flattened at the base of the cells, indicating that the cells are filled with secretion.

The diagram in the center illustrates the appearance of sections resulting from cuts passing at different angles through various parts of the gland.

At A, the section was taken at the level of blue line a-a', which passes through the nuclear region of the surface epithelial cells in a plane parallel to the surface. In the center of the section is the orifice or opening of the gland with its wall of low columnar cells (A-1). Surrounding this area are transverse sections of the surface epithelial cell (A-2).

B represents a sagittal section of the same gland along the vertical red line b-b', which extends through the entire length of the gland. At B-1, the plane of section passes through the surface epithelium and tangentially through the wall of the duct. As a result, the lumen is not seen and the duct wall appears as a solid column of stratified epithelium. The next plane of section passes through the lumen of the duct (B-2) and the lumen of one of the secretory tubules (B-3). At the bottom of the gland, the plane of section passes transversely through the curved basal portion of the adjacent secretory tubule (B-4), which is seen as a circular structure with central lumen surrounded by pyramid-shaped cells.

C represents an oblique section through the duct along the blue line c-c'; the lumen has an elliptical shape (C-1). At both ends of the section, the epithelium has a mosaic appearance (C-2) because the oblique plane of section passed through both nucleated and non-nucleated regions of the duct cells.

D represents a sagittal section through the wall of one of the secretory tubules along the blue line d-d'. As a result, the section appears as a solid mass of cells.

E represents an oblique (E-1) and a transverse (E-2) plane of section through the lumen and wall of a secretory tubule along blue line e-e'.

F illustrates transverse planes of sections through three tubules along the red line f-f'. Each tubule shows a central lumen surrounded by cuboidal or pyramidal cells.

G represents a portion of a secretory tubule sectioned longitudinally along blue line g-g'. The plane passes through the lumen of the tubule except in the upper region where the wall was sectioned at an oblique angle.

EXAMPLES

There are probably no tubular glands in the human body that have the exact structure represented in the general diagram; however, tubular glands with similar variations occur in several locations in the body.

Unbranched simple tubular glands without ducts are represented by the intestinal glands (crypts of Lieberkühn) of the large intestine (Plate 72:20) and rectum (Plate 75:7). The glands are lined with goblet cells and columnar cells that exhibit striated borders.

Similar shorter intestinal glands are found in the small intestine (Plate 69, Fig. 1:3). These glands also contain goblet cells and cells with striated borders. In addition, cells in the bottom of the glands (Paneth cells) are specialized for enzymatic secretion (Plate 69, Fig. 2).

The simple or slightly branched tubular gastric glands, without ducts, are lined with different, modified columnar cells that are highly specialized for secreting hydrochloric acid and the precursor for the proteolytic enzyme pepsin (Plate 64:4, 15-17). The pyloric glands, in contrast, are coiled tubular glands; their columnar cells secrete mucus and are, therefore, lightly stained (Plate 66:5, 14).

A coiled tubular gland with a long, unbranched duct is a sweat gland, illustrated in Plate 47.

The highly branched tubular glands, lined with mucus-secreting columnar cells, are found in the cervix (Plate 113:2); a narrow constricted portion of the gland serves as a duct.

PLATE 5

SIMPLE BRANCHED TUBULAR GLAND (DIAGRAM)

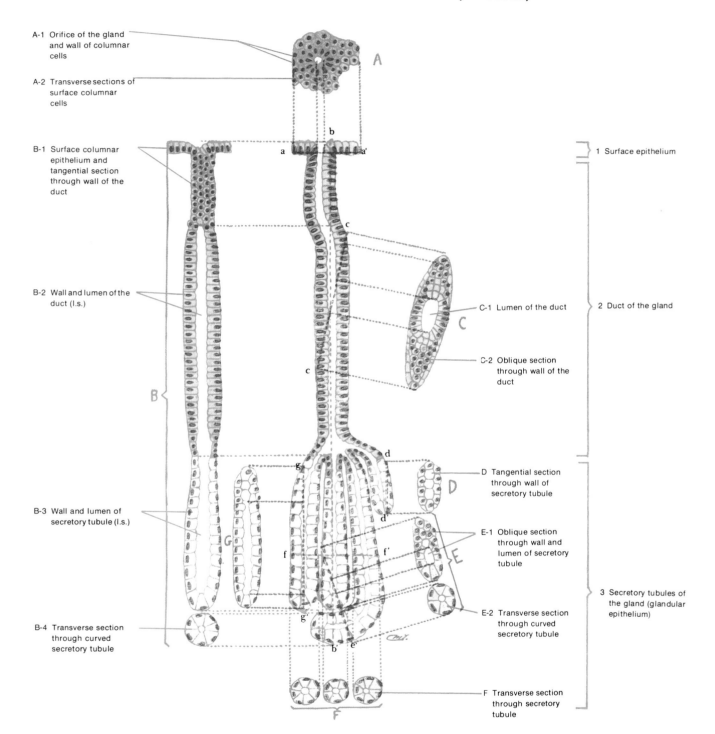

A-1 Orifice of the gland and wall of columnar cells

A-2 Transverse sections of surface columnar cells

B-1 Surface columnar epithelium and tangential section through wall of the duct

B-2 Wall and lumen of the duct (l.s.)

B-3 Wall and lumen of secretory tubule (l.s.)

B-4 Transverse section through curved secretory tubule

1 Surface epithelium

C-1 Lumen of the duct

C-2 Oblique section through wall of the duct

2 Duct of the gland

D Tangential section through wall of secretory tubule

E-1 Oblique section through wall and lumen of secretory tubule

E-2 Transverse section through curved secretory tubule

F Transverse section through secretory tubule

3 Secretory tubules of the gland (glandular epithelium)

PLATE 6

COMPOUND TUBULOALVEOLAR GLAND (DIAGRAM)

This diagram illustrates a general type of gland that is associated with the oral cavity, some parts of the digestive system, and the respiratory system. A large excretory duct (A-1) opens onto an epithelial surface (not indicated in the diagram). The duct divides or gives off successively smaller ducts (A-5, A-6) as it descends toward the secretory portion of the gland. At the terminal portion of the gland are round or elongated secretory units (alveoli) with small lumina surrounded by pyramidal or columnar cells.

Illustrated in this figure is the general structure of ducts and secretory units and their appearance when sectioned in various planes.

A illustrates the appearance of sections when the red line a-a' passes obliquely (A-2) through a large duct (A-1) and transversely through two small ducts (A-3) and two alveoli (A-4).

At B are illustrated sections of small ducts (B-1, B-3) and alveoli (B-2, B-4) when the red line b-b' passes through them in transverse or oblique planes.

At C-1 are sections when the blue line c-c' passes through different parts of two alveoli. Because these alveoli are round units, both sections appear similar. At C-2, the same blue line passes longitudinally through two small ducts and the lumen of an alveolus which opens into the smallest duct.

EXAMPLES

The major salivary glands are of this type (Plates 56, 57, 58), composed of masses of alveoli and ducts of various sizes. The salivary glands illustrate two major types of secretory alveoli: serous and mucous alveoli. Serous alveoli are described in detail on page 124 and are present in glands illustrated in Plates 56, 57, and 58. Mucous alveoli are described and compared with serous alveoli on page 126; they are illustrated in Plates 57 and 58. Ducts are distinct structures; they are lined with cuboidal, columnar, or stratified epithelium, and are named according to their location in the gland.

A less complex tubuloalveolar gland, consisting of mucous alveoli and ducts, is illustrated in Plate 59:11, 12 (esophageal glands). Similar glands consisting of ducts, mucous alveoli, and serous alveoli are found in the connective tissue of the trachea (Plate 84).

PLATE 6

COMPOUND TUBULOALVEOLAR GLAND (DIAGRAM)

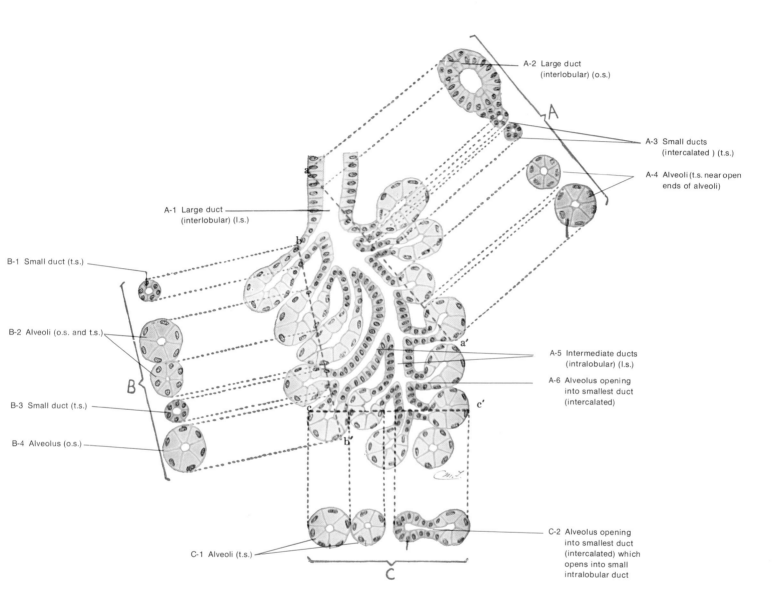

A-2 Large duct
(interlobular) (o.s.)

A-3 Small ducts
(intercalated) (t.s.)

A-4 Alveoli (t.s. near open
ends of alveoli)

A-1 Large duct
(interlobular) (l.s.)

B-1 Small duct (t.s.)

B-2 Alveoli (o.s. and t.s.)

A-5 Intermediate ducts
(intralobular) (l.s.)

A-6 Alveolus opening
into smallest duct
(intercalated)

B-3 Small duct (t.s.)

B-4 Alveolus (o.s.)

C-2 Alveolus opening
into smallest duct
(intercalated) which
opens into small
intralobular duct

C-1 Alveoli (t.s.)

PLATE 7

COMPOUND ALVEOLAR GLAND (DIAGRAM)

This is a representative illustration of a gland similar to the mammary gland. The terminal secretory units are the alveoli. In an active gland, the alveoli are large rounded sacs with large central lumina surrounded by cuboidal or low columnar cells (4, 6, 7); the alveoli may branch (1).

As described previously, the alveoli open into small ducts (2, 3) which are lined with low columnar cells. The small ducts then open into successively larger ducts (1, 5). The final excretory duct, which is even larger, is not illustrated in the diagram.

The blue line a-a' and the red line b-b' pass through the alveoli and ducts at different planes of section. The resulting appearances of such sections are shown at A and B.

EXAMPLES

The mammary gland, a good example of this type of gland, is illustrated in Plates 116 and 117. The secretory alveoli with large lumina are illustrated in the active stage (Plate 117, Fig. 2).

PLATE 7

COMPOUND ALVEOLAR GLAND (DIAGRAM)

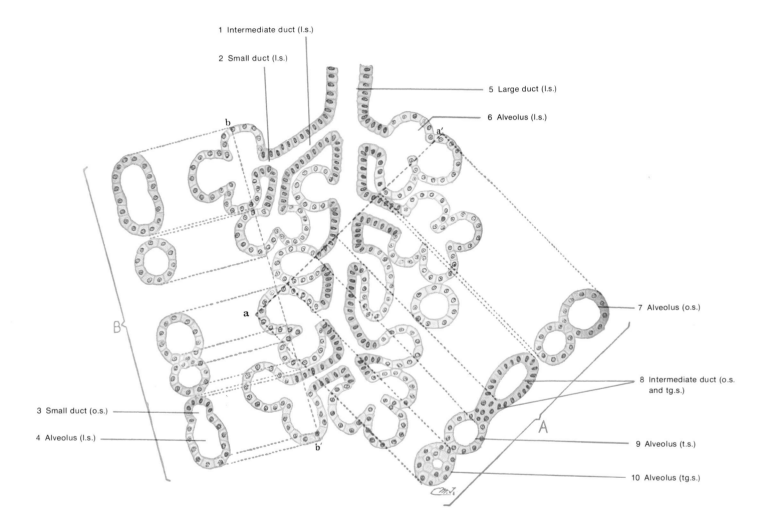

1 Intermediate duct (l.s.)

2 Small duct (l.s.)

5 Large duct (l.s.)

6 Alveolus (l.s.)

7 Alveolus (o.s.)

3 Small duct (o.s.)

4 Alveolus (l.s.)

8 Intermediate duct (o.s. and tg.s.)

9 Alveolus (t.s.)

10 Alveolus (tg.s.)

PLATE 8 (Fig. 1)

LOOSE (IRREGULAR) CONNECTIVE TISSUE: SPREAD

The plate illustrates subcutaneous connective tissue from a rat, stained by injection of a dilute solution of neutral red in saline. This solution not only permits the tissue elements to remain in their natural state but also separates them farther than would be seen under normal conditions or when they are prepared in histological sections. Under this condition, fibers and cells may be readily identified.

The unstained collagenous fibers are the most numerous and largest (2, 9). These fibers course in all directions, are thick and somewhat wavy, and exhibit faint longitudinal striations (parts of their component fibrils).

Elastic fibers are fine, single fibers (1, 10) which are usually straight; however, after the section is cut, the fibers may be wavy due to release of tension. Elastic fibers form branching and anastomosing networks. Although unstained, the fibers are highly refringent, in contrast to the dull appearance of collagenous fibers. The fine reticular fibers are also present in loose connective tissue, but are not seen in the illustration.

The fixed permanent cells of this and other connective tissue proper are fibroblasts (8, I). In this preparation, they are illustrated as flattened, branching cells with an oval nucleus in which chromatin is sparse (8) but one or two nucleoli may be present (1:14, 15). Fixed macrophages or histiocytes (4, 11, II) are always present in varying numbers. When inactive, the macrophages have an appearance like that of fibroblasts, although their processes may be more irregular and their nuclei smaller. Phagocytic inclusions, however, give their cytoplasm a varied appearance. In the illustration, the phagocytic vacuoles in the cytoplasm are filled with neutral red (small vacuoles in 4, larger vacuoles in 11 and II:17).

Mast cells (7, III) are a usual component of loose connective tissue, seen either singly or grouped along small blood vessels (7). The cells are usually ovoid, with small, pale, centrally placed nuclei (18) and cytoplasm filled with fine, closely packed granules which are stained deep red with neutral red stain (7, 19).

Present also are groups of adipose cells (fat cells) (3). Each cell is a spherical, colorless globule; the small, eccentric nucleus is not visible.

Blood and other connective tissue cells may be present in small numbers. These cells are not stained with neutral red; however, eosinophils (5) may be identified by lobulated nucleus and coarse, cytoplasmic granules. In the small round lymphocytes (6), the nucleus occupies most of the cell.

The faint background stain is the ground substance, which has been infiltrated with injected fluid.

PLATE 8 (Fig. 2)

CELLS OF LOOSE CONNECTIVE TISSUE IN SECTIONS

This figure illustrates some cells of loose connective tissue as they appear in histologic sections after fixation and hematoxylin-eosin staining.

Free macrophages (1) usually appear round with slightly irregular cell outlines. The macrophage appearance is variable; in the illustration, the macrophage exhibits a small nucleus rich in chromatin and slightly acidophilic cytoplasm. The fibroblast (2) is elongated with cytoplasmic projections, ovoid nucleus with sparse chromatin, and one or two nucleoli. The fibrocyte (3) is a more mature, smaller cell without cytoplasmic projections; the nucleus is similar but smaller than that in the fibroblast.

The large (4) and small (5) lymphocytes are round cells that differ principally in the larger amount of cytoplasm in the former. Their dark-staining nuclei have condensed chromatin clumps but no nucleoli.

Plasma cells (6) are distinguished from large lymphocytes (4) by a smaller, eccentrically placed nucleus with condensed, coarse chromatin clumps distributed in a characteristic radial pattern and one central mass in the nucleus. A prominent, clear area in the cytoplasm is seen adjacent to the nucleus.

Eosinophils (7) of the circulating blood are readily distinguished by their large size, a bilobed nucleus, and large, cytoplasmic granules that stain intensely with eosin.

Occasional pigment cells (8) may be seen. Adipose cells (9) have a narrow rim of cytoplasm and an eccentrically placed nucleus. In histologic sections, the large globule of fat in the living cell has been dissolved by reagents used in section preparation, leaving a large, empty space.

PLATE 8

LOOSE (IRREGULAR) CONNECTIVE TISSUE

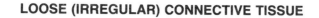

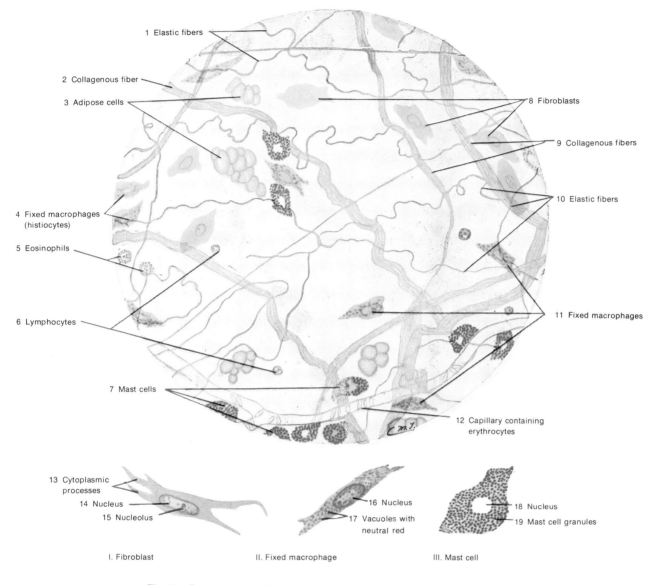

1 Elastic fibers

2 Collagenous fiber

3 Adipose cells

8 Fibroblasts

9 Collagenous fibers

10 Elastic fibers

4 Fixed macrophages
  (histiocytes)

5 Eosinophils

6 Lymphocytes

11 Fixed macrophages

7 Mast cells

12 Capillary containing
   erythrocytes

13 Cytoplasmic
   processes

14 Nucleus

15 Nucleolus

16 Nucleus

17 Vacuoles with
   neutral red

18 Nucleus

19 Mast cell granules

I. Fibroblast   II. Fixed macrophage   III. Mast cell

Fig. 1. *Spread:* supravital staining with neutral red. 320 × and 1200 ×.

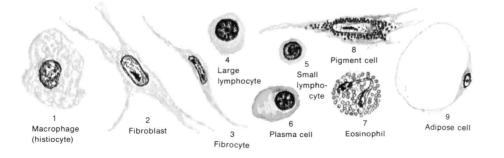

1
Macrophage
(histiocyte)

2
Fibroblast

3
Fibrocyte

4
Large
lymphocyte

5
Small
lympho-
cyte

6
Plasma cell

7
Eosinophil

8
Pigment cell

9
Adipose cell

Fig. 2. *Individual cells of loose connective tissue.* Stain: hematoxylin-eosin. 1200 ×.

PLATE 9 (Fig. 1)

LOOSE (IRREGULAR) CONNECTIVE TISSUE

The area in the illustration represents a small section of loose connective tissue.

Collagenous fibers (6) predominate in loose connective tissue, course in different directions, and form a loose meshwork. These fibers are sectioned in various planes and transverse sections of cut ends may be seen. Collagenous fibers have different diameters (6) and appear longitudinally striated because of their fibrillar structure. The fibers are acidophilic and stain pink with eosin. Thin elastic fibers are also present in loose connective tissue but are not easily distinguished with this stain and at this magnification.

Fibroblasts (1) are the most numerous cells in loose connective tissue and may be sectioned in various planes, so that only parts of the cells may be seen. Also, during section preparation, the cytoplasm of these cells may shrink. A typical fibroblast (1) shows an oval nucleus with sparse chromatin and lightly acidophilic cytoplasm with few short processes. The fibroblasts may be seen in profile, in surface view without much cytoplasm, and in transverse section in which the nucleus is spherical.

Also occasionally present in loose connective tissue are different blood cells such as the neutrophils (3) with lobulated nuclei and small lymphocytes (2) with dense nuclei and sparse cytoplasm. Fat or adipose cells appear characteristically empty, with a thin rim of cytoplasm (11) and peripherally displaced flat nuclei (12).

The connective tissue is highly vascular. Capillaries (7, 13) appear cut in different planes and are lined with endothelium. Larger blood vessels such as the arterioles (4, 9) and venules (5, 8), sectioned in different planes, are also illustrated in the loose connective tissue.

Other examples of loose connective tissue in organs are illustrated in Plate 25, Fig. 1:9, and Plate 90, Fig. 2:6.

PLATE 9 (Fig. 2)

DENSE IRREGULAR CONNECTIVE TISSUE
(DENSE FIBROELASTIC CONNECTIVE TISSUE)

This figure illustrates dense irregular connective tissue from the dermis of the skin. Arrangement of fibers and cells is similar to that in loose connective tissue; however, this is modified for areas in the body where more firm support and strength are required.

Collagenous fibers are large, found typically in thick bundles (1, 2), and sectioned in different planes because they course in various directions. This type of fiber arrangement is compact. Also present are thin, wavy elastic fibers (10), which form fine networks.

Fibroblasts (5) are often found compressed among the collagenous fibers. Also illustrated is an undifferentiated mesenchymal cell (6) along a small blood vessel and a few blood cells: neutrophils with lobulated nuclei (3) and lymphocytes (9) with large round nuclei but no visible cytoplasm. Small blood vessels are also illustrated (4, 8).

Dense irregular connective tissue in the dermis of the skin is also illustrated in Plate 46, Fig. 1:3.

PLATE 9

CONNECTIVE TISSUE

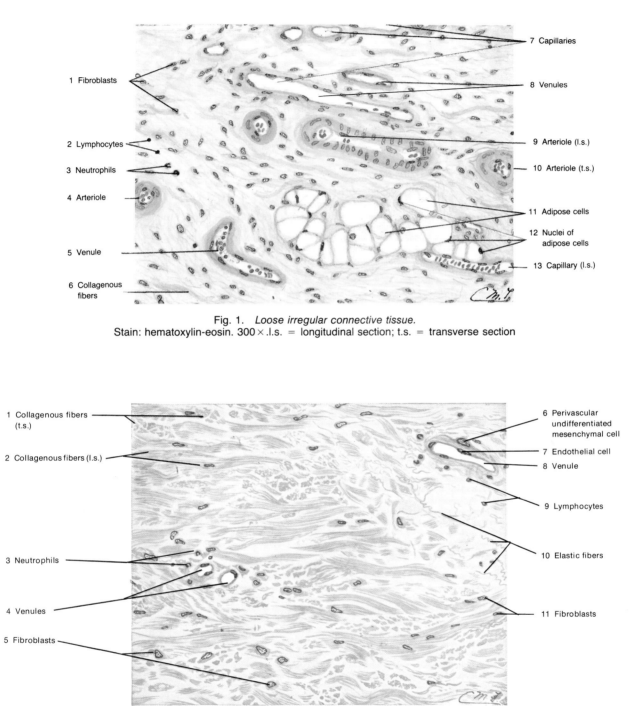

Fig. 1. *Loose irregular connective tissue.*
Stain: hematoxylin-eosin. 300×.l.s. = longitudinal section; t.s. = transverse section

Fig. 2. *Dense irregular connective tissue (dense fibroelastic connective tissue).*
Stain: hematoxylin-eosin. 300 ×.

PLATE 10 (Fig. 1)

DENSE REGULAR CONNECTIVE TISSUE: TENDON
(LONGITUDINAL SECTION)

Dense regular connective tissue is found where great tensile strength is required, such as in ligaments and tendons. A section of a tendon is illustrated at a high magnification.

Collagenous fibers are arranged in compact, parallel bundles (2, 3). Between these bundles are thin partitions of looser connective tissue that contain parallel rows of fibroblasts (1, 4, 5). These cells have short processes (not visible here) and nuclei that are ovoid when seen in surface view (4) and rod-like in lateral view (5).

Dense regular connective tissue with less regular arrangement also forms fibrous membranes or capsules around various organs in the body. Examples of such connective tissue are peri-chondrium around the tracheal cartilage (Plate 84, Fig. 1:2), the dura mater around the spinal cord (Plate 34, Fig. 1:13), and the tunica albuginea surrounding the testis (Plate 97, Fig. 1:1).

PLATE 10 (Fig. 2)

DENSE REGULAR CONNECTIVE TISSUE: TENDON
(TRANSVERSE SECTION)

A tendon in transverse section is illustrated at a lower magnification than that in Figure 1. Within each large bundle of collagenous fibers (1) are fibroblasts (nuclei) sectioned transversely (2). The fibroblasts are located between small bundles of collagenous fibers. Their cut ends are not distinguishable at this magnification and are separately illustrated in the insert (10).

Between the large collagenous bundles are thin partitions of connective tissue (3). Collagen bundles are grouped into fascicles, between which course larger partitions (septa or trabeculae) of interfascicular connective tissue (4, 8). These partitions contain blood vessels (5), nerves, and occasionally lamellar Pacinian corpuscles (6), which are sensitive pressure receptors.

Also illustrated in the figure is a transverse section of a skeletal muscle (7) which is adjacent to the tendon but separated from it by connective tissue septa.

At a higher magnification, the small bundles of collagenous fibers (10) and the branched shape of fibroblasts (9) are illustrated in transverse section.

PLATE 10

CONNECTIVE TISSUE

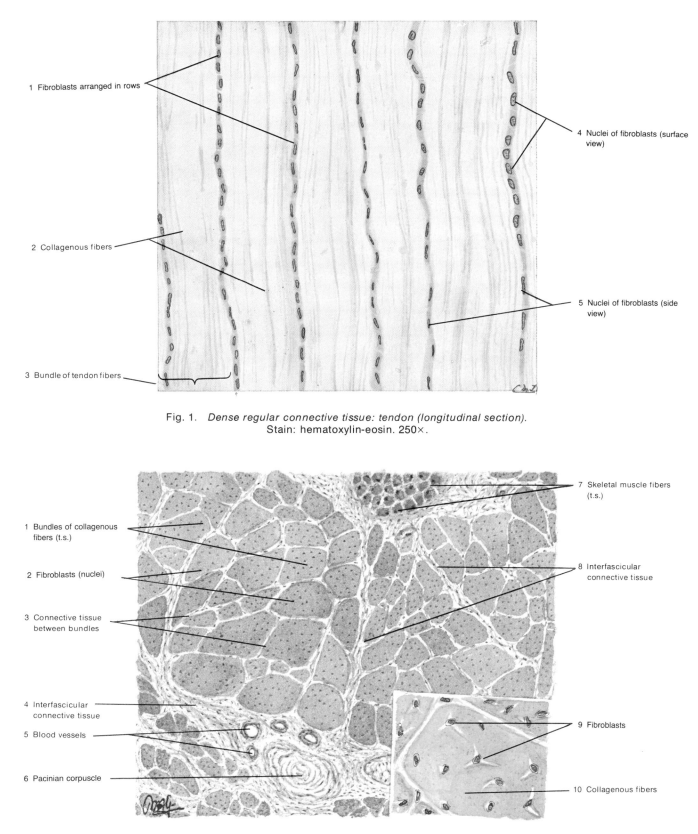

1 Fibroblasts arranged in rows

2 Collagenous fibers

3 Bundle of tendon fibers

4 Nuclei of fibroblasts (surface view)

5 Nuclei of fibroblasts (side view)

Fig. 1. *Dense regular connective tissue: tendon (longitudinal section).*
Stain: hematoxylin-eosin. 250×.

1 Bundles of collagenous fibers (t.s.)

2 Fibroblasts (nuclei)

3 Connective tissue between bundles

4 Interfascicular connective tissue

5 Blood vessels

6 Pacinian corpuscle

7 Skeletal muscle fibers (t.s.)

8 Interfascicular connective tissue

9 Fibroblasts

10 Collagenous fibers

Fig. 2. *Dense regular connective tissue: tendon (transverse section).*
Stain: hematoxylin-eosin. 80× and 300×.

PLATE 11 (Fig. 1)

DENSE IRREGULAR AND LOOSE CONNECTIVE TISSUE

This figure illustrates an area with dense irregular connective tissue on the left side, a transition zone in the middle, and loose connective tissue on the right.

Using Verhoeff's method, elastic fibers are selectively stained a deep blue (1, 4). Using Van Gieson's as a counterstain, acid fuchsin stains collagenous fibers red (2, 5). Cytoplasmic details of the fibroblasts are not revealed, but the nuclei stain deep blue (3, 6).

The characteristic features of dense irregular and loose connective tissues become apparent with this technique. In dense irregular connective tissue (2), the collagenous fibers are larger, more numerous, and more concentrated. Elastic fibers are also somewhat larger and more numerous (1). In contrast, in the loose connective tissue, both fiber types are smaller (4, 5) and more loosely arranged. Fine elastic networks are seen in both types of connective tissue.

PLATE 11 (Fig. 2)

ADIPOSE TISSUE

A small section of a mesentery is illustrated in which large accumulations of adipose (fat) cells are organized into adipose tissue. The connective tissue of the peritoneum (6) serves as a capsule around the adipose tissue.

Adipose cells (2) are packed close together and separated only by thin strips of connective tissue in which the fibroblasts (7) are compressed. Lobules of adipose tissue are separated by connective tissue septa (3) in which are found blood vessels (1, 4) and nerves; capillaries (5) are distributed in the intercellular connective tissue.

Individual adipose cells are illustrated as empty cells (2) because the fat was dissolved during routine section preparation. Their nuclei are compressed in the peripheral rim of the cytoplasm (8), and in sections, it is difficult to distinguish between fibroblast nuclei (7) and adipose cell nuclei (8).

PLATE 11 (Fig. 3)

EMBRYONIC CONNECTIVE TISSUE

Illustrated is a portion of embryonic connective tissue, which structurally resembles the mesenchyme or mucous connective tissue, which is loose and irregular in type. The difference in ground substance (semi-fluid versus jelly-like) is not apparent in these sections.

Fibroblasts (2) are numerous and fine collagenous fibers (3) are found between them, some coming in close contact with fibroblasts. Embryonic connective tissue is also vascular (1, 4).

At a higher magnification, a primitive fibroblast (5) is seen as a large, branching cell with abundant cytoplasm, prominent cytoplasmic processes, an oval nucleus with fine chromatin, and one or more nucleoli. The widely separated collagenous fibers (6) are more apparent at this magnification.

PLATE 11

CONNECTIVE TISSUE

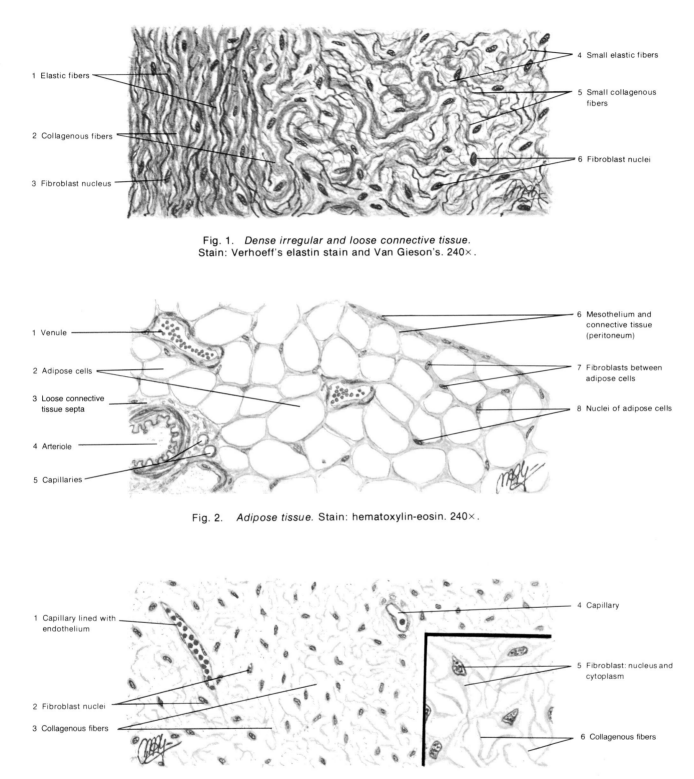

1 Elastic fibers

2 Collagenous fibers

3 Fibroblast nucleus

4 Small elastic fibers

5 Small collagenous fibers

6 Fibroblast nuclei

Fig. 1. *Dense irregular and loose connective tissue.*
Stain: Verhoeff's elastin stain and Van Gieson's. 240×.

1 Venule

2 Adipose cells

3 Loose connective tissue septa

4 Arteriole

5 Capillaries

6 Mesothelium and connective tissue (peritoneum)

7 Fibroblasts between adipose cells

8 Nuclei of adipose cells

Fig. 2. *Adipose tissue.* Stain: hematoxylin-eosin. 240×.

1 Capillary lined with endothelium

2 Fibroblast nuclei

3 Collagenous fibers

4 Capillary

5 Fibroblast: nucleus and cytoplasm

6 Collagenous fibers

Fig. 3. *Embryonic connective tissue.* Stain: hematoxylin-eosin. 240× and 900×.

PLATE 12 (Fig. 1)

FETAL CARTILAGE:
EARLY DEVELOPMENT OF HYALINE CARTILAGE

This figure illustrates a cartilage model of a short bone in an early stage of development. Most of the model consists of young chondroblasts that still resemble mesenchymal cells, having spherical nuclei and cytoplasmic processes (1). Lacunae have not developed at this stage. The chondroblasts are numerous, crowded into a specific area, and randomly distributed in the cartilage matrix without forming isogenous groups. At this stage of development, cartilage matrix is being secreted (3).

On the periphery of the cartilage model (left side), mesenchymal cells are concentrated and exhibit a parallel arrangement (2). The nuclei of these cells are elongated and flattened, and the cell membranes indistinct. This peripheral area of the cartilage will develop into perichondrium, a sheath of dense connective tissue that will surround hyaline and elastic cartilage. The inner portion of perichondrium will be the chondrogenic layer from which chondroblasts (2) can develop; there is some indication of such transition in the illustration.

PLATE 12 (Fig. 1-A)

FETAL CARTILAGE: SECTIONAL VIEW

A higher magnification of a region from the middle of the cartilage in Figure 1 illustrates early chondroblasts with round nuclei and cytoplasmic processes (2). A few cells from the superficial portion of the cartilage exhibit more elongated nuclei and indistinct cell outlines (1).

In a routine histologic section, the collagenous fibers in the matrix are not visible and the matrix appears homogeneous (3) in both areas; however, it is more acidophilic in the superficial zone.

PLATE 12 (Fig. 2)

MATURE HYALINE CARTILAGE

This section illustrates an area in the interior or central region of the hyaline cartilage. Distributed throughout the homogeneous ground substance, the matrix (5, 6), are ovoid spaces called lacunae (2), which contain mature cartilage cells, the chondrocytes (1).

In the intact cartilage, chondrocytes fill the lacunae. Each cell has a granular cytoplasm and a nucleus (3). In histologic sections, the chondrocytes usually shrink and the lacunae are seen as clear spaces (2). Cartilage cells in the matrix are observed either singly or in isogenous groups.

The matrix (6) appears homogeneous and is usually basophilic, but can vary under different conditions. The matrix between cells or groups of cells is called interterritorial matrix (6). The more basophilic matrix around groups of cartilage cells is the territorial matrix (5). Around each lacuna, the matrix forms a thin cartilage capsule (4).

PLATE 12 (Fig. 3)

NEWLY FORMED HYALINE CARTILAGE OF THE TRACHEA

A plate of hyaline cartilage from the trachea illustrates lacunae with either single (12) chondrocytes or isogenous groups (13). Because the chondrocytes appear to fill their lacunae, only margins of lacunae are visible (16). Lacunae and chondrocytes in the middle of the cartilage are large and spherical (12, 13), but become progressively flatter (11) in the periphery; these flat cells are young chondrocytes (11).

The interterritorial (intercellular) matrix stains lighter (14), whereas the territorial matrix stains deeper (15).

A perichondrium of dense connective tissue (4, 9, 18) surrounds the entire cartilage plate. Its inner layer is chondrogenic (10) where the chondrocytes are formed by proliferation and differentiation of mesenchymal cells (17).

Other examples of hyaline cartilage are illustrated in Plates 83 and 84.

PLATE 12

HYALINE CARTILAGE

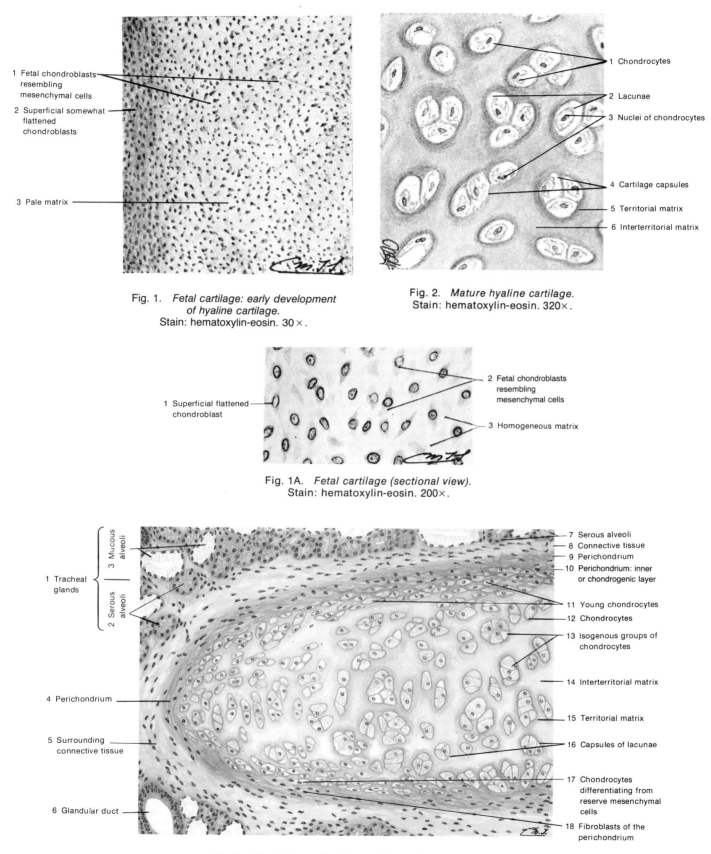

1 Fetal chondroblasts resembling mesenchymal cells

2 Superficial somewhat flattened chondroblasts

3 Pale matrix

Fig. 1. *Fetal cartilage: early development of hyaline cartilage.*
Stain: hematoxylin-eosin. 30 ×.

1 Chondrocytes

2 Lacunae

3 Nuclei of chondrocytes

4 Cartilage capsules

5 Territorial matrix

6 Interterritorial matrix

Fig. 2. *Mature hyaline cartilage.*
Stain: hematoxylin-eosin. 320×.

1 Superficial flattened chondroblast

2 Fetal chondroblasts resembling mesenchymal cells

3 Homogeneous matrix

Fig. 1A. *Fetal cartilage (sectional view).*
Stain: hematoxylin-eosin. 200×.

1 Tracheal glands
  3 Mucous alveoli
  2 Serous alveoli

4 Perichondrium

5 Surrounding connective tissue

6 Glandular duct

7 Serous alveoli
8 Connective tissue
9 Perichondrium
10 Perichondrium: inner or chondrogenic layer

11 Young chondrocytes
12 Chondrocytes

13 Isogenous groups of chondrocytes

14 Interterritorial matrix

15 Territorial matrix

16 Capsules of lacunae

17 Chondrocytes differentiating from reserve mesenchymal cells

18 Fibroblasts of the perichondrium

Fig. 3. *Newly formed hyaline cartilage of the trachea.*
Stain: hematoxylin-eosin. 120×.

PLATE 13 (Fig. 1)

FIBROUS CARTILAGE: INTERVERTEBRAL DISK

In fibrous cartilage, the matrix (6) is permeated with collagenous fibers (5), which frequently exhibit parallel fiber arrangement as is seen in tendons.

Small chondrocytes in lacunae (1, 2, 4) are usually distributed in rows (3) within the fibrous matrix and not at random or in isogenous groups as is usually seen in hyaline or elastic cartilage. All chondrocytes and lacunae are of similar size; there is no gradation from larger central chondrocytes to smaller and flatter peripheral cells.

A perichondrium, normally present around hyaline and elastic cartilage, is absent because fibrous cartilage usually forms a transition area between hyaline cartilage and tendon or ligament.

The proportion of fibers to matrix, the number of chondrocytes, and their arrangement may vary. Fibers may be so dense that matrix becomes invisible; in such cases, chondrocytes and lacunae appear flattened. Fibers within a bundle may be parallel, but different fibers may course in different directions.

PLATE 13 (Fig. 2)

ELASTIC CARTILAGE: EPIGLOTTIS

Elastic cartilage differs from hyaline cartilage principally by the presence of elastic fibers in its matrix (1). These can be demonstrated as deep purple fibers after staining the cartilage with orcein (3). The fibers enter the cartilagenous matrix from the perichondrium (4), usually as small fibers, and are distributed in the interior as branching and anastomosing fibers of varying size (3); some of the fibers exhibit considerable thickness (3, middle leader). The density of fibers in the matrix varies in different elastic cartilages and in different areas of the same cartilage.

As in hyaline cartilage, larger chondrocytes in lacunae are seen in the interior of the plate while the smaller ones are more peripheral (2, 5); the latter finally become fibroblasts in the perichondrium.

CARTILAGE

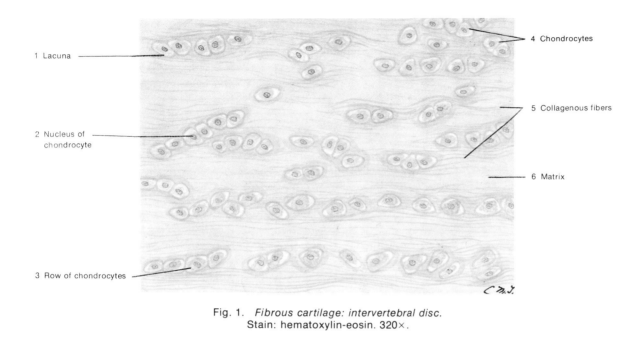

1 Lacuna

4 Chondrocytes

2 Nucleus of
chondrocyte

5 Collagenous fibers

6 Matrix

3 Row of chondrocytes

Fig. 1. *Fibrous cartilage: intervertebral disc.*
Stain: hematoxylin-eosin. 320×.

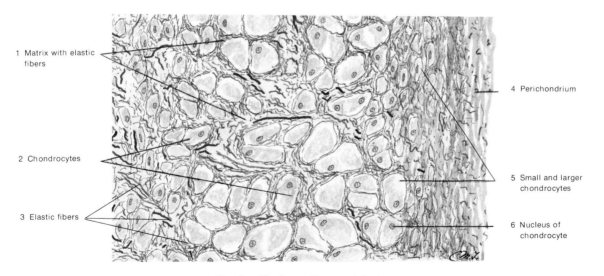

1 Matrix with elastic
fibers

4 Perichondrium

2 Chondrocytes

5 Small and larger
chondrocytes

3 Elastic fibers

6 Nucleus of
chondrocyte

Fig. 2. *Elastic cartilage: epiglottis.*
Stain: hematoxylin-orcein. 320 ×.

PLATE 14 (Fig. 1)

COMPACT BONE, DRIED: DIAPHYSIS OF THE TIBIA
(TRANSVERSE SECTION)

The characteristic feature of a compact bone is the arrangement of mineralized bone matrix into layers called lamellae. These are thin plates of bony tissue containing osteocytes or bone cells in almond-shaped lacunae (11, 15) from which radiate in all directions small canals, the canaliculi (12). These penetrate the lamellae and anastomose with canaliculi from other lacunae, while some canaliculi open into Haversian canals (2) and marrow cavities of the bone. Lamellae exhibit variety of shapes.

The outer wall of the compact bone (beneath the periosteum) is formed of external circumferential lamellae (10), which run parallel to each other and to the long axis of the bone. The inner wall (along the marrow cavity) is composed of internal circumferential lamellae (6). Between the internal and external circumferential lamellae are the osteons (Haversian systems) (4, 8), which are illustrated in transverse or oblique sections. The small irregular areas of bone between osteons are the interstitial lamellae (7, 9).

The osteons or Haversian systems are the structural units of bone. Each osteon (4, 8) consists of a number of concentric lamellae (3) that surround a central Haversian canal (2, 14). In a living bone, the Haversian canal contains reticular connective tissue, blood vessels and nerves (a miniature marrow cavity). The boundary of each osteon is sharply outlined by a refractile line called the cement line (5), which consists of modified matrix. Connections or anastomoses between Haversian canals are often visible (13).

PLATE 14 (Fig. 2)

COMPACT BONE, DRIED: DIAPHYSIS OF THE TIBIA
(LONGITUDINAL SECTION)

The figure represents a small area of a longitudinal section taken from the diaphysis of a compact bone.

Because the Haversian canals course longitudinally in the bone, each canal (3) is seen as a tube, often branched, sectioned parallel to the long axis of the bone. It is surrounded by numerous lamellae (1), within or between which are the lacunae (4) from which radiate the canaliculi (6). Lamellae, lacunae, and the osteon boundaries (the cement lines) (2) are, in general, parallel to the corresponding Haversian canals. The cement lines (2) indicate the extent of an osteon, as seen in longitudinal section.

PLATE 14

COMPACT BONE, DRIED

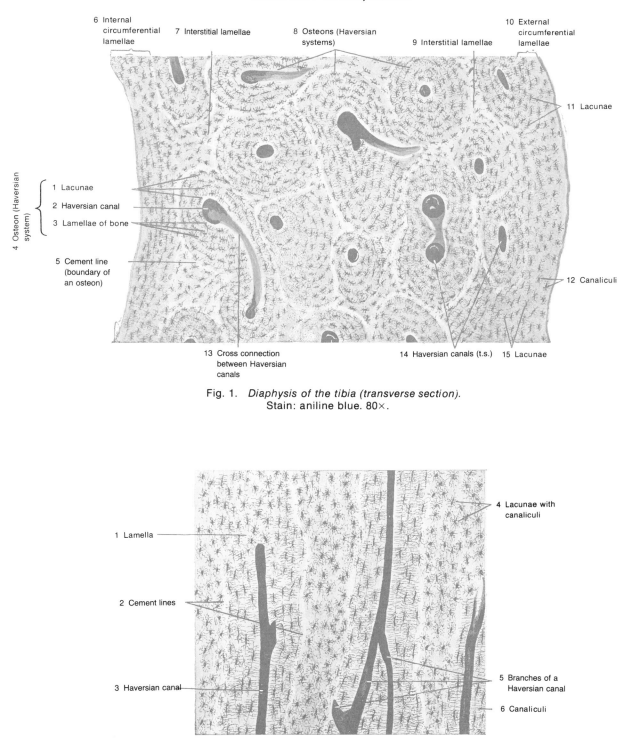

Fig. 1. *Diaphysis of the tibia (transverse section).*
Stain: aniline blue. 80×.

Fig. 2. *Diaphysis of the tibia (longitudinal section).*
Stain: aniline blue. 80×.

PLATE 15 (Fig. 1)

CANCELLOUS BONE: ADULT STERNUM
(TRANSVERSE SECTION, DECALCIFIED)

Cancellous bone consists primarily of slender, bony trabeculae which ramify, anastomose (6), and enclose irregular marrow cavities of various sizes (5). Peripherally, these trabeculae merge with a thin shell of compact bone (3) which contains scattered osteons (Haversian systems) (4, 7). The surrounding periosteum (2) may descend into the bone at intervals and merge with adjacent loose connective tissue (1), which is highly vascularized.

Except for concentric lamellae in the osteons (7), the peripheral rim of bone and the trabeculae are composed of parallel lamellae, which (in this figure) are more apparent on the margins of bony areas (8). Lacunae with osteocytes (9) are present throughout the bone.

The framework of reticular connective tissue in the marrow cavities is obscured by adipose cells (10) and groups of hemopoietic cells (11). Arteries are visible but sinusoids are not distinguishable in this illustration. Marrow fills the cavities, but a thin, inner layer of cells, the endosteum, becomes visible when marrow separates from the bone (12).

PLATE 15 (Fig. 2)

INTRAMEMBRANOUS OSSIFICATION:
MANDIBLE OF FIVE-MONTH FETUS
(TRANSVERSE SECTION, DECALCIFIED)

The upper part of the illustration shows the gum covering the developing mandible. The mucosa of the gum consists of stratified squamous epithelium (1) and a wide lamina propria (2) containing blood vessels and nerves.

Below the lamina propria is the developing bone. The periosteum (3) is differentiated, and numerous anastomosing trabeculae constitute the bone. These trabeculae surround the primitive marrow cavities of various sizes (14), which consist of embryonic connective tissue, blood vessels, and nerves (16). Peripherally, collagenous fibers of the inner periosteum are in continuity with the fibers of the embryonic connective tissue of adjacent marrow cavities (6) and with collagenous fibers within the bony trabeculae (10).

Osteoblasts (7, 15) are associated with bone deposition and are seen in linear arrangement along the developing trabeculae. Osteoclasts (5, 8) are multinucleated giant cells associated with bone resorption and remodeling.

The bony trabeculae contain osteocytes in lacunae (4, 9). Although collagenous fibers embedded in the bony matrix are obscured, the continuity with fibers of embryonic connective tissue in the marrow cavities may be seen at the margins of numerous trabeculae (13).

Formation of new bone is not a continuous process. Inactive areas appear where ossification has temporarily ceased: osteoid (newly synthesized bony matrix) and osteoblasts are not present. In some of the primitive marrow cavities, fibroblasts enlarge and differentiate into osteoblasts (12). In other areas, osteoid is seen on the margins of bony trabeculae (11, 17); osteoblasts may (11) or may not (17) be present.

PLATE 15

CANCELLOUS BONE AND INTRAMEMBRANOUS OSSIFICATION

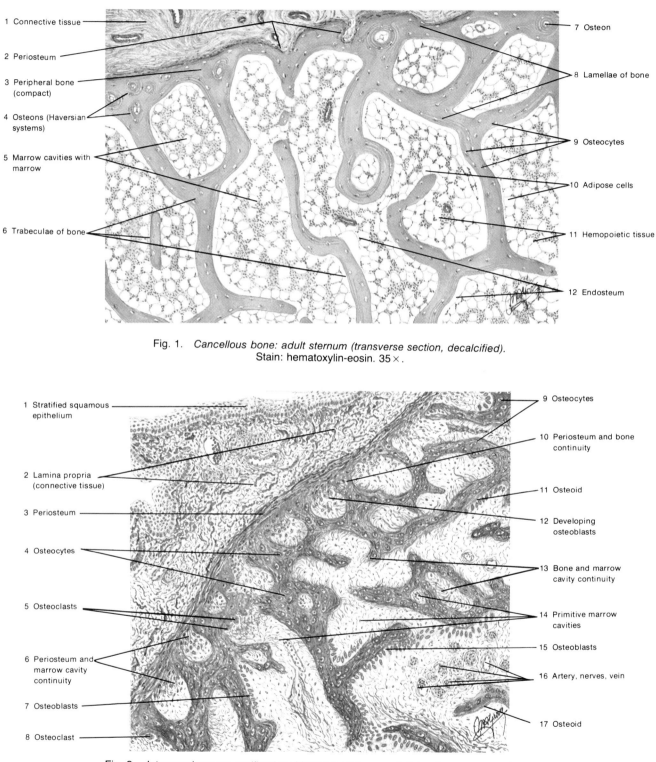

1 Connective tissue

2 Periosteum

3 Peripheral bone (compact)

4 Osteons (Haversian systems)

5 Marrow cavities with marrow

6 Trabeculae of bone

7 Osteon

8 Lamellae of bone

9 Osteocytes

10 Adipose cells

11 Hemopoietic tissue

12 Endosteum

Fig. 1. *Cancellous bone: adult sternum (transverse section, decalcified).*
Stain: hematoxylin-eosin. 35 ×.

1 Stratified squamous epithelium

2 Lamina propria (connective tissue)

3 Periosteum

4 Osteocytes

5 Osteoclasts

6 Periosteum and marrow cavity continuity

7 Osteoblasts

8 Osteoclast

9 Osteocytes

10 Periosteum and bone continuity

11 Osteoid

12 Developing osteoblasts

13 Bone and marrow cavity continuity

14 Primitive marrow cavities

15 Osteoblasts

16 Artery, nerves, vein

17 Osteoid

Fig. 2. *Intramembranous ossification: Mandible of five-month fetus (transverse section, decalcified)*
Stain: Mallory-azan. 50 ×.

PLATE 16

ENDOCHONDRAL OSSIFICATION:
DEVELOPING METACARPAL BONE
(PANORAMIC VIEW, LONGITUDINAL SECTION)

This illustration depicts endochondral ossification, in which the future bone is first formed as a model of embryonic hyaline cartilage. The cartilage model is then gradually replaced by a deposition of bone. In the center of the illustrated model, this process has already occurred. In addition, most of the original spongy bone so formed has been replaced and resorbed to form the central marrow cavity, leaving only scattered, thin spicules of bone of endochondral origin (11, 30). Red marrow (13) fills the cavity of newly formed bone. The stroma of reticular connective tissue is obscured by masses of developing erythrocytes, granulocytes, and megakaryocytes (14), numerous sinusoids (12), capillaries, and other blood vessels.

The process of endochondral ossification can be followed from the upper part of the illustration downward to the central marrow cavity. In the uppermost region is seen the zone of reserve hyaline cartilage (17), in which the chondrocytes in their lacunae are distributed singly or in small groups (2). Chondrocytes then proliferate rapidly and become arranged in columns (3, 18); cells and lacunae increase in size toward the lower area of this zone of proliferating cartilage (18). The chondrocytes then hypertrophy due to the swelling of nucleus and cytoplasm (19). The lacunae enlarge (4), the cells then degenerate, and the thin partitions of intervening matrix calcify (20); the calcified cartilage stains a deep purple.

Tufts of vascular marrow invade the area of calcifying cartilage (5, 21), erode the lacunar walls and calcified cartilage (5, 21), and form new, small marrow cavities. Osteoprogenitor cells differentiate into osteoblasts and deposit osteoid and bone around the remaining spicules of calcified cartilage (6). This region is the zone of ossification (21).

The lower, lateral two thirds of the illustration show the development of periosteal bone. Osteoblasts differentiate from osteoprogenitor cells in the inner layer of the periosteum (9) and form a bone collar (10) by the intramembranous method. Formation of new periosteal bone (22) keeps pace with formation of new endochondral bone. The bone collar increases in thickness and compactness as development of bone proceeds. The thickest portion of the collar is seen in the central part of the diaphysis at the initial site of periosteal bone formation (29) around the primary ossification center.

Surrounding the shaft of the developing bone are soft tissues: muscle (7), subcutaneous connective tissue and dermis of skin (15, 25) with hair follicles (26), sebaceous glands (28), sweat glands (16), and the epidermis (24).

PLATE 16

ENDOCHONDRAL OSSIFICATION:
DEVELOPING METACARPAL BONE
(PANORAMIC VIEW, LONGITUDINAL SECTION)

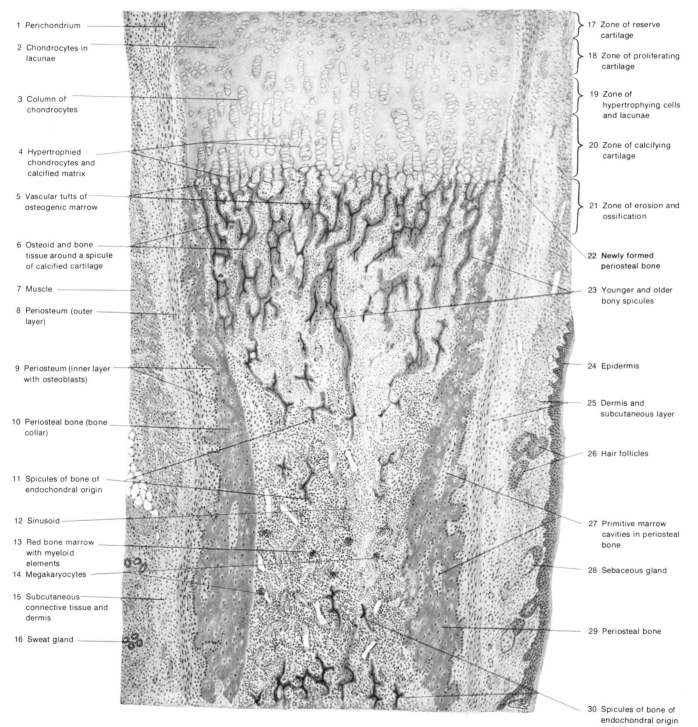

1 Perichondrium

2 Chondrocytes in lacunae

3 Column of chondrocytes

4 Hypertrophied chondrocytes and calcified matrix

5 Vascular tufts of osteogenic marrow

6 Osteoid and bone tissue around a spicule of calcified cartilage

7 Muscle

8 Periosteum (outer layer)

9 Periosteum (inner layer with osteoblasts)

10 Periosteal bone (bone collar)

11 Spicules of bone of endochondral origin

12 Sinusoid

13 Red bone marrow with myeloid elements

14 Megakaryocytes

15 Subcutaneous connective tissue and dermis

16 Sweat gland

17 Zone of reserve cartilage

18 Zone of proliferating cartilage

19 Zone of hypertrophying cells and lacunae

20 Zone of calcifying cartilage

21 Zone of erosion and ossification

22 Newly formed periosteal bone

23 Younger and older bony spicules

24 Epidermis

25 Dermis and subcutaneous layer

26 Hair follicles

27 Primitive marrow cavities in periosteal bone

28 Sebaceous gland

29 Periosteal bone

30 Spicules of bone of endochondral origin

Stain: hematoxylin-eosin. 60×.

PLATE 17

ENDOCHONDRAL OSSIFICATION
(SECTIONAL VIEW)

This preparation shows in greater detail the processes of endochondral ossification at the zone of ossification and adjacent areas that correspond approximately to labels 3 through 6 in Plate 16.

Proliferating chondrocytes are arranged in columns (2, 10). The cells in the lower part of this zone hypertrophy due to increased glycogen accumulation in the cytoplasm and nuclear swelling; lacunae also hypertrophy simultaneously. Cytoplasm then exhibits vacuolations, the nuclei become pyknotic (3), and the thin partitions of cartilagenous matrix become calcified (4, 11).

Tufts of vascular marrow invade this area (5) and produce the zone of erosion. Osteoblasts are formed, line up along remaining spicules of calcified cartilage (14), and lay down osteoid (15) and bone. Osteoblasts trapped in the osteoid or bone become osteocytes (7).

The marrow (17) contains cells belonging to the erythrocytic (18) and granulocytic (19) series as well as megakaryocytes (8). Multinucleated osteoclasts (16), which lie in shallow depressions called the Howship's lacunae, are situated adjacent to bone which is being resorbed.

On the right side of the illustration is an area of periosteal cancellous bone (13) with osteocytes and bone marrow cavities. The new bone is added peripherally by osteoblasts derived from osteoprogenitor cells of the inner periosteum (12). The outer layer of periosteum continues upward over the cartilage as the perichondrium (9).

PLATE 17

ENDOCHONDRAL OSSIFICATION (SECTIONAL VIEW)

1 Basophilic matrix

2 Columns of chondrocytes

3 Hypertrophied
   chondrocytes
   (vacuolized cytoplasm,
   pyknotic nuclei)

4 Degenerating chondrocytes
   surrounded by calcified
   matrix

5 Invading capillaries
   and embryonic bone
   marrow in zone of
   erosion

6 Spicules of calcified
   cartilage surrounded
   by osteoid

7 Newly formed
   osteocytes

8 Megakaryocytes

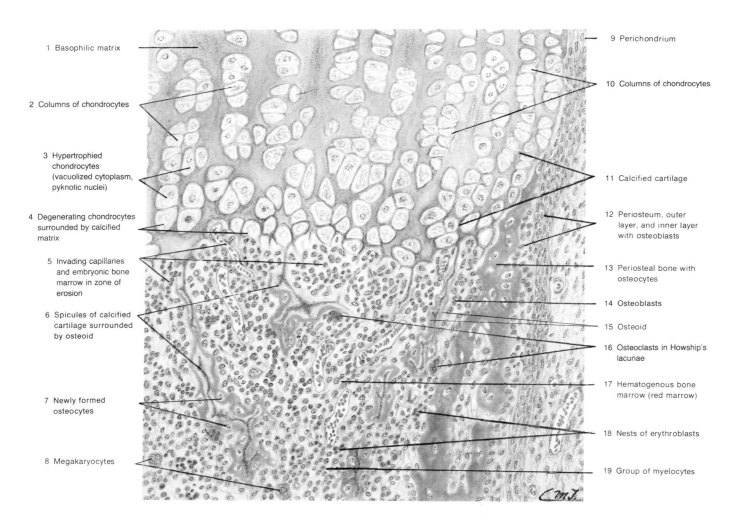

9 Perichondrium

10 Columns of chondrocytes

11 Calcified cartilage

12 Periosteum, outer
   layer, and inner layer
   with osteoblasts

13 Periosteal bone with
   osteocytes

14 Osteoblasts

15 Osteoid

16 Osteoclasts in Howship's
   lacunae

17 Hematogenous bone
   marrow (red marrow)

18 Nests of erythroblasts

19 Group of myelocytes

Stain: hematoxylin-eosin. 200×.

PLATE 18

FORMATION OF BONE: DEVELOPMENT OF OSTEONS (HAVERSIAN SYSTEMS) (DECALCIFIED, TRANSVERSE SECTION)

This illustration represents a late stage in the development of compact bone. Primitive osteons (Haversian systems) have already formed and others are in the process of development. In a metacarpal bone, such as that seen in Plate 16, or in a long bone, the first compact bone will be formed by deposition in the subperiosteal region (Plate 16:29). Vascular tufts of connective tissue from periosteum or endosteum will erode this bone and form primitive osteons, as seen in this illustration. Bone reconstruction will continue by breakdown of these first and later osteons and formation of new ones.

This plate illustrates a section of immature compact bone whose matrix (11) is stained deep with eosin. Primitive osteons are seen in transverse sections, with large Haversian canals (8) surrounded by a few concentric lamellae of bone (3) and osteocytes (1). The Haversian canals contain primitive connective tissue and blood vessels (6, 8). Bone deposition is continuing in some of these osteons, as indicated by the presence of osteoblasts along the periphery of the Haversian canal (9) and the margin of the innermost bone lamella. In some of the primitive osteons, the osteoclasts (2) are in the process of resorbing and remodeling the bone.

A longitudinal channel of osteogenic connective tissue (10) passes through the bone. From it arise tufts of vascular connective tissue which give rise to Haversian canals (4); osteoblasts already line the periphery of the canal.

In the lower part of the figure is a large bone marrow cavity (14) in which hemopoiesis is in progress; this is the red marrow. Also present in the marrow are developing erythrocytes and granulocytes, megakaryocytes (16), blood vessels (6), bone spicule (15), and osteoclasts (13) in Howship's lacunae (12) along the wall of the bone.

PLATE 18

FORMATION OF BONE: DEVELOPMENT OF OSTEONS
(HAVERSIAN SYSTEMS) (DECALCIFIED, TRANSVERSE SECTION)

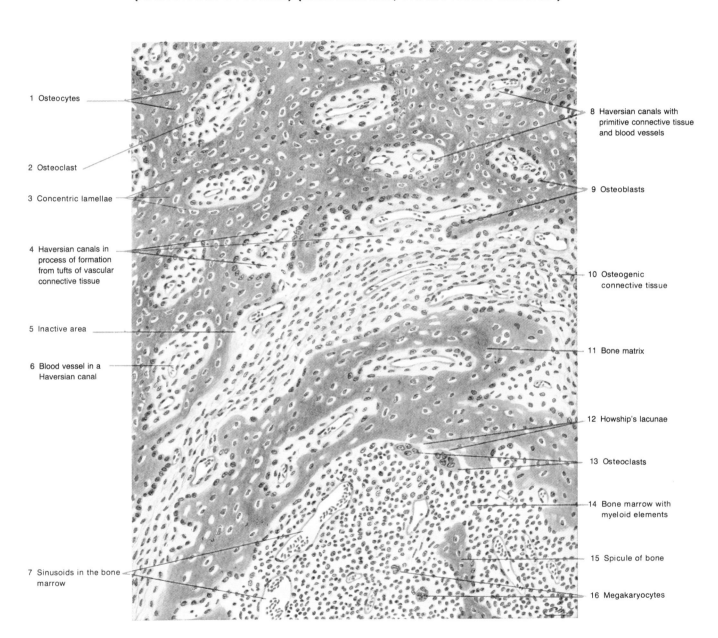

1 Osteocytes

2 Osteoclast

3 Concentric lamellae

4 Haversian canals in
process of formation
from tufts of vascular
connective tissue

5 Inactive area

6 Blood vessel in a
Haversian canal

7 Sinusoids in the bone
marrow

8 Haversian canals with
primitive connective tissue
and blood vessels

9 Osteoblasts

10 Osteogenic
connective tissue

11 Bone matrix

12 Howship's lacunae

13 Osteoclasts

14 Bone marrow with
myeloid elements

15 Spicule of bone

16 Megakaryocytes

Stain: hematoxylin-eosin. 140×.

PLATE 19

FORMATION OF BONE: SECONDARY (EPIPHYSEAL) OSSIFICATION CENTERS (DECALCIFIED, LONGITUDINAL SECTION)

The cartilagenous epiphyseal ends (articular cartilages) of two fetal finger bones are illustrated. Both bones contain a secondary center of ossification. The ossification center in the upper bone (2) exhibits an earlier stage of development than that in the lower bone (6). Located between the two developing cartilage models is the synovial or joint cavity (5, 11).

In the upper epiphysis is seen the peripheral or superficial zone of cartilage with flattened chondrocytes and lacunae (3). Toward the center, the chondrocytes and lacunae are rounder (1). Deeper and at the margin of the established center of calcification, the chondrocytes show hypertrophy (10) in preparation for ossification. Small spicules of red-stained bone (2) and primitive marrow cavities are seen in the center.

Similar structural components are also seen in the secondary center of ossification in the lower bone (6; 13–15). Bony spicules (13) are larger and more numerous than above. A small area of metaphysis, a transitional zone where cartilage is being replaced by bone, is present (9), illustrating typical features of the zone of ossification in this region (8, 9, 16, 17). Periosteum is seen on the right side (18) and on the left side (unlabeled) (8, 9).

The synovial or joint cavity (5, 11) is covered by a joint capsule (a diarthritic joint). A portion of the outer fibrous layer of the articular capsule is illustrated (7). The inner synovial membrane of flattened cells lines the cavity except over the articulating cartilages. The synovial membrane, together with the connective tissue of the capsule, may extend into the joint cavity as simple projections (12) or more complex synovial folds (4).

PLATE 19

FORMATION OF BONE: SECONDARY (EPIPHYSEAL) OSSIFICATION CENTERS (DECALCIFIED, LONGITUDINAL SECTION)

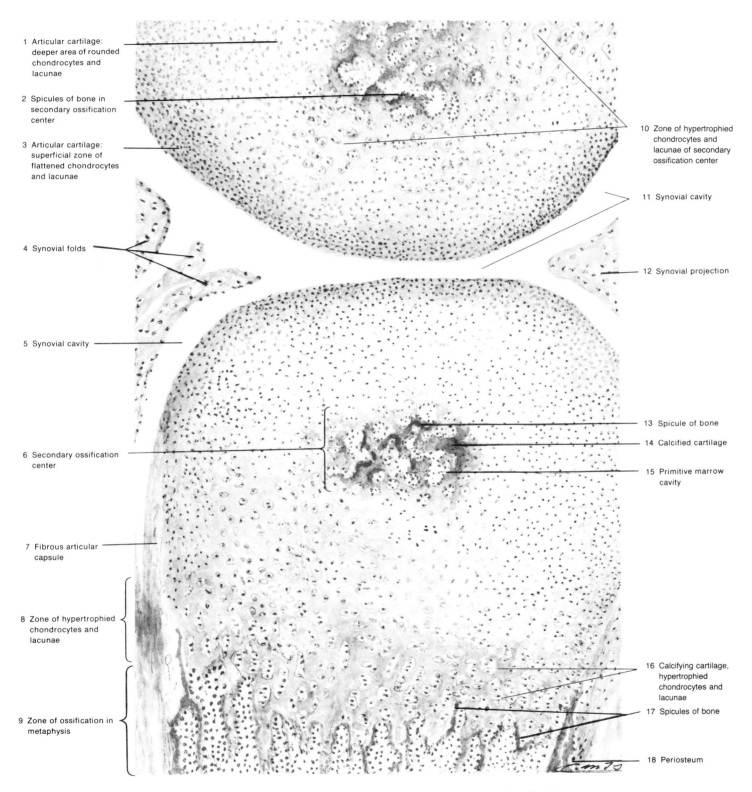

1 Articular cartilage: deeper area of rounded chondrocytes and lacunae

2 Spicules of bone in secondary ossification center

3 Articular cartilage: superficial zone of flattened chondrocytes and lacunae

4 Synovial folds

5 Synovial cavity

6 Secondary ossification center

7 Fibrous articular capsule

8 Zone of hypertrophied chondrocytes and lacunae

9 Zone of ossification in metaphysis

10 Zone of hypertrophied chondrocytes and lacunae of secondary ossification center

11 Synovial cavity

12 Synovial projection

13 Spicule of bone

14 Calcified cartilage

15 Primitive marrow cavity

16 Calcifying cartilage, hypertrophied chondrocytes and lacunae

17 Spicules of bone

18 Periosteum

Fetal fingertip: epiphyses of two adjacent bones in early stages of ossification.
Stain: hematoxylin-eosin. 20×.

PLATE 20

PERIPHERAL BLOOD SMEAR

The circular area in the illustration represents an idealized blood smear, stained with May-Grünwald-Giemsa stain. Erythrocytes, leucocytes, and blood platelets are shown.

The erythrocytes (6) are enucleated cells that stain pink with eosin. They are uniform in size, about 7.5 μm in diameter, and can be used as a size reference for other cell types.

The blood platelets (7), the smallest of the formed elements, are irregular masses of basophilic cytoplasm containing azurophilic granules. Platelets tend to form clumps in blood smears.

The leukocytes are subdivided into different categories according to the shape of the nucleus, the absence or presence of cytoplasmic granules, and the staining affinities of their granules.

Leukocytes with numerous granules and a lobulated nucleus are polymorphonuclear granulocytes, of which the neutrophils (3) are most numerous. Their cytoplasm contains very fine violet or pink granules. The nucleus consists of several lobes connected by narrow chromatin strands; the presence of fewer lobes indicates less mature cells.

Eosinophils (1) have large, bright pink granules which fill the cytoplasm. The nucleus is typically bilobed, but a small third lobe may be present. In basophils (2), the granules are not as numerous as in eosinophils but are more variable in size, less densely packed, and stain dark blue or brown. The nucleus is not markedly lobulated and stains pale basophilic.

Agranular leukocytes have few or no cytoplasmic granules and round to horseshoe-shaped nuclei. Lymphocytes show more variation in size, ranging from smaller than erythrocytes to almost twice as large (4). The nucleus occupies a large portion of the cytoplasm and stains intensely with chromatin, which is arranged in dense blocks intermingled with less dense areas. The narrow rim of basophilic cytoplasm is agranular but may contain a few azurophilic granules.

The monocytes (5) are the largest leukocytes. The nucleus varies from round or oval to indented or horseshoe-shaped and stains lighter than in lymphocytes. The chromatin is more finely dispersed; the abundant cytoplasm is lightly basophilic and often contains a few fine azurophilic granules.

PLATE 20

PERIPHERAL BLOOD SMEAR

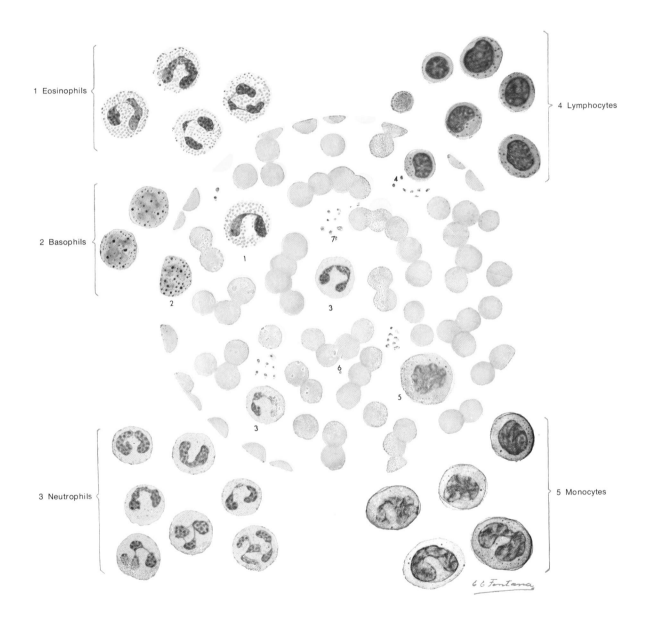

1 Eosinophils

2 Basophils

3 Neutrophils

4 Lymphocytes

5 Monocytes

Stain: May-Grünwald-Giemsa. 1100×.

PLATE 21 (Fig. 1)

SUPRAVITAL STAIN: BLOOD CELLS

The formation of phagocytic vacuoles within leukocytes can be easily demonstrated. A dilute solution of neutral red stain is placed on a slide, a drop of blood is added, and a cover slip placed over the solution. In 15 to 50 minutes, vacuoles of different sizes appear in the cytoplasm (1, 2, 3:a). The smallest and slowest vacuoles to appear are in the cytoplasm of the small lymphocytes (2:a).

Mitochondria are demonstrated by using essentially the same technique and employing the Janus green stain. Mitochondria stain a bluish green in the cell cytoplasm (1, 2, 3:b).

In reticulated erythrocytes, which are the youngest erythrocytes after extrusion of the nucleus, the reticulum can be demonstrated by placing a drop of blood on a slide on which a solution of cresyl blue has dried. The reticulum is then seen as a filamentous network of dark-staining granular material (4:c).

PLATE 21 (Fig. 2)

PAPPENHEIM'S AND CELANI'S STAINS: BLOOD SMEARS

The various types of blood cells are clearly differentiated by staining a blood film with Pappenheim's stain (May–Grünwald's stain followed by Giemsa's stain). Nuclear structures, the more or less intense basophilic nature of the cytoplasm, and the various types of granules are well demonstrated (a) by this method.

Benzidine is oxidized by hydrogen peroxide activated by the peroxides in the blood cells (Celani's stain). Granules which have oxidases stain blue. Polymorphs and monocytes in circulating blood have peroxidases (b), whereas the lymphocytes do not.

PLATE 21

BLOOD CELLS: SUPRAVITAL STAIN

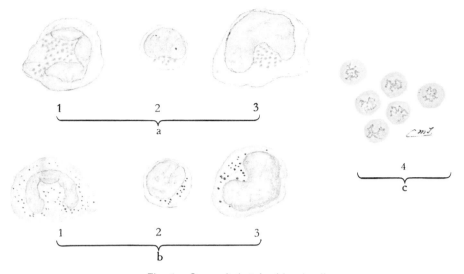

Fig. 1. *Supravital stain: blood cells.*
1. Neutrophilic granulocyte; 2. lymphocyte; 3. monocyte; 4. erythrocytes
  a) Vacuoles stained with neutral red.
  b) Mitochondria stained with Janus green.
  c) Reticulum stained with cresyl blue.

BLOOD SMEARS: PAPPENHEIM'S AND CELANI'S STAINS

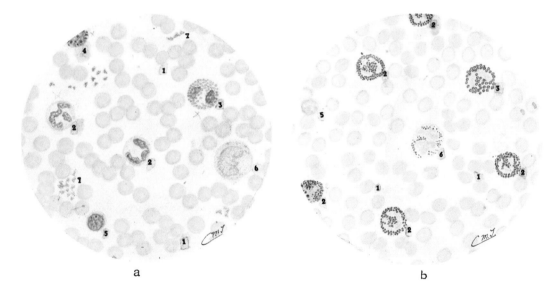

Fig. 2. *Pappenheim's and Celani's stains: blood smears.*
a) Pappenheim's method (May-Grünwald and Giemsa stains). Nuclei: reddish violet; basophilic cytoplasm: blue of varying intensity according to degree of basophilia; acidophilic cytoplasm: more or less deep red; neutrophilic granules: violet; eosinophilic granules: orange-red; basophilic granules: dark violet; azurophilic granules: brilliant purple.
b) Peroxidase reaction. Celani's technique. Nuclei: light red; cytoplasm of leukocytes: pale pink; erythrocytes: yellow; granules with peroxidases: blue.
1. erythrocytes; 2. neutrophilic granulocyte; 3. eosinophil granulocyte; 4. basophil granulocyte; 5. lymphocyte; 6. monocyte; 7. platelets.

PLATE 22 (Fig. 1)

BONE MARROW OF A RABBIT

In a section of a red bone marrow, it is difficult to distinguish all types of developing blood cells. The cells are densely packed and different cell types are intermixed, although some of the erythrocytic forms often occur in groups or "nests" (6, 20). Structural details of different cells are not as apparent in a section as in a smear due to cell shrinkage during slide preparation; only parts of cells, rather than entire cells, may be present.

This section is stained with hematoxylin–eosin. At low magnification, little differentiation of cytoplasm is visible, except for bright-staining eosinophilic granules (4). For a comparison, the individual cells illustrated below the figure are from a marrow smear where a more detailed structure is visible.

The reticular connective tissue stroma of the marrow is largely obscured by hemopoietic cells. In less dense areas (8), the reticular connective tissue can be seen and the elongated reticular cells often recognized (24). Different types of blood vessels are also seen (9, 10, 19, 25).

Conspicuous in marrow are large adipose cells (14) with large vacuoles (due to fat removal during section preparation) and small, peripheral cytoplasm surrounding the nucleus (2).

Other cells easily identified are the large megakaryocytes (5, 23) with varied nuclear lobulation.

Erythrocytes are abundant (12). The most easily recognizable of the earlier erythrocytic cells are the normoblasts (20), characterized by small, dark-staining nuclei (as in f); also, numerous cells exhibit mitotic activity (18). Polychromatophilic erythroblasts may also occur in groups or "nests" (22). These cells are larger than normoblasts, with a larger nucleus exhibiting a more evident "checkerboard" distribution of the chromatin (as in e). Basophilic erythroblasts (3) are still larger cells exhibiting a large, less dense nuclei and basophilic cytoplasm (as in d).

In the granulocytic series, the most easily recognizable cells are the polymorphonuclear heterophils (16) (corresponding to neutrophils in man) and eosinophils. Their earlier forms, the metamyelocytes (21), have bean- or horseshoe-shaped nuclei (as in c). Heterophilic myelocytes (1, 4, b) have larger, round or ovoid nuclei.

Less easily recognizable in a section are the pale-staining primitive reticular cells (11) and hemocytoblasts (13, 17, a).

An alternate terminology for the developing erythrocytic forms, in wide use clinically, is as follows:

Proerythroblast = rubriblast
Basophilic erythroblast = prorubricyte
Polychromatophilic erythroblast = rubricyte
Normoblast (orthochromatophilic erythroblast) = metarubricyte

PLATE 22 (Fig. 2)

BONE MARROW OF A RABBIT, INDIA INK PREPARATION (SECTION)

Illustrated is a section of a hemopoietic bone marrow from a rabbit, injected with India ink.

Carbon particles have been ingested by the stromal macrophages (1, 8) and by fixed macrophages (3), situated adjacent to the endothelium that lines the sinusoids. Dense carbon inclusions in some phagocytic cells can obscure the nucleus (1).

Reticular cells of the connective tissue may be seen occasionally (12) but are frequently obscured by developing blood cells. Various cells of the erythrocytic and granulocytic series (4, 6, 7, 11, 13) as well as megakaryocytes (10) can be identified.

PLATE 22

BONE MARROW (SECTION)

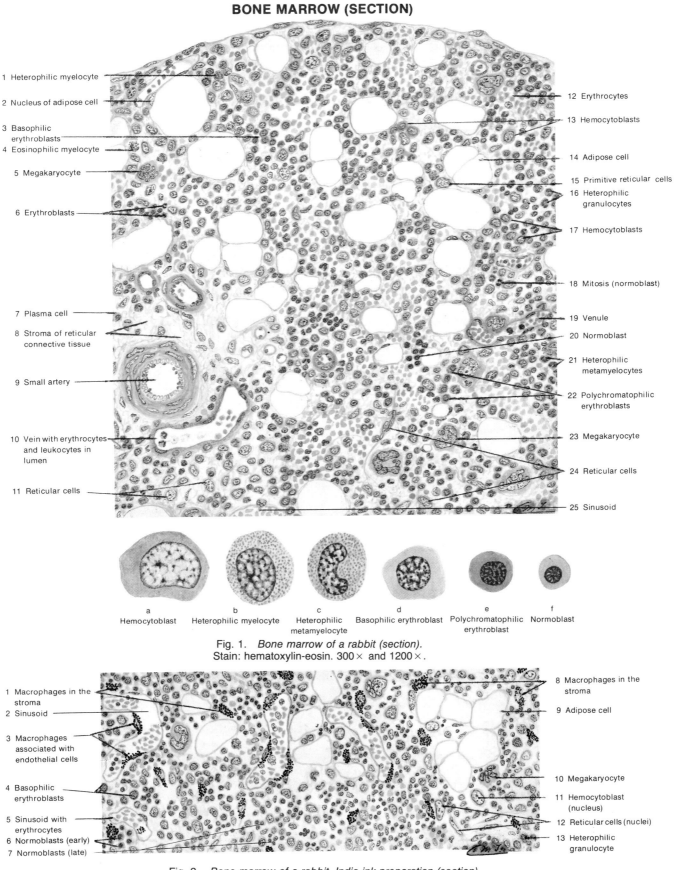

1 Heterophilic myelocyte

2 Nucleus of adipose cell

3 Basophilic erythroblasts

4 Eosinophilic myelocyte

5 Megakaryocyte

6 Erythroblasts

7 Plasma cell

8 Stroma of reticular connective tissue

9 Small artery

10 Vein with erythrocytes and leukocytes in lumen

11 Reticular cells

12 Erythrocytes

13 Hemocytoblasts

14 Adipose cell

15 Primitive reticular cells

16 Heterophilic granulocytes

17 Hemocytoblasts

18 Mitosis (normoblast)

19 Venule

20 Normoblast

21 Heterophilic metamyelocytes

22 Polychromatophilic erythroblasts

23 Megakaryocyte

24 Reticular cells

25 Sinusoid

a	b	c	d	e	f
Hemocytoblast	Heterophilic myelocyte	Heterophilic metamyelocyte	Basophilic erythroblast	Polychromatophilic erythroblast	Normoblast

Fig. 1. *Bone marrow of a rabbit (section).*
Stain: hematoxylin-eosin. 300 × and 1200 ×.

1 Macrophages in the stroma

2 Sinusoid

3 Macrophages associated with endothelial cells

4 Basophilic erythroblasts

5 Sinusoid with erythrocytes

6 Normoblasts (early)

7 Normoblasts (late)

8 Macrophages in the stroma

9 Adipose cell

10 Megakaryocyte

11 Hemocytoblast (nucleus)

12 Reticular cells (nuclei)

13 Heterophilic granulocyte

Fig. 2. *Bone marrow of a rabbit, India ink preparation (section).*
Stain: hematoxylin-eosin. 250 ×.

PLATE 23

BONE MARROW: SMEAR

In the center of the illustration is a representative microscopic field of human bone marrow smear obtained by sternal puncture. Distributed peripherally are typical bone marrow cells showing their detailed structure. Formed elements normally found in the peripheral blood are easily recognized: erythrocytes (18, 31), granulocytes (eosinophil, 32; neutrophil, 33), and platelets (24).

Recent evidence indicates that a common, free pluripotential stem cell is capable of differentiating into stem cells for different hemopoietic cell lines such as the erythrocytes, granulocytes, lymphocytes, and megakaryocytes. Because the existence of this stem cell was first demonstrated on the basis of colonies in the spleen, this cell has been termed the colony-forming unit (CFU). It is currently believed that these stem cells appear similar to a large lymphocyte. In adults, the greatest concentration of such stem cells is found in the bone marrow.

In the erythrocytic series, the precursor is the proerythroblast* (3, 8), which is 20 to 30 μm in diameter and contains a thin rim of basophilic cytoplasm and a large, oval nucleus that occupies most of the cell. Azurophilic granules are absent in all cells of this series. The chromatin is uniformly dispersed and two or more nucleoli may be present. Early proerythroblast undergoes a series of divisions to produce smaller basophilic erythroblasts whose size varies from 15 to 17 μm.

Basophilic erythroblasts (4, 7) exhibit less intensely basophilic cytoplasm; however, sufficient basophilia is present in the cytoplasm to obscure the small amount of hemoglobin that is being synthesized by these cells. The nucleus has decreased in size; the chromatin is coarse and exhibits the characteristic "checkerboard" pattern; nucleoli are either inconspicuous or absent. The progeny of mitotic divisions of basophilic erythroblasts are the polychromatophilic erythroblasts (5, 13, 14). These cells are recognized by their smaller size (12 to 15 μm) whose cytoplasm becomes progressively less basophilic and more acidophilic as a result of increased hemoglobin accumulation. The nuclei are smaller and exhibit the coarse "checkerboard" pattern.

When the cells acquire an acidophilic cytoplasm due to increased amount of hemoglobin, they are called normoblasts (6, 11) and their size is about 8 to 10 μm. Initially, the nucleus still exhibits a concentrated "checkerboard" chromatin pattern (6, 11) and the cell division continues. The nucleus then decreases in size, becomes pyknotic, and is extruded from the cytoplasm. The resulting flattened cell is the reticulocyte or young erythrocyte, which exhibits a bluish-pink cytoplasm (9, 16, 17). With special supravital staining, a delicate reticulum is demonstrated in the cytoplasm (see Plate 21, Fig. 1, 4c). Mature erythrocytes are smaller and have a homogeneous acidophilic cytoplasm (18, 31).

The granulocytes also originate from the pluripotential stem cell or the colony-forming unit (CFU), and the myeloblast (2, 25) is the first recognizable precursor in the granulocytic series. The myeloblast is a relatively small cell (10 to 13 μm in diameter) with a large nucleus containing two or three nucleoli and a distinctly basophilic cytoplasm that lacks specific granules. In its further development, the cell enlarges, acquires azurophilic granules, and is now called a promyelocyte (19, early; 23, later). The cell measures about 15 to 20 μm. The chromatin in the oval nucleus exhibits a dispersed pattern and multiple nucleoli are still evident. In more advanced promyelocytes, the cells are smaller, nucleoli become inconspicuous, azurophilic granules increase, and there is an appearance of specific granules with different staining properties in the perinuclear region (23, neutrophilic promyelocyte).

Myelocytes are smaller than promyelocytes. The nucleus is eccentric and the chromatin more condensed. The cytoplasm is less basophilic, with few azurophilic granules evident, and there is an increase of specific granules (neutrophilic early myelocyte, 26; basophilic early myelocyte, 20). More mature myelocytes have an abundance of specific granules, slightly acidophilic cytoplasm, and a smaller nucleus (12, 21, 22, 27, 29, 34, 35). The myelocyte is the last cell of the granulocytic series capable of mitosis; myelocytes then mature into metamyelocytes.

In the metamyelocytes, the configuration of the nucleus changes from an oval, eccentric form to that of deep indentation seen in mature cells; the greatest change takes place in the neutrophilic forms (in succession: 30 and 36, 28, the two cells in line with erythrocytes 31, 33). Similar structural alterations in eosinophils and basophils can be also followed in the illustrations (27 lower leader, 27 upper leader, 32; 20, 12).

Megakaryoblasts (37) are large cells about 40 to 60 μm in diameter. The cytoplasm is basophilic and largely free of specific granules. The voluminous nucleus is ovoid or indented, and exhibits a loose chromatin pattern and poorly defined nucleoli. The mature cells, megakaryocytes, are giant cells approximately 80 to 100 μm in diameter, and have a larger volume of slightly acidophilic cytoplasm filled with fine azurophilic granules (15, 38). The nucleus of these cells is large and convoluted, and contains multiple irregular lobes of variable size, interconnected by constricted regions. The chromatin is condensed and coarse, and there are no visible nucleoli. In mature megakaryocytes, plasma membrane invaginates the cytoplasm and forms demarcation membranes. This delimits the area of the megakaryocyte cytoplasm that is then shed into the blood as platelets (39).

*For alternate terminology, see page 56, Figure 1, paragraph 9.

PLATE 23

BONE MARROW: SMEAR

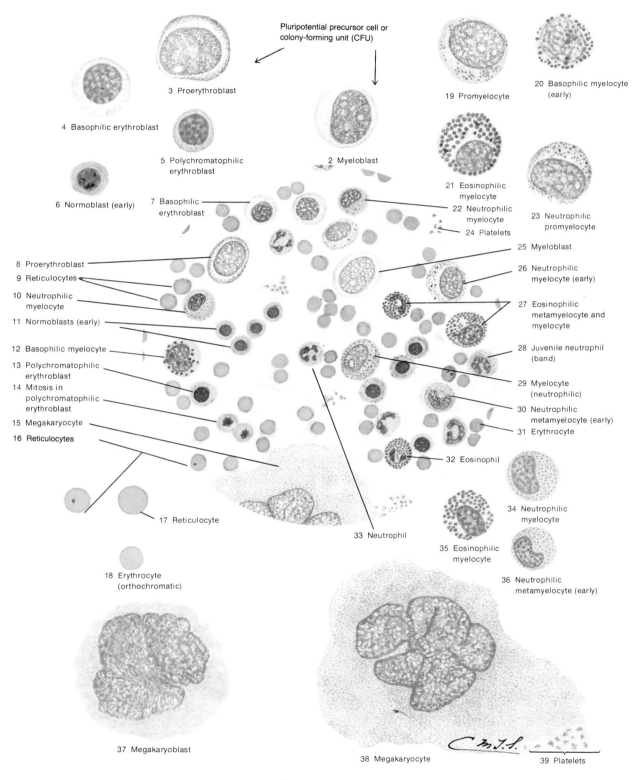

Pluripotential precursor cell or colony-forming unit (CFU)

3 Proerythroblast

4 Basophilic erythroblast

5 Polychromatophilic erythroblast

2 Myeloblast

6 Normoblast (early)

7 Basophilic erythroblast

8 Proerythroblast

9 Reticulocytes

10 Neutrophilic myelocyte

11 Normoblasts (early)

12 Basophilic myelocyte

13 Polychromatophilic erythroblast

14 Mitosis in polychromatophilic erythroblast

15 Megakaryocyte

16 Reticulocytes

17 Reticulocyte

18 Erythrocyte (orthochromatic)

37 Megakaryoblast

19 Promyelocyte

20 Basophilic myelocyte (early)

21 Eosinophilic myelocyte

22 Neutrophilic myelocyte

23 Neutrophilic promyelocyte

24 Platelets

25 Myeloblast

26 Neutrophilic myelocyte (early)

27 Eosinophilic metamyelocyte and myelocyte

28 Juvenile neutrophil (band)

29 Myelocyte (neutrophilic)

30 Neutrophilic metamyelocyte (early)

31 Erythrocyte

32 Eosinophil

33 Neutrophil

34 Neutrophilic myelocyte

35 Eosinophilic myelocyte

36 Neutrophilic metamyelocyte (early)

38 Megakaryocyte

39 Platelets

Stain: May-Grünwald-Giemsa. 800× and 1200×.

PLATE 24 (Fig. 1)

SMOOTH MUSCLE FIBERS

This illustration represents the wall of the distended bladder of a toad, in which the smooth muscles are distributed in small bundles of various sizes (2, 5). Individual muscle fibers can be distinguished in some of the smaller bundles (5). Each muscle fiber is a spindle-shaped cell with deeply stained cytoplasm (called sarcoplasm in the muscle) and an elongated or ovoid nucleus (3) in the center.

The loose connective tissue that surrounds the bundles of muscle fibers contains fibroblasts with their processes (1, 6) and a capillary with erythrocytes (4); mature erythrocytes in the toad remain nucleated.

Single and small groups of smooth muscle fibers are also illustrated on Plate 2, Figure 2 (4, 11).

PLATE 24 (Fig. 2)

SKELETAL (STRIATED) MUSCLE FIBERS (DISSOCIATED)

In this illustration, the muscle fibers from the leg of a toad have been separated and stained with hematoxylin-eosin. The skeletal muscle fibers (1) are much longer and larger in diameter than the smooth muscle fibers. Each fiber shows distinct cross-striations, which are visible as alternating dark or A bands (4) and light or I bands (5). With higher magnification, additional details are visible in Plate 25, Figure 4. Each muscle fiber is multinucleated, with the nuclei situated immediately below the sarcolemma (6). (Sarcolemma is not illustrated in the figure).

A muscle fiber that has been dissociated exhibits thin bundles of myofibrils (2). Each myofibril has the characteristic cross-striations which are aligned adjacent to each other in the myofibrils, thus giving the appearance of continuous cross-striations across the entire muscle fiber.

Numerous capillaries (3) are present in the connective tissue (endomysium) which surrounds each muscle fiber.

PLATE 24

MUSCLE TISSUE

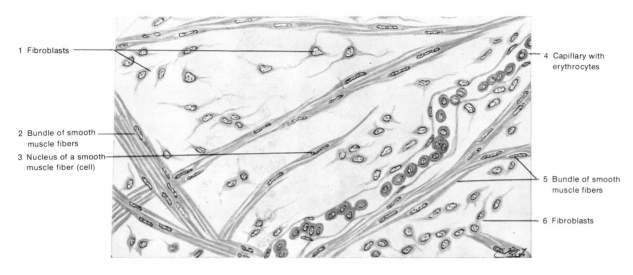

1 Fibroblasts

2 Bundle of smooth muscle fibers

3 Nucleus of a smooth muscle fiber (cell)

4 Capillary with erythrocytes

5 Bundle of smooth muscle fibers

6 Fibroblasts

Fig. 1. *Smooth muscle fibers.*
Stain: hematoxylin-eosin. 360×.

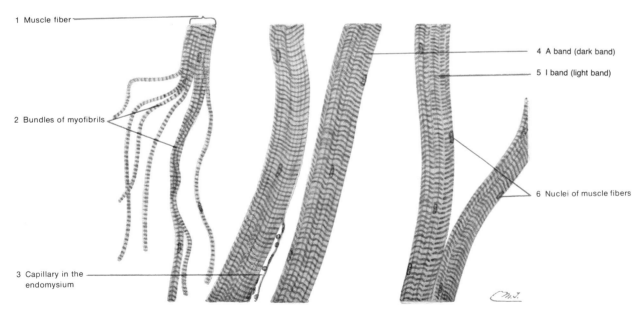

1 Muscle fiber

2 Bundles of myofibrils

3 Capillary in the endomysium

4 A band (dark band)

5 I band (light band)

6 Nuclei of muscle fibers

Fig. 2. *Skeletal (striated) muscle fibers (dissociated).*
Stain: hematoxylin-eosin. 250×.

PLATE 25 (Fig. 1)
SKELETAL MUSCLES OF THE TONGUE

A section taken from the central part of the tongue shows skeletal muscle fibers that have been cut longitudinally (3, 5) or transversely (4, 7). The fibers are aggregated into fascicles (3, 5) and are bound by connective tissue sheath (9). The connective tissue sheath around each muscle fascicle is the perimysium (2). From the perimysium, thin partitions of connective tissue, the endomysium (1, 11) extend into each fascicle and invest individual muscle fibers. Small blood vessels (6) are present throughout the connective tissue sheaths.

The muscle fibers that have been sectioned longitudinally show cross-striations (5); fibers sectioned transversely exhibit cross sections of myofibril bundles (4, 7). Nuclei of skeletal muscle fibers are located peripherally (8, 10), as demonstrated in transverse sections (8).

PLATE 25 (Fig. 2)
SMOOTH MUSCLE LAYERS OF THE INTESTINE

In the upper muscle layer, the smooth muscle fibers have been sectioned longitudinally (1), exhibiting the spindle shape of individual fibers. The nucleus (2) is located in the widest part of each fiber. The muscle fibers in this compact layer are arranged so that wide portions of some fibers are adjacent to the tapered ends of others.

In the lower muscle layer, the fibers have been sectioned transversely (5). The cross sections are of different diameters, depending on whether the plane of section passed through the central or the tapering ends of each fiber. The widest sections of the fibers contain nuclei, as seen in the transverse section (5, upper leader).

Fine reticular and elastic fibers envelop individual muscle fibers, whereas larger amounts of connective tissue are seen between the muscle layers (3) and around blood vessels (4).

PLATE 25 (Fig. 3)
CARDIAC MUSCLE: MYOCARDIUM

Although resembling skeletal muscle, the cardiac muscle fibers branch without much change in diameter. Cross striations (1) and intercalated disks (2) are clearly visible in fibers sectioned longitudinally. The intercalated disks are irregular and broader than the normal cross striations, and represent specialized junctions between cardiac muscle fibers; they are characteristic features of cardiac muscle.

Nuclei of cardiac muscle fibers are centrally placed (5, 8) and are clearly visible in fibers sectioned transversely (8). A clear zone of perinuclear sarcoplasm, free of myofibrils (9), may be seen in some sections.

Numerous small blood vessels (6, 7) lie in the interfascicular connective tissue (4), and capillaries are abundant in the endomysium.

PLATE 25 (Fig. 4)
SKELETAL MUSCLE (LONGITUDINAL SECTION)

Several muscle fibers are illustrated at high magnification and stained with iron hematoxylin to demonstrate the cross-striations. The A or anisotropic bands (2) are the prominent, dark-staining bands; a lighter, middle region or the H band is not visible. The I or isotropic bands are equally prominent and are lightly stained acidophilic bands. Crossing each central portion of the I bands are distinct, narrow lines, the Z lines (3).

The closely arranged parallel myofibrils give a faint, longitudinally striated appearance to the muscle fibers. Where the myofibrils (6) are separated because of rupture of the sarcolemma, the A, I, and Z lines are visible on the myofibrils, aligned next to each other on adjacent myofibrils.

Slender ovoid or elongated nuclei (4) of muscle fibers are seen at the periphery of the fibers. In the endomysium (1) between muscle fibers are seen fibroblasts (5) and a capillary (7).

PLATE 25 (Fig. 5)
CARDIAC MUSCLE (LONGITUDINAL SECTION)

Comparison of cardiac muscle with skeletal muscle at the same high magnification and the same stain clearly illustrates the similarities and differences between the two types of muscles.

Branching cardiac fibers (3) are in distinct contrast to individual skeletal fibers. Cross-striations are similar in both but less prominent in cardiac muscle fibers (2, 5). The prominence of the intercalated disks (7) and their irregular structure are better seen at higher magnification. The area between two intercalated disks represents one cardiac muscle cell.

Large, oval nuclei (1), usually one per cell, occupy the central position and much of the width of the cardiac fibers, in contrast to the many elongated peripheral nuclei of the skeletal fibers. The perinuclear sarcoplasm region (6) is distinct. Endomysium (4) fills the spaces between fibers.

PLATE 25

MUSCLE

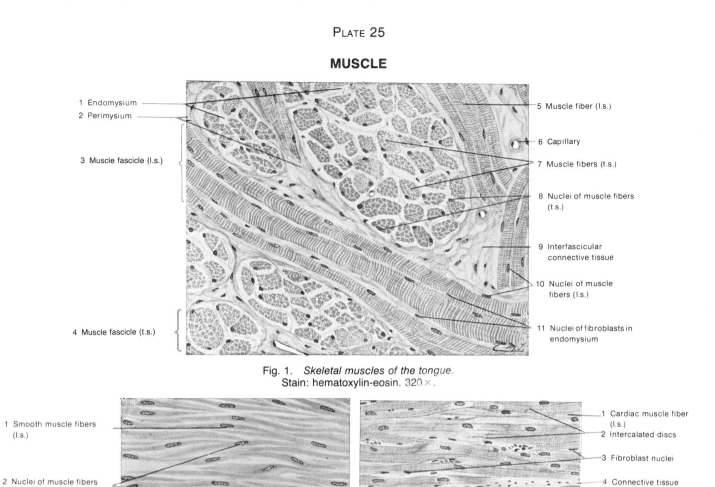

1 Endomysium
2 Perimysium

3 Muscle fascicle (l.s.)

4 Muscle fascicle (t.s.)

5 Muscle fiber (l.s.)

6 Capillary

7 Muscle fibers (t.s.)

8 Nuclei of muscle fibers (t.s.)

9 Interfascicular connective tissue

10 Nuclei of muscle fibers (l.s.)

11 Nuclei of fibroblasts in endomysium

Fig. 1. *Skeletal muscles of the tongue.*
Stain: hematoxylin-eosin. 320×.

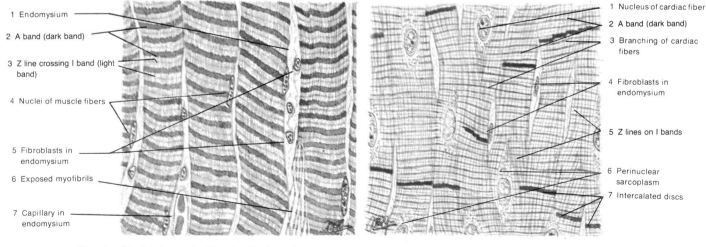

1 Smooth muscle fibers (l.s.)

2 Nuclei of muscle fibers

3 Connective tissue

4 Venule

5 Smooth muscle fibers (t.s.)

Fig. 2. *Smooth muscle layers of intestine.* 320×.

1 Cardiac muscle fiber (l.s.)
2 Intercalated discs

3 Fibroblast nuclei

4 Connective tissue

5 Nuclei of muscle fibers (l.s.)

6 Venule

7 Capillary and venule

8 Nuclei of muscle fibers (t.s.)

9 Perinuclear sarcoplasm

Fig. 3. *Cardiac muscle: Myocardium.* 320×.

1 Endomysium

2 A band (dark band)

3 Z line crossing I band (light band)

4 Nuclei of muscle fibers

5 Fibroblasts in endomysium

6 Exposed myofibrils

7 Capillary in endomysium

1 Nucleus of cardiac fiber

2 A band (dark band)

3 Branching of cardiac fibers

4 Fibroblasts in endomysium

5 Z lines on I bands

6 Perinuclear sarcoplasm

7 Intercalated discs

Fig. 4. *Skeletal muscle (longitudinal section).* 1000×. Fig. 5. *Cardiac muscle (longitudinal section).* 1000×.
Stain: Iron hematoxylin-eosin.

PLATE 26 (Fig. 1)

NERVE TERMINATIONS IN SKELETAL MUSCLE:
SKELETAL MUSCLE AND MUSCLE SPINDLE
(TRANSVERSE SECTION)

A typical transverse section of the skeletal muscle shows individual muscle fibers (1) grouped into fascicles by interfascicular connective tissue septa, the perimysium (2). In one of such septa is seen a muscle spindle (3) and a very small artery (4), in transverse section. The muscle spindle is an encapsulated sensory end organ.

At a higher magnification, the muscle spindle is surrounded by an ovoid connective tissue capsule (5), which is derived from the perimysium (9). The capsule encloses several components of the spindle, all of which are surrounded by loose connective tissue. The specialized muscle fibers (intrafusal fibers) (7) are present in the capsule. These muscle fibers are smaller in diameter and stain somewhat lighter (more sarcoplasm) than the ordinary muscle fibers (extrafusal fibers) (10). Small nerves (6) associated with the muscle spindles represent incoming myelinated and terminal unmyelinated fibers (axons). Very small blood vessels are also present in the capsule of the muscle spindle. These have penetrated the capsule of the spindle from nerves and blood vessels that are located in the connective tissue septa of the muscle proper.

PLATE 26 (Fig. 2)

NERVE TERMINATIONS IN THE SKELETAL MUSCLE:
MOTOR END PLATES

Illustrated is a portion of a skeletal muscle sectioned longitudinally (4, 7). The distal part of the motor nerve (somatic efferent) (1) courses over the muscle and distributes axonal branches that subdivide and terminate on individual muscle fibers as specialized junctional regions called the motor end plates (2, 6). The round structures seen in the motor end plates represent terminal axonal expansions and muscle nuclei which accumulate in this region but remain separated from the axon terminals.

Also seen in this figure are an end plate whose terminal fibril is in another plane of section (5) and an axon terminal whose end plate is not present in this section (3).

PLATE 26

NERVE TERMINATIONS IN SKELETAL MUSCLE

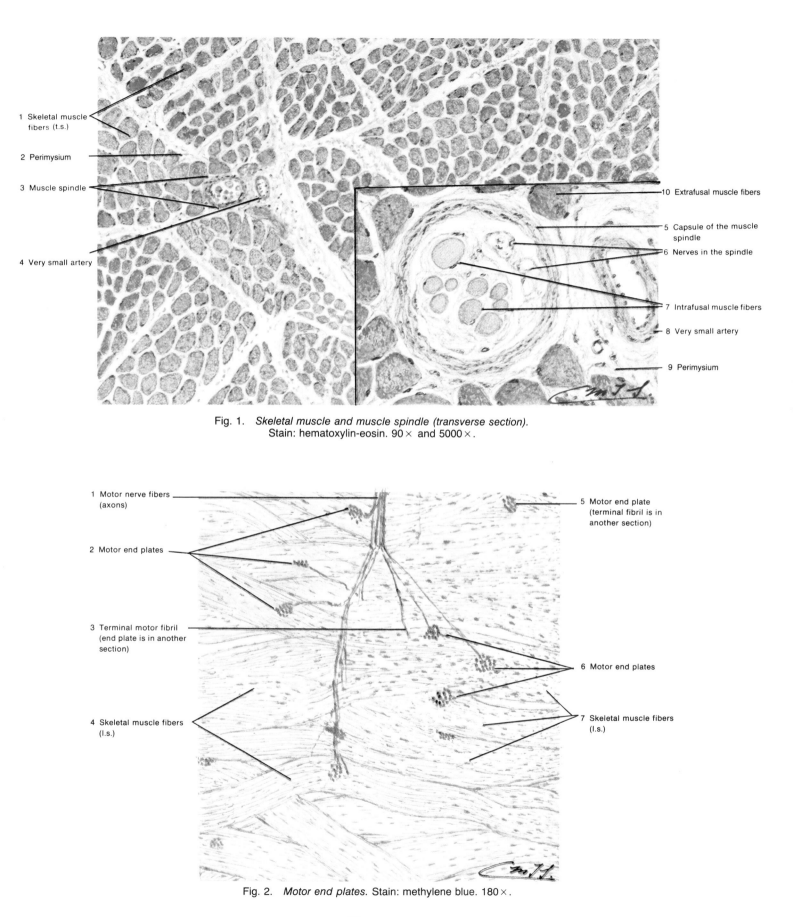

1 Skeletal muscle
fibers (t.s.)

2 Perimysium

3 Muscle spindle

4 Very small artery

10 Extrafusal muscle fibers

5 Capsule of the muscle
spindle

6 Nerves in the spindle

7 Intrafusal muscle fibers

8 Very small artery

9 Perimysium

Fig. 1. *Skeletal muscle and muscle spindle (transverse section).*
Stain: hematoxylin-eosin. 90× and 5000×.

1 Motor nerve fibers
(axons)

2 Motor end plates

3 Terminal motor fibril
(end plate is in another
section)

4 Skeletal muscle fibers
(l.s.)

5 Motor end plate
(terminal fibril is in
another section)

6 Motor end plates

7 Skeletal muscle fibers
(l.s.)

Fig. 2. *Motor end plates.* Stain: methylene blue. 180×.

PLATE 27 (Fig. 1)

GRAY MATTER: ANTERIOR HORN OF THE SPINAL CORD

The large, multipolar anterior horn cells or motor neurons (2) of the anterior gray matter of the spinal cord have a proportionately large central nucleus (7, 14), a prominent nucleolus (6, 13), and several radiating cell processes, the dendrites (8, 9). A single axon (1) arises from a clear area of the cell, the axon hillock (5).

The cytoplasm or the perikaryon of the neuron contains numerous clumps of coarse, granular substance (basophilic masses), the Nissl bodies (12), which stain a deep blue with basic aniline of Nissl's method. The Nissl bodies extend into the dendrites (8, 9) but not into the axon hillock (5) or the axon (1). The nucleus (7, 14) is distinctly outlined and stains lightly because of uniform dispersion of the chromatin in fine network often described as "vesicular." The nucleolus (6, 13) is large, dense, and stains deep.

Nuclei of neuroglia cells are stained, whereas the small amount of cytoplasm remains unstained. Protoplasmic astrocytes (3, 17) have spherical nuclei with a somewhat loose chromatin network. Nuclei of oligodendrocytes (16) are smaller and round, and stain deeper. Microglia (11) have elongated dark nuclei.

PLATE 27 (Fig. 2)

GRAY MATTER: ANTERIOR HORN OF THE SPINAL CORD

This section was prepared by silver impregnation (Cajal's method) to demonstrate neurofibrils. In the large anterior horn cells or motor neurons, typical neurofibril arrangements are seen in the nerve cell bodies (2, 3, 6, 11, 13) and the dendrites (7, 12). Axons are not illustrated, but neurofibrils would be seen in parallel arrangement.

Other details of cell structure are not revealed with silver impregnation technique. The nucleus of the neuron is seen as a lightly stained or almost clear space (14, and in neurons 3 and 11). The nucleolus may stain either lightly (11) or deeply (15).

In the intercellular areas are seen many fibrillar processes, some of which are anterior horn neurons or associated neuroglia.

Neuroglial nuclei are stained (1, 4, 5, 8, 9, 10) and show the same characteristics as described in Figure 1.

PLATE 27

NERVOUS TISSUE

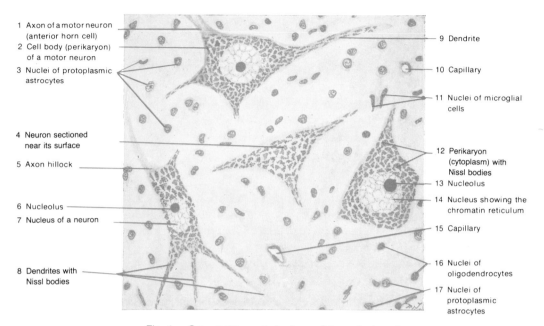

1 Axon of a motor neuron (anterior horn cell)
2 Cell body (perikaryon) of a motor neuron
3 Nuclei of protoplasmic astrocytes
4 Neuron sectioned near its surface
5 Axon hillock
6 Nucleolus
7 Nucleus of a neuron
8 Dendrites with Nissl bodies

9 Dendrite
10 Capillary
11 Nuclei of microglial cells
12 Perikaryon (cytoplasm) with Nissl bodies
13 Nucleolus
14 Nucleus showing the chromatin reticulum
15 Capillary
16 Nuclei of oligodendrocytes
17 Nuclei of protoplasmic astrocytes

Fig. 1. *Gray matter: anterior horn of the spinal cord.*
Nissl's method for chromophilic substance (Nissl bodies). 350 ×.

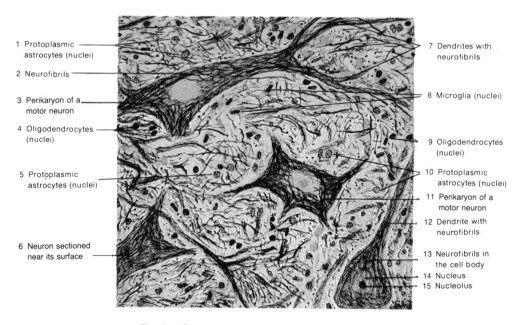

1 Protoplasmic astrocytes (nuclei)
2 Neurofibrils
3 Perikaryon of a motor neuron
4 Oligodendrocytes (nuclei)
5 Protoplasmic astrocytes (nuclei)
6 Neuron sectioned near its surface

7 Dendrites with neurofibrils
8 Microglia (nuclei)
9 Oligodendrocytes (nuclei)
10 Protoplasmic astrocytes (nuclei)
11 Perikaryon of a motor neuron
12 Dendrite with neurofibrils
13 Neurofibrils in the cell body
14 Nucleus
15 Nucleolus

Fig. 2. *Gray matter: anterior horn of the spinal cord.*
Cajal's method for neurofibrils. 350 ×.

PLATE 28 (Fig. 1)

GRAY MATTER: ANTERIOR HORN OF THE SPINAL CORD

With Golgi's method of silver impregnation, neurons, their processes, and their finest branches stain a homogeneous dark brown (2, 4). Structural details of different cells as seen in Plate 27, however, are not well demonstrated with this method.

Protoplasmic astrocytes are also stained (1, 3). The small cell body and numerous short, thick, branching processes are characteristic features of these cells.

PLATE 28 (Fig. 2)

GRAY MATTER: ANTERIOR HORN OF THE SPINAL CORD

This staining method, using mordanted sections and hematoxylin demonstrates different nerve fibers (axons). In the gray matter, nerve fibers of different sizes course in various directions. The myelin in the myelinated fibers stains deep blue or reddish-blue (2).

Neurons are visible but without structural details. The cells appear shrunken and retracted, and stain only pale yellow or green (1, 4). The nucleus is outlined but shows shrinkage (3).

PLATE 28

NERVOUS TISSUE

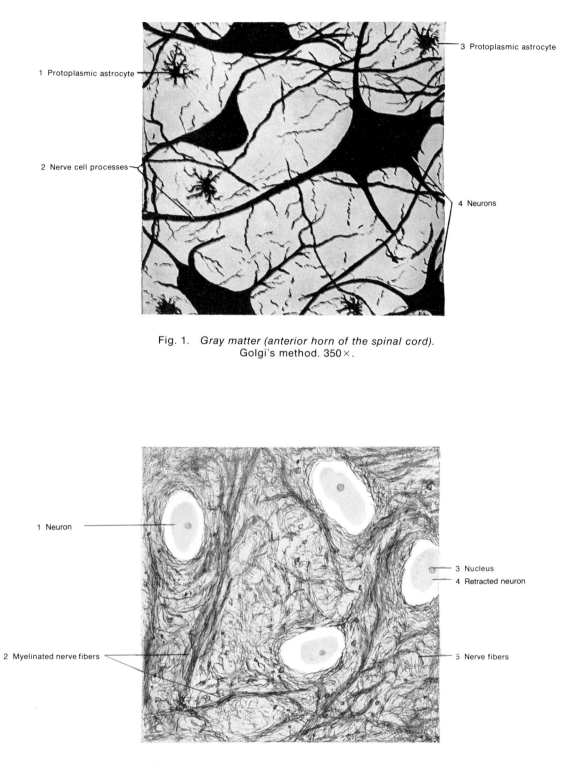

3 Protoplasmic astrocyte

1 Protoplasmic astrocyte

2 Nerve cell processes

4 Neurons

Fig. 1. *Gray matter (anterior horn of the spinal cord).*
Golgi's method. 350×.

1 Neuron

3 Nucleus
4 Retracted neuron

2 Myelinated nerve fibers

5 Nerve fibers

Fig. 2. *Gray matter (anterior horn of the spinal cord).*
Modified Weigert-Pal's method. 350×.

PLATE 29 (Fig. 1)

FIBROUS ASTROCYTES OF THE BRAIN

This section has been stained by Del Rio Hortega's method for astrocytes (i.e., macroglia), which demonstrates their cell outline, processes, and glial fibers.

In the center of the figure is a fibrous astrocyte with a small cell body and a large nucleus (5), and numerous long, smooth, slightly branched processes extending in all directions. One of the processes terminates on a blood vessel (4) as a vascular pedicle or foot plate.

In the upper left of the figure, the processes of another fibrous astrocyte are seen associated with a blood vessel (1); one foot plate or pedicle is indicated (2, lower leader).

PLATE 29 (Fig. 2)

OLIGODENDROCYTES OF THE BRAIN

This section has been stained with Del Rio Hortega's modification of Golgi's method.

A protoplasmic astrocyte (4) is seen with its small cell body, large nucleus, and numerous, thick, greatly branched processes.

Oligodendrocytes (2, 5) have smaller oval cell bodies and nuclei than the astrocytes, and exhibit few, thin, short processes without much branching. The processes may be either very thin (5), or somewhat thicker (2).

Oligodendrocytes are found in both the gray and white matter of the central nervous system. In the white matter, the oligodendrocytes form myelin sheaths around numerous axons (6), and are analogous to the Schwann cells on the peripheral nerves. The neuron (1) provides a size contrast with the astrocytes and oligodendrocytes.

PLATE 29 (Fig. 3)

MICROGLIA OF THE BRAIN

In this section, Del Rio Hortega's method was used to demonstrate microglia. The cell bodies are small, vary in shape, and often have irregular contours (1, 4). The small, deeply stained nucleus almost fills the entire cell. The cell processes are few, short, slender, tortuous, and covered with small "spines" (5). The neuron (3), located at the top of the figure, provides a size contrast with the microglia.

Microglia are normally not numerous, but are found in both white and gray matter of the central nervous system. Microglia are believed to be the main source of phagocytic cells in the central nervous system. It is also believed that microglia may represent a variety of oligodendrocyte. In case of injury and when there is a great demand for phagocytic cells, mesodermal cells migrate to the damaged areas of the central nervous system and become active macrophages.

PLATE 29

NEUROGLIA

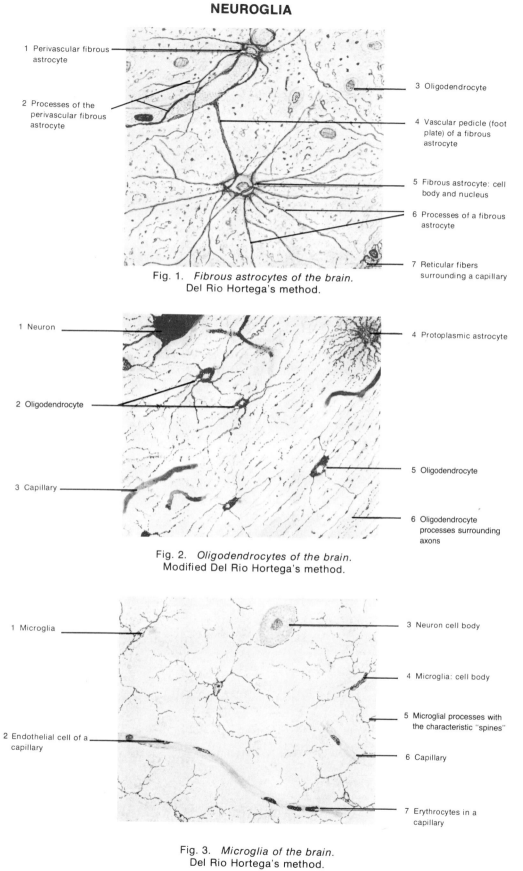

1 Perivascular fibrous astrocyte

2 Processes of the perivascular fibrous astrocyte

3 Oligodendrocyte

4 Vascular pedicle (foot plate) of a fibrous astrocyte

5 Fibrous astrocyte: cell body and nucleus

6 Processes of a fibrous astrocyte

7 Reticular fibers surrounding a capillary

Fig. 1. *Fibrous astrocytes of the brain.*
Del Rio Hortega's method.

1 Neuron

2 Oligodendrocyte

3 Capillary

4 Protoplasmic astrocyte

5 Oligodendrocyte

6 Oligodendrocyte processes surrounding axons

Fig. 2. *Oligodendrocytes of the brain.*
Modified Del Rio Hortega's method.

1 Microglia

2 Endothelial cell of a capillary

3 Neuron cell body

4 Microglia: cell body

5 Microglial processes with the characteristic "spines"

6 Capillary

7 Erythrocytes in a capillary

Fig. 3. *Microglia of the brain.*
Del Rio Hortega's method.

PLATE 30 (Fig. 1)

MYELINATED NERVE FIBERS (DISSOCIATED)

A section of the sciatic nerve of a toad has been fixed in osmic acid and teased apart to show individual nerve fibers. The axon occupies the center of each fiber (2, 5); the constituent neurofibrils of the axon, however, are not distinguishable with this staining method. The myelin sheath (4) stains as a thick, dark band on the fiber periphery. At intervals, the myelin sheath is discontinuous along its path and exhibits intervals between adjacent Schwann cells called the nodes of Ranvier (1, 6).

The Schwann sheath (neurolemma) envelops the entire nerve fiber (axon) forming its peripheral boundary; this is not illustrated in the figure as a separate membrane. Between the two nodes of Ranvier are the Schwann cells containing a single Schwann cell nucleus.

In the internodal segments, the myelin sheath contains many small, oblique, unstained incisures or clefts of Schmidt-Lanterman (3, 8). These clefts represent areas of loosened or local separation of myelin lamellae.

PLATE 30 (Fig. 2)

NERVE (TRANSVERSE SECTION)

Several bundles (fascicles) of nerve fibers have been sectioned transversely (1) or obliquely (8). Each nerve fascicle is surrounded by a connective tissue sheath, the perineurium (2), which merges with surrounding interfascicular connective tissue (17). Perineurial septa may separate larger nerve fascicles. From these or directly from perineurium, delicate connective tissue strands surround individual nerve fibers of a fascicle and form the endoneurium (5).

Numerous nuclei are seen between individual nerve fibers. Most of these are Schwann cell nuclei; others are fibroblasts of the endoneurium (3, 5). (See Plate 31, Fig. 2).

Blood vessels coursing in the interfascicular connective tissue (9, 10–11, 12–15, 16) send branches into each fascicle that ultimately divide into capillaries in the endoneurium.

PLATE 30

NERVOUS TISSUE: NERVE FIBERS AND NERVES

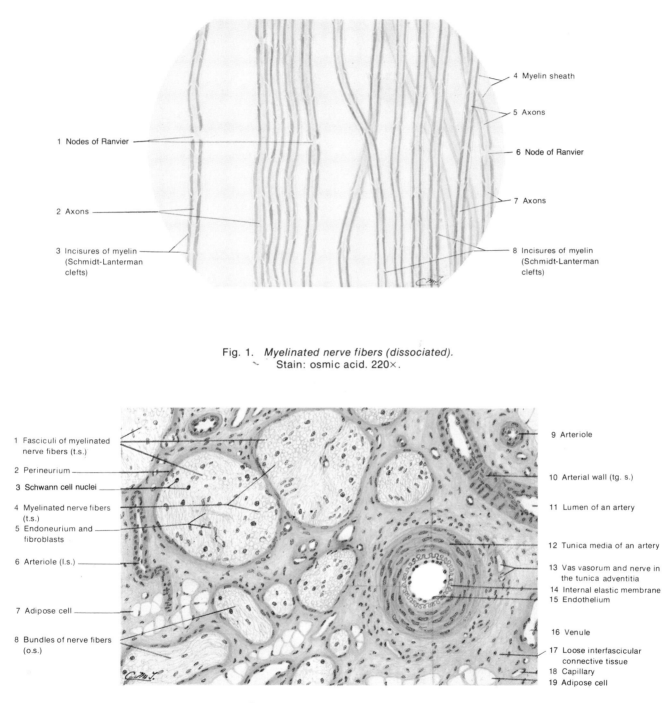

1 Nodes of Ranvier

2 Axons

3 Incisures of myelin
(Schmidt-Lanterman
clefts)

4 Myelin sheath

5 Axons

6 Node of Ranvier

7 Axons

8 Incisures of myelin
(Schmidt-Lanterman
clefts)

Fig. 1. *Myelinated nerve fibers (dissociated).*
Stain: osmic acid. 220×.

1 Fasciculi of myelinated
nerve fibers (t.s.)

2 Perineurium

3 Schwann cell nuclei

4 Myelinated nerve fibers
(t.s.)

5 Endoneurium and
fibroblasts

6 Arteriole (l.s.)

7 Adipose cell

8 Bundles of nerve fibers
(o.s.)

9 Arteriole

10 Arterial wall (tg. s.)

11 Lumen of an artery

12 Tunica media of an artery

13 Vas vasorum and nerve in
the tunica adventitia
14 Internal elastic membrane
15 Endothelium

16 Venule

17 Loose interfascicular
connective tissue
18 Capillary
19 Adipose cell

Fig. 2. *Nerve (transverse section).*
Stain: hematoxylin-eosin. 250×.

PLATE 31 (Fig. 1)
NERVE (SCIATIC), PANORAMIC VIEW, LONGITUDINAL SECTION

A portion of sciatic nerve is illustrated at a low magnification, as it appears in a routine histologic preparation stained with hematoxylin-eosin. The complete outer layer of dense connective tissue, the epineurium, is not shown in the illustration; the deeper part of the epineurium contains adipose tissue (2) and blood vessels (1). Extensions of the epineurium (3) pass around large nerve fascicles (5). Perineurium (4) forms a connective tissue sheath around individual nerve fascicles. The numerous nuclei that are arranged along nerve fibers are the Schwann cell nuclei (neurolemma nuclei) or fibroblast nuclei of the endoneurium connective tissue. It is not possible to differentiate between the Schwann cells and fibroblasts at this magnification.

PLATE 31 (Fig. 2)
NERVE (SCIATIC), LONGITUDINAL SECTION

A small portion of the nerve illustrated in Figure 1 is shown at a higher magnification. The axons appear as slender threads stained lightly with hematoxylin (1). The surrounding myelin sheath has been dissolved, leaving a distinct neurokeratin network of protein (3). The sheath of Schwann cells is not always distinguishable from the surrounding connective tissue; however, it may be seen in certain areas as a thin, peripheral boundary (4) and at the node of Ranvier (2) as it descends toward the axon. Two Schwann cell nuclei are seen (5) in the illustration as the endoneurium (7) surrounds each fiber. The fibroblasts in the endoneurium (6) can now be distinguished from the Schwann cell nuclei (5).

PLATE 31 (Fig. 3)
NERVE (SCIATIC), TRANSVERSE SECTION

The transverse section of sciatic nerve, as seen in Figure 2, illustrates the central axons (2), the neurokeratin network (3) of protein as peripheral radial lines that do not reach the axons, and the peripheral Schwann cell sheath (4). Schwann cell nucleus (1) appears to encircle the axon (2).

Collagenous fibers of the endoneurium are faintly distinguishable; however, the fibroblasts (5) are clearly seen. Perineurium (6) surrounds a fascicle of nerve fibers and contains a small blood vessel (7).

PLATE 31 (Fig. 4)
NERVE (SCIATIC), LONGITUDINAL SECTION

This section is stained with Protargol and aniline blue. Axons (1) are prominent due to silver impregnation of the neurofibrils. The scattered black droplets probably represent remnants of neurofibrils remaining after axon shrinkage. The neurokeratin network is not stained; other structures are stained with aniline blue.

PLATE 31 (Fig. 5)
NERVE (SCIATIC), TRANSVERSE SECTION

As described in Figure 4, Protargol stains the axon black (1), as seen in cross section. The surrounding gray area and small, black droplets probably indicate the original axon diameter. Endoneurium is well demonstrated by aniline blue staining of collagenous fibers (4, 6).

PLATE 31 (Fig. 6)
NERVE (BRANCH OF THE VAGUS), TRANSVERSE SECTION

This figure illustrates still another staining method for nerve fibers and shows myelinated axons of varying size in a branch of the vagus nerve. Nuclei, axons, and neurokeratin network stain red with azocarmine (1, 3, 4, 6). Endoneurium is again clearly demonstrated, especially in areas where axons are close together (7) and within groups of small nerve fibers (8).

PLATE 31

NERVOUS TISSUE: NERVES AND NERVE FIBERS

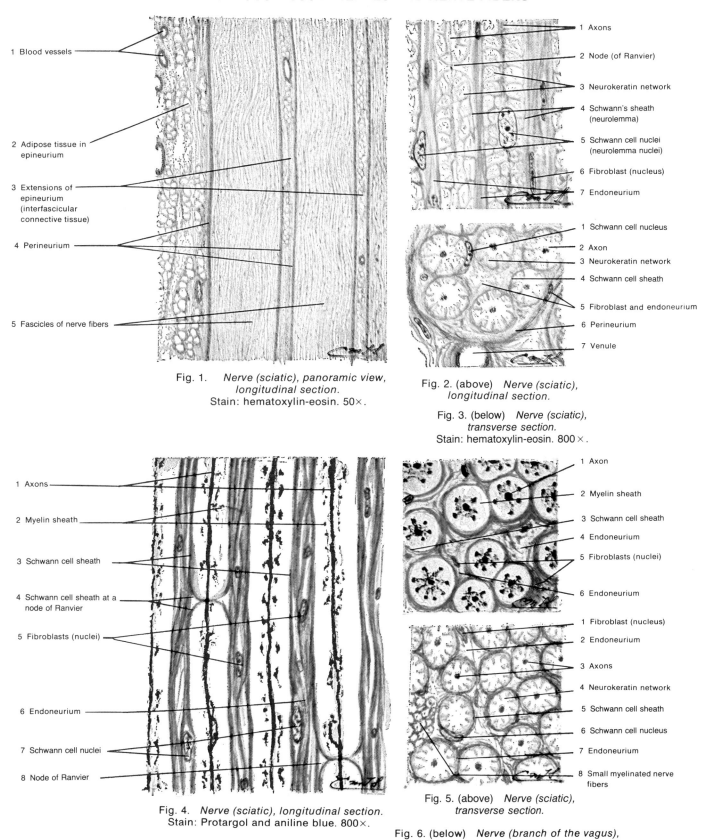

1 Blood vessels

2 Adipose tissue in epineurium

3 Extensions of epineurium (interfascicular connective tissue)

4 Perineurium

5 Fascicles of nerve fibers

Fig. 1. *Nerve (sciatic), panoramic view, longitudinal section.*
Stain: hematoxylin-eosin. 50×.

1 Axons
2 Node (of Ranvier)
3 Neurokeratin network
4 Schwann's sheath (neurolemma)
5 Schwann cell nuclei (neurolemma nuclei)
6 Fibroblast (nucleus)
7 Endoneurium

Fig. 2. (above) *Nerve (sciatic), longitudinal section.*

1 Schwann cell nucleus
2 Axon
3 Neurokeratin network
4 Schwann cell sheath
5 Fibroblast and endoneurium
6 Perineurium
7 Venule

Fig. 3. (below) *Nerve (sciatic), transverse section.*
Stain: hematoxylin-eosin. 800×.

1 Axons
2 Myelin sheath
3 Schwann cell sheath
4 Schwann cell sheath at a node of Ranvier
5 Fibroblasts (nuclei)
6 Endoneurium
7 Schwann cell nuclei
8 Node of Ranvier

Fig. 4. *Nerve (sciatic), longitudinal section.*
Stain: Protargol and aniline blue. 800×.

1 Axon
2 Myelin sheath
3 Schwann cell sheath
4 Endoneurium
5 Fibroblasts (nuclei)
6 Endoneurium

1 Fibroblast (nucleus)
2 Endoneurium
3 Axons
4 Neurokeratin network
5 Schwann cell sheath
6 Schwann cell nucleus
7 Endoneurium
8 Small myelinated nerve fibers

Fig. 5. (above) *Nerve (sciatic), transverse section.*

Fig. 6. (below) *Nerve (branch of the vagus), transverse section.*
Stain: Mallory-azan. 800×.

PLATE 32 (Fig. 1)

DORSAL ROOT GANGLION: PANORAMIC VIEW
(LONGITUDINAL SECTION)

A connective tissue layer, rich in adipose cells and blood vessels, surrounds the mass of nervous tissue (1, 5, 13). It merges with the external capsule of the ganglion, the epineurium (2), which is continuous with the epineurium of the dorsal root (3) and with that of the spinal neve (10). The perineurium and the endoneurium are not distinguishable at this magnification.

Many round pseudounipolar neurons of varying size make up the bulk of the ganglion (8); they are conspicuous because of their size and staining capacity. Their vesicular nuclei with nucleoli are better visible at higher magnification in Figure 2. Fascicles of nerve fibers are seen between groups of ganglion cells. The larger fascicles run in a longitudinal direction (9) and will either enter the dorsal root (4) or the spinal nerve (11). These nerve fibers represent, respectively, the central processes and peripheral processes formed by bifurcation of a single axon process which emerges from each ganglion cell.

The ventral root (7) joins the nerve fibers that emerge from the ganglion (12) to form the spinal nerve (11).

PLATE 32 (Fig. 2)

SECTION OF A DORSAL ROOT GANGLION

With a higher magnification, the pseudounipolar neurons are variable in size. The characteristic vesicular nucleus with its prominent nucleolus (2) is conspicuous and the cytoplasm is filled with Nissl bodies (3). Some cells display a small clump of lipofuscin pigment (5). Each cell has an axon hillock (not visible in this illustration).

Within the perineuronal space and in close association with the ganglion cells are the satellite cells. These cells have spherical nuclei, are of neuroectodermal origin, and form a loose inner layer of the capsule (6) around the ganglion cells. An outer capsule of more flattened fibroblasts and connective tissue fibers (7) is continuous with the endoneurium. In sections, these two layers are not always clearly distinguishable; often the two cell types appear intermingled, as seen around the cell with the lipofuscin pigment (5).

Between ganglion cells are seen many fibroblasts (4), randomly arranged in the connective tissue framework, or in rows in the endoneurium between nerve fibers (1, 8). With hematoxylin-eosin stain, small axons and connective tissue fibers are not clearly defined. Large myelinated fibers are recognizable when sectioned longitudinally (1).

PLATE 32 (Fig. 3)

SECTION OF A SYMPATHETIC TRUNK GANGLION

Similar to the dorsal root ganglion cells, sympathetic trunk ganglion cells contain a characteristic nucleus and a nucleolus (sometimes multiple nucleoli) and Nissl bodies throughout the cytoplasm.

In contrast to the dorsal root ganglion cells, these cells are multipolar neurons and are smaller in size. As a result, cell outlines are often irregular and remnants of processes may be present (6). Nuclei are often eccentric (6) and binucleated cells are common. Most neurons contain lipofuscin pigment. The neurons are more uniform in size than the dorsal root ganglion cells.

Satellite cells (2, 5) are usually less numerous than in the dorsal root ganglion cells and the connective tissue capsule may or may not be well defined (3).

In the intercellular areas (4) are fibroblasts, supportive connective tissue, blood vessels, and unmyelinated and myelinated axons. Nerve fibers aggregate into bundles (1, 7) which course through the sympathetic trunk; they represent preganglionic fibers, postganglionic visceral efferent fibers, and visceral afferent fibers.

PLATE 32

NERVOUS TISSUE: GANGLIA

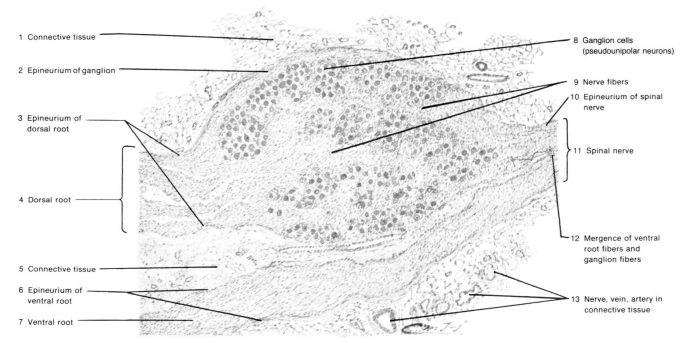

1 Connective tissue

2 Epineurium of ganglion

3 Epineurium of dorsal root

4 Dorsal root

5 Connective tissue

6 Epineurium of ventral root

7 Ventral root

8 Ganglion cells (pseudounipolar neurons)

9 Nerve fibers

10 Epineurium of spinal nerve

11 Spinal nerve

12 Mergence of ventral root fibers and ganglion fibers

13 Nerve, vein, artery in connective tissue

Fig. 1. *Dorsal root ganglion: panoramic view (longitudinal section).*
Stain: hematoxylin-eosin. 25×.

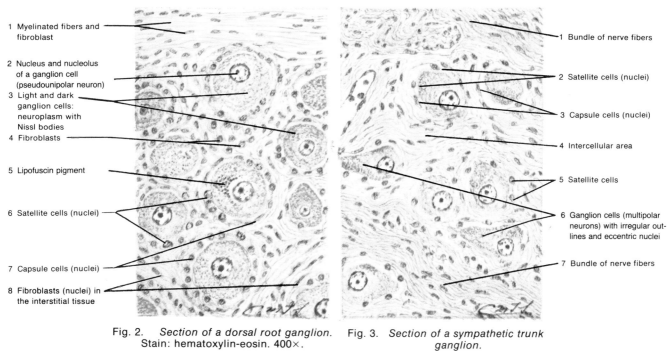

1 Myelinated fibers and fibroblast

2 Nucleus and nucleolus of a ganglion cell (pseudounipolar neuron)

3 Light and dark ganglion cells: neuroplasm with Nissl bodies

4 Fibroblasts

5 Lipofuscin pigment

6 Satellite cells (nuclei)

7 Capsule cells (nuclei)

8 Fibroblasts (nuclei) in the interstitial tissue

1 Bundle of nerve fibers

2 Satellite cells (nuclei)

3 Capsule cells (nuclei)

4 Intercellular area

5 Satellite cells

6 Ganglion cells (multipolar neurons) with irregular outlines and eccentric nuclei

7 Bundle of nerve fibers

Fig. 2. *Section of a dorsal root ganglion.*
Stain: hematoxylin-eosin. 400×.

Fig. 3. *Section of a sympathetic trunk ganglion.*
Stain: hematoxylin-eosin. 400×.

PLATE 33 (Fig. 1)

SPINAL CORD: CERVICAL REGION (PANORAMIC VIEW), TRANSVERSE SECTION

In a transverse section of a fresh spinal cord, the cord can be divided into outer white and inner gray matter. After staining, the two areas are readily recognized, but the significance of the "white" and "gray" terms is lost. Cajal's silver impregnation method demonstrates the neurofibrils.

The inner gray matter in the spinal cord is H-shaped, and the two symmetrical halves are joined across the midline by a transverse commissure of gray substance (15). The anterior (ventral) gray horn (column) (18) is thicker and shorter than the posterior (dorsal) gray horn (column) (14). The anterior horn contains two groups of neurons: motor neurons of the anteromedial horn (8) and anterolateral horn (7). Unmyelinated axons (18) are seen in this area. Some of the axons (9) from these neurons cross the white matter to enter the periphery of the cord, at which point they emerge obliquely from the cord as components of the anterior (ventral) roots (21). The posterior horn contains groups of isolated large neurons (5) and groups of smaller ones.

The spinal cord on the dorsal surface has a longitudinal groove in the middle, the posterior median sulcus (10). A neuroglial membrane, the posterior median septum (13), extends inward and divides the posterior white matter into right and left halves. Each half, in turn, is divided by a less conspicuous postero-intermediate septum (12) into a postero-medial column, the fasciculus gracilis (11) and a postero-lateral column, the fasciculus cuneatus (1).

A transverse section of the central canal (16) is seen in the middle of the gray commissure. Located above and below the central canal is a gray matter called posterior (15) and anterior gray commissure (not illustrated), respectively. An anterior white commissure (17) is usually seen below the anterior gray commissure.

The most peripheral part of the spinal cord is the external glial limiting membrane (4), an area free of nerve fibers. Pia mater is indicated by a yellow zone around the cord; it is seen best in the anterior median fissure (20).

PLATE 33 (Fig. 2)

SPINAL CORD: ANTERIOR GRAY HORN AND
ADJACENT ANTERIOR WHITE MATTER

The anterior gray matter contains multipolar anterior horn cells or motor neurons (10) and their dendrites (2). The higher magnification illustrates typical characteristics, described previously. In the neurons (8, 10), the neurofibrils are arranged in a network, whereas in the dendrites (2), the arrangement is more parallel. The large, distinct, and spherical nucleus shows its prominent nucleolus (7). The surrounding small cells are the neuroglia cells (6).

In the intercellular areas of the anterior gray are seen different-sized axons (9) sectioned in various planes.

Axons of the anterior horn cells aggregate into groups and enter the white matter (1). As the axons pass through the white matter, they are myelinated and leave the cord as anterior (ventral) root fibers.

The white matter is composed primarily of myelinated axons that are closely packed, as illustrated in the transverse sections (5). The dark-stained and shrunken axons (3) are surrounded by a clear space which was occupied by myelin sheaths in unstained sections. These axons compose the ascending and descending tracts that course the length of the spinal cord.

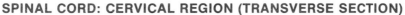

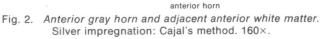

PLATE 33

SPINAL CORD: CERVICAL REGION (TRANSVERSE SECTION)

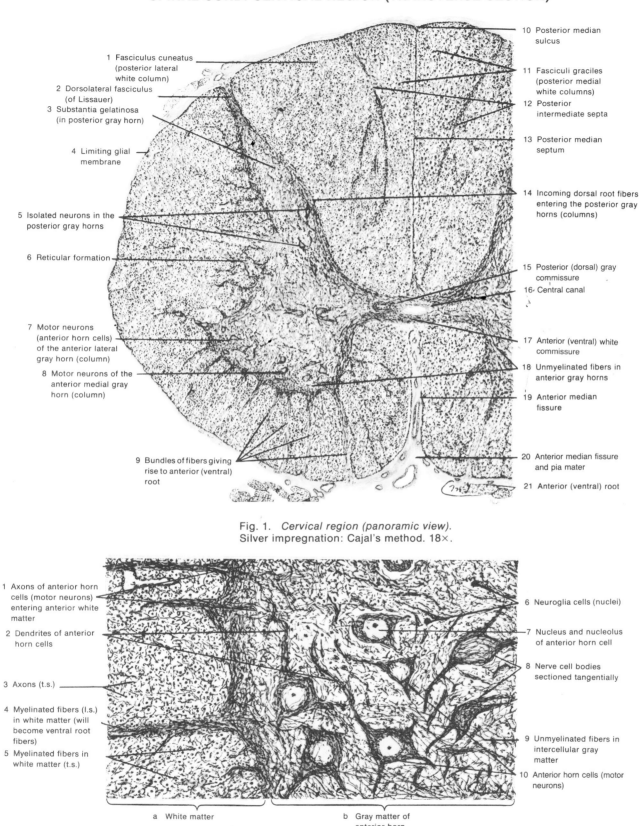

1 Fasciculus cuneatus
(posterior lateral
white column)

2 Dorsolateral fasciculus
(of Lissauer)

3 Substantia gelatinosa
(in posterior gray horn)

4 Limiting glial
membrane

5 Isolated neurons in the
posterior gray horns

6 Reticular formation

7 Motor neurons
(anterior horn cells)
of the anterior lateral
gray horn (column)

8 Motor neurons of the
anterior medial gray
horn (column)

9 Bundles of fibers giving
rise to anterior (ventral)
root

10 Posterior median
sulcus

11 Fasciculi graciles
(posterior medial
white columns)

12 Posterior
intermediate septa

13 Posterior median
septum

14 Incoming dorsal root fibers
entering the posterior gray
horns (columns)

15 Posterior (dorsal) gray
commissure

16 Central canal

17 Anterior (ventral) white
commissure

18 Unmyelinated fibers in
anterior gray horns

19 Anterior median
fissure

20 Anterior median fissure
and pia mater

21 Anterior (ventral) root

Fig. 1. *Cervical region (panoramic view).*
Silver impregnation: Cajal's method. 18×.

1 Axons of anterior horn
cells (motor neurons)
entering anterior white
matter

2 Dendrites of anterior
horn cells

3 Axons (t.s.)

4 Myelinated fibers (l.s.)
in white matter (will
become ventral root
fibers)

5 Myelinated fibers in
white matter (t.s.)

6 Neuroglia cells (nuclei)

7 Nucleus and nucleolus
of anterior horn cell

8 Nerve cell bodies
sectioned tangentially

9 Unmyelinated fibers in
intercellular gray
matter

10 Anterior horn cells (motor
neurons)

a White matter

b Gray matter of
anterior horn

Fig. 2. *Anterior gray horn and adjacent anterior white matter.*
Silver impregnation: Cajal's method. 160×.

PLATE 34 (Fig. 1)

SPINAL CORD: MID-THORACIC REGION
(TRANSVERSE SECTION, PANORAMIC VIEW)

This illustration represents a transverse section of a spinal cord in mid-thoracic region, as seen in a routine hematoxylin-eosin preparation. It differs in several ways from the section of the cervical cord illustrated in Plate 33. The posterior gray horns (columns) are slender (5). At the ventromedial basal portion of the horn is seen the nucleus dorsalis (of Clarke), a prominent structure because of the number and size of the neurons (22). The lateral gray columns are well developed and contain small neurons of the sympathetic nucleus (23). The anterior gray horns are small, and the number of motor neurons is reduced to only a few cells in both the medial and lateral motor nuclei regions (24).

Other structures in the mid-thoracic section of the cord are represented in corresponding areas of the cervical cord illustrated in Plate 33, differing only in appearance because of the type of stain used.

Also illustrated in this section are the meninges of the spinal cord. The fibrous pia mater (9), the innermost layer of the meninges, adheres closely to the external glial limiting membrane of the spinal cord, which is not clearly seen in the figure. Pia mater contains both small and larger blood vessels (1, 15) which supply and drain the cord. Fine trabeculae in the subarachnoid space (10) connect the pia mater with the arachnoid (11); the subarachnoid space is normally filled with cerebrospinal fluid. External to the arachnoid is the thick, fibrous dura mater (13), separated from the arachnoid by the subdural space (12). In this preparation, the subdural space is unusually large because of artifactual retraction of the arachnoid.

PLATE 34 (Fig. 2)

NERVE CELLS OF SOME TYPICAL REGIONS
OF THE SPINAL CORD

Nerve cells situated in the gray matter exhibit different characteristics according to the region they occupy and the function that they perform.

This figure illustrates several anterior horn cells (a), whose typical characteristic features have been described in Plate 27, Figure 1. The only difference in this figure is the type of stain that was used. The typical vesicular nucleus, with its prominent nucleolus, is centrally located. When the plane of section passes through the superficial portion of the cell, the nucleus is normally not observed (2). Nissl substance appears as large clumps (1), uniformly distributed throughout the cytoplasm and partially into the dendrites (4). The clear axon hillock and the initial segment of the axon may be seen in some of the cells (3). These axons contribute to the formation of the ventral roots and terminate by innervating skeletal muscles.

The two cells in (b) are posterior horn cells from the substantia gelatinosa. They are much smaller than the anterior horn cells, are spherical or polygonal in shape, exhibit fine Nissl bodies, and contain a nucleus that is usually deep-staining. These cells are believed to function as association cells, especially for incoming pain and temperature impulses.

At (c) are illustrated two cells of the lateral sympathetic nucleus, which is located in the lateral gray horns of the thoracic and upper lumbar segments of the spinal cord. These are small cells, somewhat larger than those of the substantia gelatinosa, but with similar features. Their axons enter the ventral roots and pass by way of white rami to the vertebral or prevertebral ganglia.

The last illustration (d) represents cells from the nucleus dorsalis (of Clarke); its location is seen at (22) in Figure 1. They are large multipolar cells, similar in size to anterior horn cells. The Nissl substance is in coarse clumps and characteristically situated at the cell periphery (5). The typical vesicular nucleus with its nucleolus is eccentric (7). As usual, the nucleus is not seen when the section passes through the periphery of the cell (6). These cells receive incoming proprioceptive fibers.

Plate 34

SPINAL CORD: MID-THORACIC REGION (TRANSVERSE SECTION)

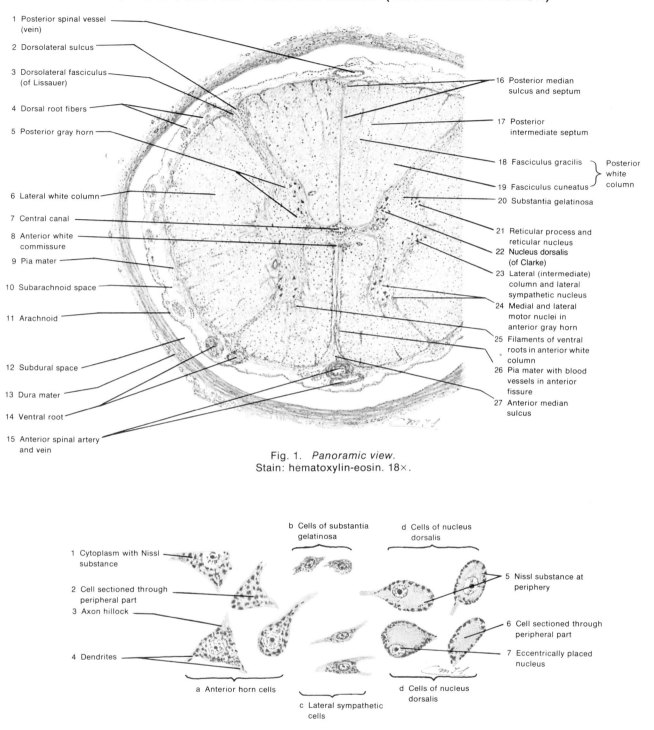

1 Posterior spinal vessel (vein)

2 Dorsolateral sulcus

3 Dorsolateral fasciculus (of Lissauer)

4 Dorsal root fibers

5 Posterior gray horn

6 Lateral white column

7 Central canal

8 Anterior white commissure

9 Pia mater

10 Subarachnoid space

11 Arachnoid

12 Subdural space

13 Dura mater

14 Ventral root

15 Anterior spinal artery and vein

16 Posterior median sulcus and septum

17 Posterior intermediate septum

18 Fasciculus gracilis ⎫ Posterior
19 Fasciculus cuneatus ⎭ white column

20 Substantia gelatinosa

21 Reticular process and reticular nucleus

22 Nucleus dorsalis (of Clarke)

23 Lateral (intermediate) column and lateral sympathetic nucleus

24 Medial and lateral motor nuclei in anterior gray horn

25 Filaments of ventral roots in anterior white column

26 Pia mater with blood vessels in anterior fissure

27 Anterior median sulcus

Fig. 1. *Panoramic view.*
Stain: hematoxylin-eosin. 18×.

b Cells of substantia gelatinosa

d Cells of nucleus dorsalis

1 Cytoplasm with Nissl substance

2 Cell sectioned through peripheral part

3 Axon hillock

4 Dendrites

5 Nissl substance at periphery

6 Cell sectioned through peripheral part

7 Eccentrically placed nucleus

a Anterior horn cells

c Lateral sympathetic cells

d Cells of nucleus dorsalis

Fig. 2. *Nerve cells of some typical regions of the spinal cord.*
Stain: hematoxylin-eosin. 380×.

PLATE 35 (Fig. 1)

CEREBELLUM: SECTIONAL VIEW, TRANSVERSE SECTION

The cerebellum consists of an inner medullary center of white matter (4) and an outer cortex of gray matter (3).

The white matter (4, 10) is composed of myelinated fibers; its ramifications (10) form the core of the numerous cerebellar folds. These fibers are the afferent and efferent fibers of the cerebellar cortex.

The gray matter constitutes the cortex and three distinct cell layers can be distinguished; an outer molecular layer (6) with relatively few cells and horizontally directed fibers; an inner granular layer (7) with numerous small cells with intensely stained nuclei; and a central layer of Purkinje cells (8). The Purkinje cells are pyriform in shape with ramified dendrites that extend into the molecular layer (see Figure 2 below).

PLATE 35 (Fig. 2)

CEREBELLUM: CORTEX

Purkinje cells (9) are typically arranged in a single row at the junction of the molecular and granular cell layers. Their large "flask-shaped" bodies give off one or more thick dendrites (3) which extend through the molecular layer to the surface, giving off complex branchings along their course. The thin axon (5) leaves the base of the Purkinje cell, passes through the granular layer, and becomes myelinated as it enters the white matter (12).

The molecular layer contains scattered stellate cells (8) whose unmyelinated axons normally course in a horizontal direction. Descending collaterals of more deeply placed basket cells arborize around the Purkinje cells (4) in a "basket-like" arrangement. Axons of the granule cells in the granular layer extend into the molecular layer and also course horizontally (2) as unmyelinated fibers.

In the granular layer are found numerous small granule cells (6) with dark-staining nuclei (an exception to the usual vesicular nucleus of nerve cells) and very little cytoplasm. Also present in the granular layer are scattered larger stellate cells or Golgi type II cells (7) with typical vesicular nuclei and more cytoplasm. Throughout the granular layer are small, irregularly dispersed, clear spaces called the glomeruli (11), in which cells are absent and synaptic complexes occur.

PLATE 35

CEREBELLUM

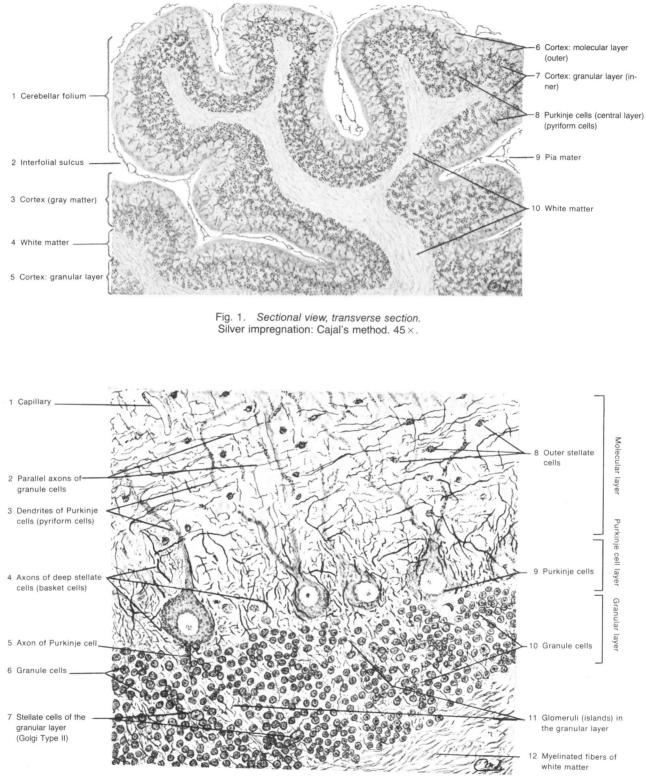

1 Cerebellar folium

2 Interfolial sulcus

3 Cortex (gray matter)

4 White matter

5 Cortex: granular layer

6 Cortex: molecular layer (outer)

7 Cortex: granular layer (inner)

8 Purkinje cells (central layer) (pyriform cells)

9 Pia mater

10 White matter

Fig. 1. *Sectional view, transverse section.*
Silver impregnation: Cajal's method. 45×.

1 Capillary

2 Parallel axons of granule cells

3 Dendrites of Purkinje cells (pyriform cells)

4 Axons of deep stellate cells (basket cells)

5 Axon of Purkinje cell

6 Granule cells

7 Stellate cells of the granular layer (Golgi Type II)

8 Outer stellate cells

9 Purkinje cells

10 Granule cells

11 Glomeruli (islands) in the granular layer

12 Myelinated fibers of white matter

Molecular layer

Purkinje cell layer

Granular layer

Fig. 2. *Cortex.*
Silver impregnation: Cajal's method. 300×.

PLATE 36 (Fig. 1)

CEREBRAL CORTEX: SECTION PERPENDICULAR TO THE CORTICAL SURFACE

The staining method used for this section of cerebral cortex demonstrates neurofibrils.

The various cell types that constitute the cerebral cortex are distributed in layers, with one or more cell types predominant in each layer. Horizontal fibers associated with each layer give the cortex a laminated appearance. Fibers exhibiting radial arrangement (14) are also present.

Although there are variations in arrangement of cells in different parts of the cerebral cortex, six distinct layers are recognized; these layers are labeled on the left side of the figure.

Starting at the periphery of the cortex, the outermost layer is the molecular layer (1). Its peripheral portion is composed predominantly of horizontally directed neuronal processes, both dendrites and axons. In its deeper region lie the infrequent horizontal cells of Cajal (10) which exhibit a stellate or spindle shape; their axons contribute to the horizontal fibers. Overlying and covering the molecular layer is the pia mater (8).

In the next four layers, the predominant cells are the characteristic pyramidal cells of the cerebral cortex; these cells vary in size. The figure illustrates that the pyramidal cells get progressively larger (11, 13) in layers 2, 3, 4, and 5. Their dendrites (13) are directed toward the periphery and the axon extends from the cell base. In the internal granular layer (4), numerous smaller and larger stellate cells (12) form numerous and complex connections with the pyramidal cells.

The multiform layer (6) lacks the pyramidal cells; however, the fusiform cells predominate and the granule cells, stellate cells, and cells of Martinotti are intermixed. All of these cells vary in size. Axons of the cells of Martinotti are directed peripherally, whereas the axons from other cells enter the white matter (16).

PLATE 36 (Fig. 2)

CEREBRAL CORTEX: CENTRAL AREA OF THE CORTEX

Higher magnification of the cerebral cortex illustrates the large pyramidal cells (1, 8). Neurofibrils in the cell bodies have the characteristic network arrangement (1, 8), whereas neurofibrils in the dendrites (6) and the axons (7) exhibit a more parallel arrangement. The typical large vesicular nucleus (3) with its prominent nucleolus (3, lower leader) is outlined. The most prominent cell process is the apical dendrite (6), which is directed toward the surface of the cortex. Several collaterals (5) are given off along its course through the cortex. Smaller dendrites (6, middle leader) arise from other parts of the cell body. The axon (7) arises from the base of the cell body and passes into the white matter.

The intercellular area is occupied by nerve fibers (2) of various cells in the cortex, small astrocytes (4), and blood vessels.

PLATE 36

CEREBRAL CORTEX

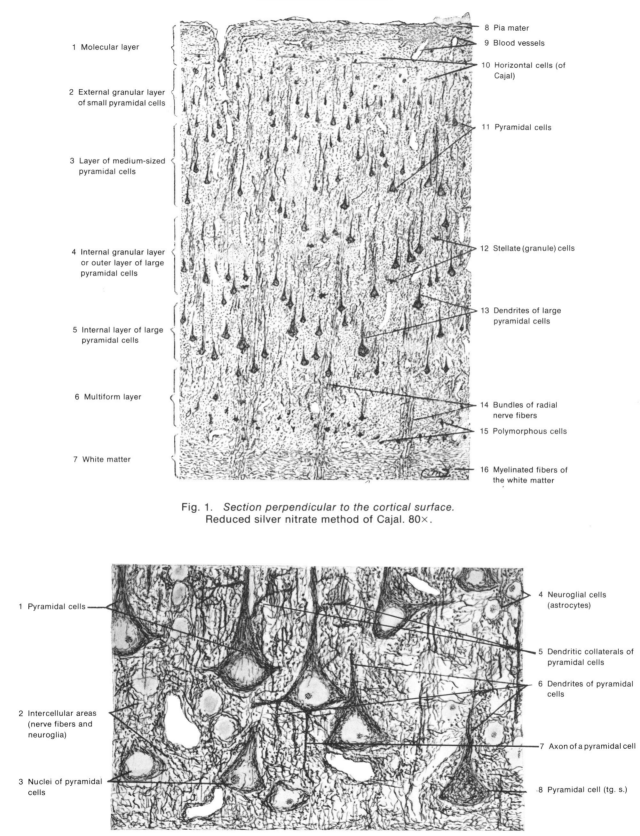

1 Molecular layer

2 External granular layer of small pyramidal cells

3 Layer of medium-sized pyramidal cells

4 Internal granular layer or outer layer of large pyramidal cells

5 Internal layer of large pyramidal cells

6 Multiform layer

7 White matter

8 Pia mater

9 Blood vessels

10 Horizontal cells (of Cajal)

11 Pyramidal cells

12 Stellate (granule) cells

13 Dendrites of large pyramidal cells

14 Bundles of radial nerve fibers

15 Polymorphous cells

16 Myelinated fibers of the white matter

Fig. 1. *Section perpendicular to the cortical surface.*
Reduced silver nitrate method of Cajal. 80×.

1 Pyramidal cells

2 Intercellular areas (nerve fibers and neuroglia)

3 Nuclei of pyramidal cells

4 Neuroglial cells (astrocytes)

5 Dendritic collaterals of pyramidal cells

6 Dendrites of pyramidal cells

7 Axon of a pyramidal cell

8 Pyramidal cell (tg. s.)

Fig. 2. *Central area of the cortex.*
Reduced silver nitrate method of Cajal. 300×.

PLATE 37 (Fig. 1)

BLOOD AND LYMPHATIC VESSELS

This plate illustrates various types of blood and lymphatic vessels, surrounded by loose connective and adipose tissue (13, 28). Most vessels have been cut in transverse or oblique sections.

A small artery is shown at the top center of the plate, illustrating the basic structure of its wall. In contrast to a vein, an artery has a relatively thick wall and a small lumen. In cross section, the wall of an artery shows the following layers:

a. tunica intima, composed of an inner layer of endothelium (16), a subendothelial layer of connective tissue (17), and an internal elastic lamina (membrane) (19) which marks the boundary between the tunica intima and tunica media.

b. tunica media (4), composed predominantly of circular smooth muscle fibers. A loose network of fine elastic fibers is interspersed among the smooth muscle cells.

c. tunica adventitia (6), composed of connective tissue which contains small nerves (14) and blood vessels (15). The blood vessels in the adventitia are collectively called vasa vasorum (15), or "blood vessels of blood vessels."

When arteries acquire about 25 or more layers of smooth muscle in tunica media, they are called muscular or distributing arteries. Elastic fibers become more numerous, but are still present as thin fibers and networks.

A medium-sized vein (22) is illustrated at the lower center of the plate. It has a relatively thin wall and a large lumen. In cross section, the wall of the vein shows the following layers:

a. tunica intima, composed of endothelium (24) and a very thin layer of fine collagenous and elastic fibers which blend with the connective tissue of the media.

b. tunica media (25), consisting of a thin layer of circularly arranged smooth muscle loosely embedded in connective tissue. This layer is much thinner in veins than in arteries.

c. tunica adventitia (26), consisting of a wide layer of connective tissue. This layer in veins is much thicker than the tunica media.

Arterioles are also illustrated (1, 5, 8) in the figure. The smallest arteriole (1) has a thin internal elastic lamina and one layer of smooth muscle cells in the media. One arteriole with a branching capillary is sectioned longitudinally (8). Also illustrated are smaller veins (18, 27), venules (3, 10), capillaries (9, 11, 20) and small nerves (2, 23).

A lymphatic vessel (12) can be recognized by the thinness of its walls and the flaps of a valve in the lumen. Many veins in the body have similar valves.

PLATE 37 (Fig. 2)

LARGE VEIN: PORTAL VEIN (TRANSVERSE SECTION)

In large veins, the outstanding feature is the thick, muscular adventitia, with the smooth muscle fibers exhibiting a longitudinal orientation. In the illustrated transverse section of the portal vein, the typical arrangement is observed: the smooth muscle is segregated into bundles and seen mainly in cross section (1), with varying amounts of connective tissue dispersed among them (2). Vasa vasorum (3, 7) are present in the intervening connective tissue.

In contrast to the thick adventitia, the media is a thinner layer of circularly arranged smooth muscle (6) and a looser arranged connective tissue. In other large veins, the media may be thin and a more compact layer. As seen in other vessels, the tunica intima is part of the endothelium (4) and supported by a small amount of connective tissue. In addition, large veins usually exhibit an internal elastic lamina (5), not as well developed as in arteries.

PLATE 37

BLOOD AND LYMPHATIC VESSELS AND LARGE VEIN

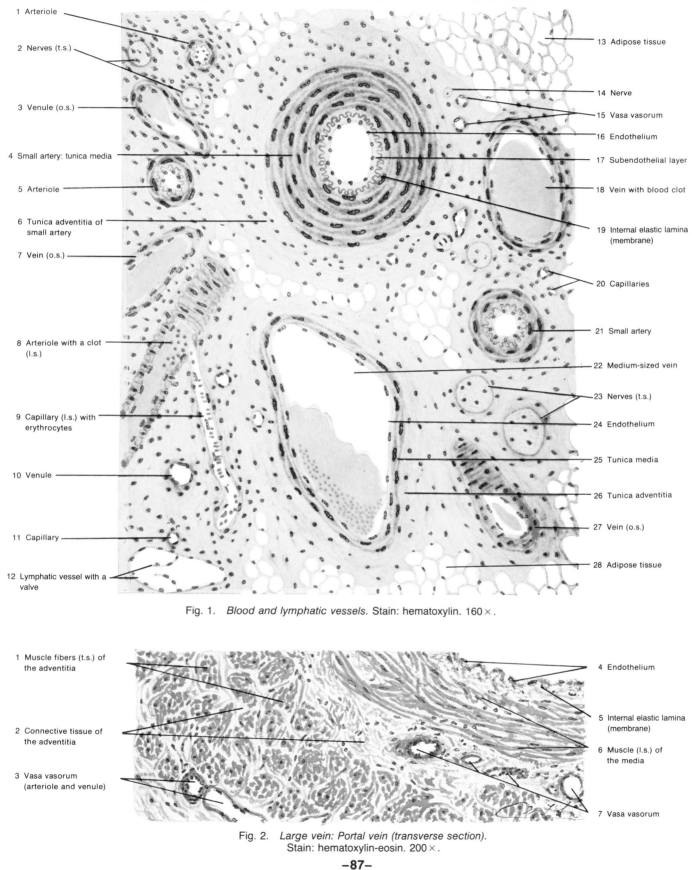

1 Arteriole

2 Nerves (t.s.)

3 Venule (o.s.)

4 Small artery: tunica media

5 Arteriole

6 Tunica adventitia of
small artery

7 Vein (o.s.)

8 Arteriole with a clot
(l.s.)

9 Capillary (l.s.) with
erythrocytes

10 Venule

11 Capillary

12 Lymphatic vessel with a
valve

13 Adipose tissue

14 Nerve

15 Vasa vasorum

16 Endothelium

17 Subendothelial layer

18 Vein with blood clot

19 Internal elastic lamina
(membrane)

20 Capillaries

21 Small artery

22 Medium-sized vein

23 Nerves (t.s.)

24 Endothelium

25 Tunica media

26 Tunica adventitia

27 Vein (o.s.)

28 Adipose tissue

Fig. 1. *Blood and lymphatic vessels.* Stain: hematoxylin. 160×.

1 Muscle fibers (t.s.) of
the adventitia

2 Connective tissue of
the adventitia

3 Vasa vasorum
(arteriole and venule)

4 Endothelium

5 Internal elastic lamina
(membrane)

6 Muscle (l.s.) of
the media

7 Vasa vasorum

Fig. 2. *Large vein: Portal vein (transverse section).*
Stain: hematoxylin-eosin. 200×.

PLATE 38 (Fig. 1)

NEUROVASCULAR BUNDLE (TRANSVERSE SECTION)

In the center of the figure is a large, elastic artery (18) with a thick tunica media (16) consisting primarily of concentric layers of elastic lamina (membrane), between which are found thin layers of smooth muscle. The tunica intima consists of endothelium (19) whose round nuclei appear to project into the lumen of the artery, and a thin layer of subendothelial connective tissue (19) containing fine collagenous and elastic fibers. The first visible elastic membrane is considered to be the internal elastic lamina (17). The tunica adventitia (15) is a thin layer of collagenous fibers, but contains vasa vasorum and the vasomotor nerves.

Several arterioles (3, 9, 26) are seen, distinguished by their thin muscular walls and relatively narrow lumina; numerous capillaries (21) are also seen in the vicinity.

Veins exhibit a varied morphology (4, 7, 22 and others); however, each vein has a thin wall and a large lumen. Some veins can contain a blood clot or hemolyzed blood (7, 22).

Nerves of various sizes (2, 8, 10, 25) accompany blood vessels. Each nerve is surrounded by perineurium and is composed primarily of unmyelinated axons. Also illustrated is a sympathetic ganglion (1) surrounded by a connective tissue capsule and containing multipolar neurons, axons and small blood vessels.

The figure also shows part of a small lymph node (5), its hilus (5), and several efferent lymphatic vessels (6). The larger lymph node (11) shows its capsule (14), the subcapsular sinus (13), cortex (12), and medulla (11).

PLATE 38 (Fig. 2)

LARGE ARTERY: AORTA (TRANSVERSE SECTION)

The structure of the illustrated artery is similar to that of the vessel illustrated in Figure 1; however, it has been stained with orcein, which specifically stains elastic fibers dark brown (2). Other tissues in the wall remain colorless or are only lightly stained. The size and arrangement of elastic lamina in the tunica media are clearly demonstrated. Smooth muscle (3) and fine elastic fibers between the laminae remain unstained.

The extent of tunica intima is indicated (4), but it remains unstained. The first elastic membrane is also considered the internal elastic lamina (membrane) (5). At times, smaller laminae appear in the subendothelial connective tissue, and a gradual transition is made to larger laminae of the tunica media.

The tunica adventitia (1), also unstained, is a narrow zone of collagenous fibers. In the aorta and pulmonary arteries, tunica media occupies most of the wall of the vessel; tunica adventitia is reduced to the proportionately small area illustrated in the figure.

PLATE 38

NEUROVASCULAR BUNDLE AND LARGE ARTERY

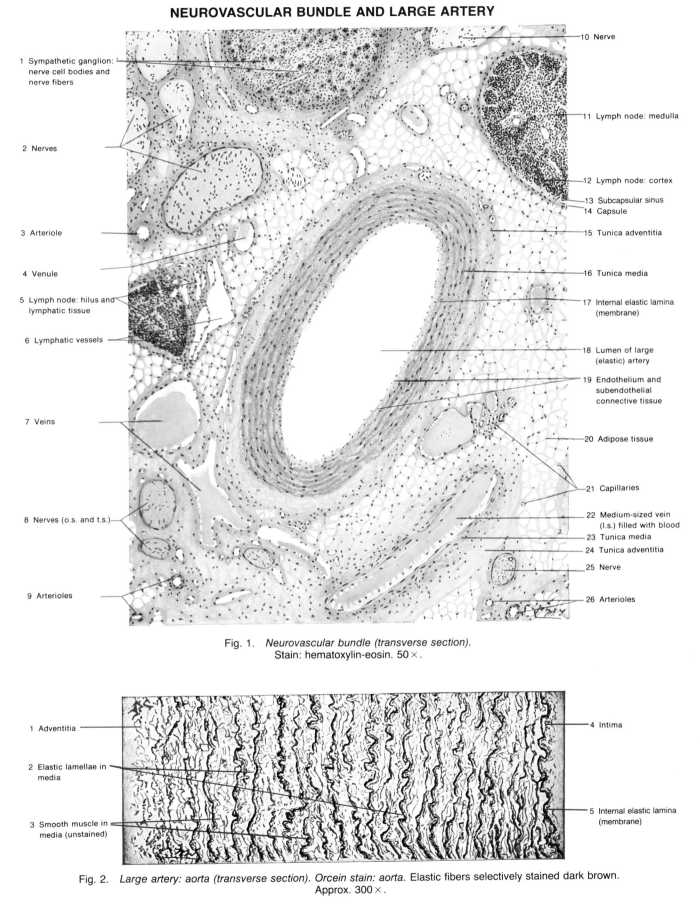

1 Sympathetic ganglion: nerve cell bodies and nerve fibers

2 Nerves

3 Arteriole

4 Venule

5 Lymph node: hilus and lymphatic tissue

6 Lymphatic vessels

7 Veins

8 Nerves (o.s. and t.s.)

9 Arterioles

10 Nerve

11 Lymph node: medulla

12 Lymph node: cortex

13 Subcapsular sinus

14 Capsule

15 Tunica adventitia

16 Tunica media

17 Internal elastic lamina (membrane)

18 Lumen of large (elastic) artery

19 Endothelium and subendothelial connective tissue

20 Adipose tissue

21 Capillaries

22 Medium-sized vein (l.s.) filled with blood

23 Tunica media

24 Tunica adventitia

25 Nerve

26 Arterioles

Fig. 1.   *Neurovascular bundle (transverse section).*
Stain: hematoxylin-eosin. 50 ×.

1 Adventitia

2 Elastic lamellae in media

3 Smooth muscle in media (unstained)

4 Intima

5 Internal elastic lamina (membrane)

Fig. 2.   *Large artery: aorta (transverse section). Orcein stain: aorta.* Elastic fibers selectively stained dark brown.
Approx. 300 ×.

PLATE 39

HEART: LEFT ATRIUM AND VENTRICLE
(PANORAMIC VIEW, LONGITUDINAL SECTION)

This figure illustrates a longitudinal section of the left side of the heart, showing a portion of the atrium, the atrioventricular (mitral) valve, and the ventricle.

In the atrial wall are seen the endocardium (1), consisting of endothelium, thick subendothelial layers of connective tissue, and the thick myocardium (2) with loosely arranged musculature. The epicardium (13) covers the heart and is lined externally by a single layer of mesothelium. A subepicardial layer contains connective tissue and fat (14) which varies in amount in different regions of the heart. This layer also extends into the coronary (atrioventricular) and interventricular sulcus of the heart.

In the ventricle, the endocardium (6) is thin in comparison with that in the atrium and the myocardium (2) is thick and more compact. The cardiac musculature is seen in various planes of section. The epicardium and subepicardial connective tissue (16) are continuous with those in the atrium.

Between the atrium and ventricle is seen the annulus fibrosus (3), which consists of dense fibrous connective tissue. The leaflet of the atrioventricular valve (mitral) (4) is formed by a double membrane of the endocardium (4a) and a core of dense connective tissue (4b), which is continuous with the annulus fibrosus (3). On the ventral surface of the valve is seen the insertion of chorda tendina (5) into the valve.

The inner surface of the ventricular wall exhibits the characteristic prominence of myocardium and endocardium: the apex of papillary muscle (18) and two trabeculae carnae (17).

The Purkinje fibers or impulse-conducting fibers (8) are located in the loose subendocardial tissue and may be distinguished by their larger size and lighter staining properties. The small area within the rectangle (9) is illustrated at a higher magnification in Plate 40, Figure 2.

The larger vessels, such as the coronary artery (10), course in the subepicardial connective tissue. Below the artery is a section through the coronary sinus (11), and entering into it is a coronary vein with its valve (12). Smaller coronary vessels may be seen in the subepicardial connective tissue and in the perimyseal septa that extend into the myocardium (15).

PLATE 39

HEART: LEFT ATRIUM AND VENTRICLE
(PANORAMIC VIEW, LONGITUDINAL SECTION)

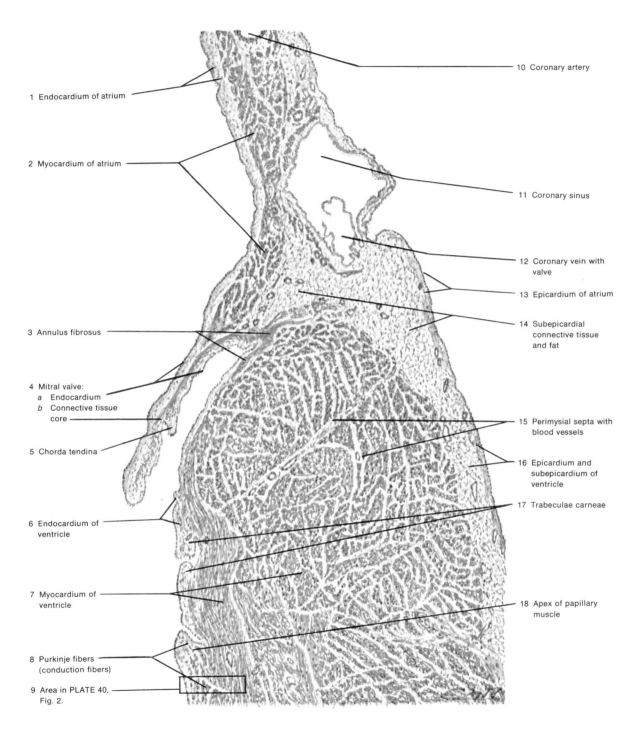

1 Endocardium of atrium

2 Myocardium of atrium

3 Annulus fibrosus

4 Mitral valve:
   a Endocardium
   b Connective tissue
      core

5 Chorda tendina

6 Endocardium of
  ventricle

7 Myocardium of
  ventricle

8 Purkinje fibers
  (conduction fibers)

9 Area in PLATE 40,
  Fig. 2.

10 Coronary artery

11 Coronary sinus

12 Coronary vein with
   valve

13 Epicardium of atrium

14 Subepicardial
   connective tissue
   and fat

15 Perimysial septa with
   blood vessels

16 Epicardium and
   subepicardium of
   ventricle

17 Trabeculae carneae

18 Apex of papillary
   muscle

Stain: hematoxylin-eosin. 6×.

PLATE 40 (Fig. 1)

HEART: PULMONARY TRUNK, PULMONARY VALVE, RIGHT VENTRICLE (PANORAMIC VIEW, LONGITUDINAL SECTION)

A portion of the right ventricle from which arises the pulmonary trunk is illustrated in Figure 1.

A section of the pulmonary trunk wall (6) is shown. The endothelium of the tunica intima is distinguishable on the right surface. Tunica media constitutes the thickest portion of its wall; however, its thick, elastic laminae are not apparent at this magnification. A thin adventitia merges into the surrounding subepicardial connective tissue (2), which contains large amounts of fat in this specimen.

The pulmonary trunk (8) arises from the annulus fibrosus (9), and one cusp of its semilunar valve (pulmonary) is illustrated (7). Like the mitral valve, it is covered with endocardium and the connective tissue from the annulus fibrosus extends into its base (10) and forms its central core.

The thick myocardium (4) of the right ventricle is covered on its internal surface by endocardium (11). The endocardium extends over the pulmonary valve and the annulus fibrosus, and blends in with tunica intima of the pulmonary trunk (8).

The external surface of the pulmonary trunk is lined with the subepicardial connective tissue and fat (2), which, in turn, is covered with epicardium (1). Both of these layers pass over the external surface of the ventricle. Coronary vessels are seen in the subepicardium (3, 5).

PLATE 40 (Fig. 2)

PURKINJE FIBERS (IMPULSE-CONDUCTING FIBERS, HEMATOXYLIN–EOSIN)

The area outlined by a rectangle (9) in Plate 39 is illustrated at higher magnification. Under the endocardium (1) are seen groups of Purkinje fibers, which are different from typical cardiac muscle fibers (5) due to their larger size and less intense staining. Some Purkinje fibers are sectioned transversely (2) and others longitudinally (4). In transverse section, the Purkinje fibers exhibit fewer myofibrils, distributed peripherally, leaving a perinuclear zone of comparatively clear sarcoplasm. A nucleus is seen in some transverse sections; in others, a central area of clear sarcoplasm is seen, with the plane of section bypassing the nucleus.

Purkinje fibers merge with cardiac fibers at a transitional fiber (3); the upper part of the fiber corresponds to a Purkinje fiber and the lower part to an ordinary cardiac muscle fiber.

PLATE 40 (Fig. 3)

PURKINJE FIBERS (IMPULSE-CONDUCTING FIBERS, MALLORY–AZAN)

This figure illustrates a cardiac region that contains an abundance of Purkinje fibers stained with Mallory–Azan; for this preparation, the same magnification as in Figure 2 was used.

The characteristic features of Purkinje fibers are adequately demonstrated in longitudinal and transverse sections (2).

With hematoxylin–eosin preparation, the connective tissue does not stain well. In this preparation, blue-stained collagenous fibers accentuate the subendocardial connective tissue (3) around the Purkinje fibers. A capillary with red blood cells (1) is seen near these fibers.

PLATE 40

HEART

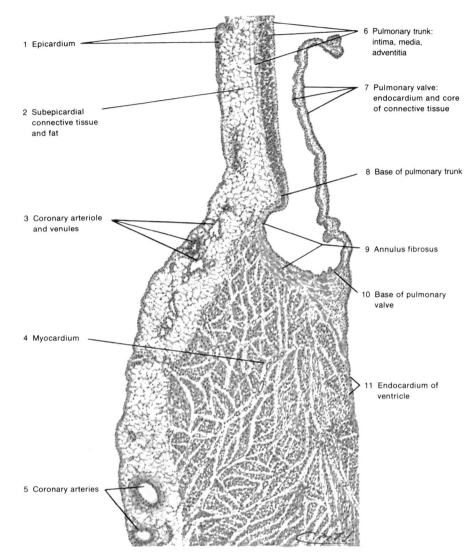

1 Epicardium

2 Subepicardial connective tissue and fat

3 Coronary arteriole and venules

4 Myocardium

5 Coronary arteries

6 Pulmonary trunk: intima, media, adventitia

7 Pulmonary valve: endocardium and core of connective tissue

8 Base of pulmonary trunk

9 Annulus fibrosus

10 Base of pulmonary valve

11 Endocardium of ventricle

Fig. 1. *Pulmonary trunk, pulmonary valve, right ventricle (panoramic view, longitudinal section).*
Stain: hematoxylin-eosin. 9 ×.

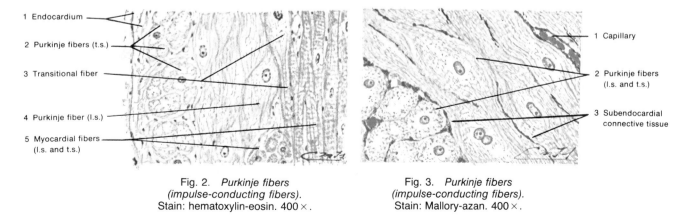

1 Endocardium

2 Purkinje fibers (t.s.)

3 Transitional fiber

4 Purkinje fiber (l.s.)

5 Myocardial fibers (l.s. and t.s.)

1 Capillary

2 Purkinje fibers (l.s. and t.s.)

3 Subendocardial connective tissue

Fig. 2. *Purkinje fibers
(impulse-conducting fibers).*
Stain: hematoxylin-eosin. 400 ×.

Fig. 3. *Purkinje fibers
(impulse-conducting fibers).*
Stain: Mallory-azan. 400 ×.

PLATE 41

LYMPH NODE (PANORAMIC VIEW)

A lymph node is an organ composed of aggregations of lymphocytes intermeshed with lymphatic sinuses, supported in a framework of reticular fibers and encased in a connective tissue capsule (2).

The cortex of the node (5) contains lymphocytes aggregated into lymphatic nodules (5, 16). In many of cortical nodules, the centers are lightly stained. These lighter areas represent the germinal centers (18) and are the active sites of lymphocyte proliferation.

In the medulla (6) of a lymph node, the lymphocytes are arranged as irregular cords of lymphatic tissue, the medullary cords (14). The medullary sinuses (13) course between these cords.

The capsule (2) of the node is surrounded by connective tissue and fat. From the capsule, connective tissue trabeculae (7) extend into the node, initially between the cortical nodules (7, upper leader) and then ramifying throughout the medulla (15) between medullary cords and sinuses. In the trabeculae are found major blood vessels (15) of the lymph node.

Afferent lymphatic vessels (4) course in the connective tissue and, at intervals, pierce the capsule to enter the subcapsular sinus (9, 17). From here, the trabecular sinuses (cortical sinuses) extend along the trabeculae to pass into medullary sinuses (13). At the upper right section of the node is an illustration of the hilus (12) and the efferent lymphatic vessels (11) which drain the lymph from the node. Also found here are nerves, small arteries, and veins which supply and drain the node.

PLATE 41

LYMPH NODE (PANORAMIC VIEW)

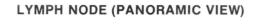

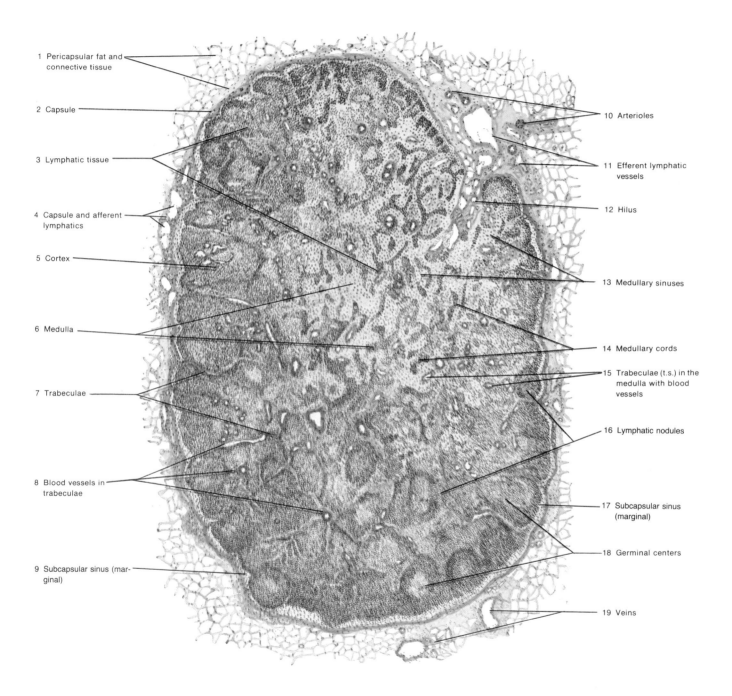

1 Pericapsular fat and connective tissue

2 Capsule

3 Lymphatic tissue

4 Capsule and afferent lymphatics

5 Cortex

6 Medulla

7 Trabeculae

8 Blood vessels in trabeculae

9 Subcapsular sinus (marginal)

10 Arterioles

11 Efferent lymphatic vessels

12 Hilus

13 Medullary sinuses

14 Medullary cords

15 Trabeculae (t.s.) in the medulla with blood vessels

16 Lymphatic nodules

17 Subcapsular sinus (marginal)

18 Germinal centers

19 Veins

Stain: hematoxylin-eosin. 32×.

PLATE 42 (Fig. 1)

LYMPH NODE (SECTIONAL VIEW)

A small section of a lymph node is illustrated at a higher magnification.

The capsule (5) is surrounded by loose connective tissue (1) containing blood vessels (2, 3, 4) and afferent lymphatic vessels (13); the latter are lined with endothelium and contain valves (14). Arising from the inner surface of the capsule (5), connective tissue trabeculae (15) extend through the cortex and medulla. Associated with these connective tissue partitions are blood vessels (18).

The cortex (7) is separated from the capsule (5) by the subcapsular (marginal) sinus (6). The cortex consists of lymphatic nodules situated adjacent to each other but incompletely separated by trabeculae (15) and trabecular (cortical) sinuses (16). In this figure, one complete lymphatic nodule (7, lower leader; 8, 17, lower leader) and portions of two other nodules (7, upper leader; 17, upper leader) are illustrated. The deep part of the cortex, the paracortical region (19), is the thymus-dependent zone and is occupied by T-lymphocytes. This is a transition area from the nodules to the medullary cords. The medulla consists of anastomosing cords of lymphatic tissue, the medullary cords (12, 20), interspersed with medullary sinuses (11, 21) which drain into the efferent lymphatic vessels located at the hilus.

Reticular connective tissue forms the stroma of the cortical nodules, the medullary cords, and all sinuses. Relatively few lymphocytes are seen in the sinuses (6, 11, 16, 21); thus, it is possible to distinguish the reticular framework (21) of the node. In the lymphatic nodules (7) and the medullary cords (12, 20), lymphocytes are so abundant that the reticulum is obscured unless specially stained, as shown in Figure 2. Most of the lymphocytes are small and contain large, deep-staining nuclei with condensed chromatin. The cells exhibit either a small amount of cytoplasm or none at all.

Lymphatic nodules often exhibit germinal centers (8) which stain less intensely than the surrounding peripheral portion of the nodule (7). In the germinal center (8), the cells are more loosely aggregated and the developing lymphocytes have larger, lighter nuclei with more cytoplasm than the small lymphocytes (see Plate 43, Fig. 1).

PLATE 42 (Fig. 2)

LYMPH NODE: RETICULAR FIBERS OF THE STROMA

A section of a lymph node has been stained with the Bielschowsky-Foot silver method to stain the reticular fibers.

The various zones illustrated in Figure 1 are readily recognized: the cortex (1), subcapsular (marginal) sinus (2), medullary cords (5), and medullary sinuses (6). All of these regions contain a stroma of delicate reticular fibers (4, 7) that form a fine meshwork.

PLATE 42

LYMPH NODE

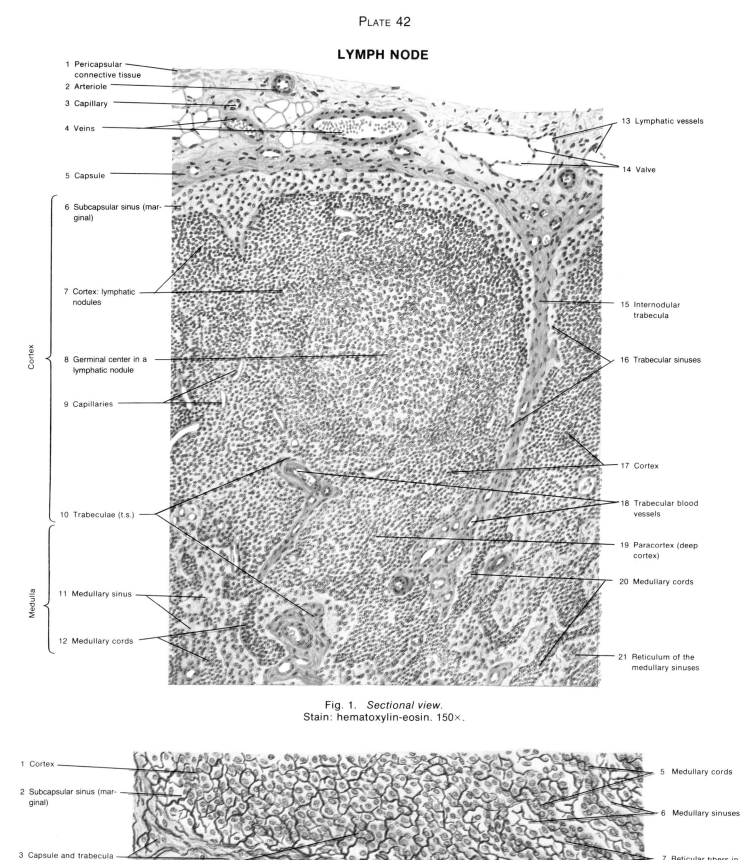

1 Pericapsular connective tissue
2 Arteriole
3 Capillary
4 Veins
5 Capsule
6 Subcapsular sinus (marginal)
7 Cortex: lymphatic nodules
8 Germinal center in a lymphatic nodule
9 Capillaries
10 Trabeculae (t.s.)
11 Medullary sinus
12 Medullary cords

Cortex
Medulla

13 Lymphatic vessels
14 Valve
15 Internodular trabecula
16 Trabecular sinuses
17 Cortex
18 Trabecular blood vessels
19 Paracortex (deep cortex)
20 Medullary cords
21 Reticulum of the medullary sinuses

Fig. 1. *Sectional view.*
Stain: hematoxylin-eosin. 150×.

1 Cortex
2 Subcapsular sinus (marginal)
3 Capsule and trabecula
4 Reticular fibers

5 Medullary cords
6 Medullary sinuses
7 Reticular fibers in sinuses

Fig. 2. *Reticular fibers of the stroma.*
Stain: Bielschowsky-Foot silver method. 240×.

PLATE 43 (Fig. 1)

LYMPH NODE: PROLIFERATION OF LYMPHOCYTES

This figure illustrates, at a higher magnification than in Plate 42, a portion of the lymph node capsule (1), the subcapsular (marginal) sinus (2), a lymphatic nodule with its peripheral zone (5), and a germinal center (6) with developing lymphocytes.

The reticular connective tissue of the node is seen in the subcapsular sinus, where reticular cells (9), their processes and associated delicate fibers are easily distinguishable. Small lymphocytes (11, upper leader) and free macrophages (3, 10) are also visible. Endothelial cells form an incomplete cover over the surface of the node (4, limiting cells). In the dense portions of the node, reticular cells are obscured but may be seen occasionally (15). Free macrophages may be seen anywhere in the node (3, 7, 10).

The peripheral zone of the lymphatic nodule contains dense accumulations of small lymphocytes (5; 11, lower leader) which are characterized by dark-stained nuclei, condensed blocks of chromatin, and either a very limited or no cytoplasm.

In the germinal center (6), the majority of cells are medium-sized lymphocytes (12) with larger, lighter nuclei and more cytoplasm than in small lymphocytes; the nuclei exhibit more variations in size and in density of chromatin. The largest lymphocytes, with less concentrated chromatin, are derived from lymphoblasts. With successive mitotic divisions (8), chromatin condenses and cell size decreases, forming small lymphocytes.

Lymphoblasts (14) are seen in small numbers in the germinal center. These are large, round cells with a broad band of cytoplasm and a large vesicular nucleus with one or more nucleoli. Mitotic divisions of these cells (13) produce other lymphoblasts and medium-sized lymphocytes.

On Plate 45 are shown developing lymphocytes and other cells formed or found in lymphatic tissues.

PLATE 43 (Fig. 2)

PALATINE TONSIL

The surface of the palatine tonsil is covered with stratified squamous epithelium (1), which also lines the deep invaginations or tonsillar crypts (3, 10). In the underlying connective tissue are numerous lymphatic nodules (2) distributed along the crypts. The nodules are embedded in reticular connective tissue stroma and diffuse lymphatic tissue. The nodules frequently merge with each other (8) and usually exhibit germinal (7) centers.

Fibroelastic connective tissue underlies the tonsil and forms its capsule (11). Septa (trabeculae) arise from the capsule (5, 9) and pass upward as a core of connective tissue between lymphatic nodules that form the walls of the crypts. Skeletal muscle fibers (6, 12) form an underlying layer and glands (not illustrated) may be seen deeper in the connective tissue.

PLATE 43

LYMPH NODE AND PALATINE TONSIL

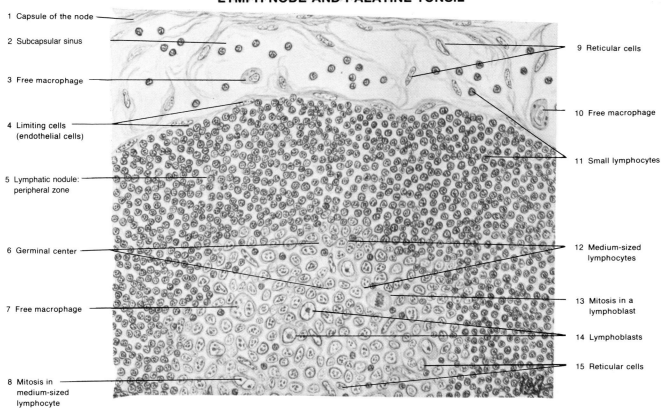

1 Capsule of the node

2 Subcapsular sinus

3 Free macrophage

4 Limiting cells
(endothelial cells)

5 Lymphatic nodule:
peripheral zone

6 Germinal center

7 Free macrophage

8 Mitosis in
medium-sized
lymphocyte

9 Reticular cells

10 Free macrophage

11 Small lymphocytes

12 Medium-sized
lymphocytes

13 Mitosis in a
lymphoblast

14 Lymphoblasts

15 Reticular cells

Fig. 1. *Lymph node: Proliferation of lymphocytes.*
Stain: hematoxylin-eosin. 450×.

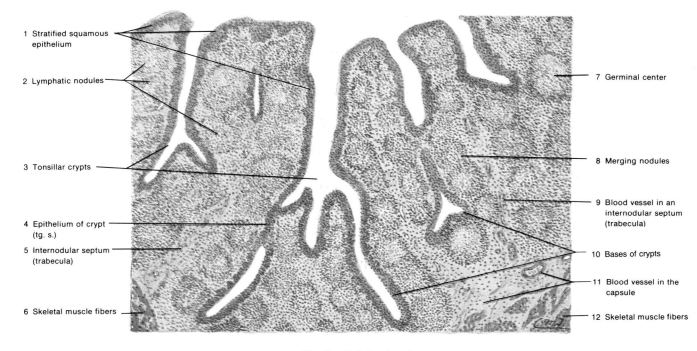

1 Stratified squamous
epithelium

2 Lymphatic nodules

3 Tonsillar crypts

4 Epithelium of crypt
(tg. s.)

5 Internodular septum
(trabecula)

6 Skeletal muscle fibers

7 Germinal center

8 Merging nodules

9 Blood vessel in an
internodular septum
(trabecula)

10 Bases of crypts

11 Blood vessel in the
capsule

12 Skeletal muscle fibers

Fig. 2. *Palatine tonsil.*
Stain: hematoxylin-eosin. 32×.

PLATE 44 (Fig. 1)

THYMUS: PANORAMIC VIEW

The thymus gland has a lobular structure. From the surrounding capsule (1) of loose connective tissue, trabeculae (2, 11) extend through the organ and divide it into lobules (5) containing a cortex (3) and a medulla (4). The lobular divisions are often incomplete (6) and the medulla is continuous with other lobules (7).

The principal cells of the thymus gland are small lymphocytes (thymic lymphocytes). In the cortex, the cells are densely packed (3) without forming nodules. In the medulla (4, 7), the lymphocytes are less densely packed and this area appears lighter. The medulla contains characteristic thymic or Hassall's corpuscles (9), which are spherical aggregations of flattened cells, often exhibiting degenerative changes in the center.

The stroma consists of branched reticular cells which are of ectodermal origin (see 6, 10 in Fig. 2) and are, therefore, called epithelial reticular cells.

PLATE 44 (Fig. 2)

THYMUS: SECTIONAL VIEW

A small portion of the cortex and the central medulla of a lobule are illustrated. The dense aggregations of thymic lymphocytes in the cortex (4) contrast with the diffuse distribution of the same cells in the medulla (5). The epithelial reticular cells are more numerous and more visible in the medulla (6) than in the cortex. Thin processes extend from their cell bodies, giving them a stellate appearance.

In the thymic (Hassall's) corpuscles (7), the epithelial reticular cells assume a concentric arrangement and form cell layers. Continuity with the stroma of the medulla is often visible (9, also seen at the upper part of the corpuscle). Cellular degenerations in the center of the corpuscle are indicated by a mass of acidophilic material (8).

An interlobular trabecula (3) with blood vessels (1, 2) is illustrated.

PLATE 44

THYMUS

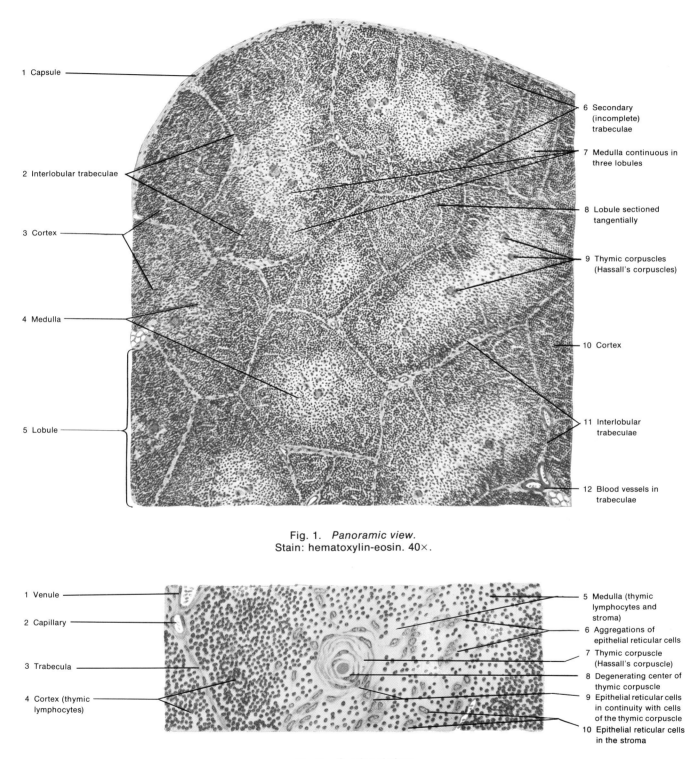

1 Capsule

2 Interlobular trabeculae

3 Cortex

4 Medulla

5 Lobule

6 Secondary (incomplete) trabeculae

7 Medulla continuous in three lobules

8 Lobule sectioned tangentially

9 Thymic corpuscles (Hassall's corpuscles)

10 Cortex

11 Interlobular trabeculae

12 Blood vessels in trabeculae

Fig. 1. *Panoramic view.*
Stain: hematoxylin-eosin. 40×.

1 Venule

2 Capillary

3 Trabecula

4 Cortex (thymic lymphocytes)

5 Medulla (thymic lymphocytes and stroma)

6 Aggregations of epithelial reticular cells

7 Thymic corpuscle (Hassall's corpuscle)

8 Degenerating center of thymic corpuscle

9 Epithelial reticular cells in continuity with cells of the thymic corpuscle

10 Epithelial reticular cells in the stroma

Fig. 2. *Sectional view.*
Stain: hematoxylin-eosin. 250×.

PLATE 45 (Fig. 1)

SPLEEN: PANORAMIC VIEW

A dense connective tissue capsule (1) encloses the spleen. From the capsule (1), connective tissue trabeculae (3) extend deep into interior of the spleen. The principal trabeculae enter at the hilus, branch throughout the spleen, and carry with them trabecular arteries (4) and veins (11). Trabeculae that are cut in transverse sections have a nodular appearance (12).

The spleen is characterized by lymphatic nodules (2, 8), which constitute the white pulp. In young individuals, the nodules contain germinal centers (7). Passing through each lymphatic nodule is an arteriole, the central artery (6, 9), which usually has an eccentric position. Central arteries are branches of trabecular arteries which become ensheathed with lymphatic tissue as they leave the trabeculae. This sheath expands to form lymphatic nodules, which then constitute the white pulp of the spleen.

Surrounding the lymphatic nodules and intermeshed with the trabeculae is a diffuse cellular meshwork which collectively forms the red or splenic pulp; it exhibits a red color in fresh preparations. Red pulp contains venous sinuses (10) and splenic cords (of Billroth) (5), which appear as diffuse strands of lymphatic tissue between the venous sinuses. The cords form a spongy meshwork of reticular connective tissue, which is usually obscured by the density of other tissue.

The spleen does not have a cortex and a medulla, as seen in lymph nodes; however, lymphatic nodules are found throughout the spleen. The spleen contains venous sinuses, in contrast to lymphatic sinuses in lymph nodes, but does not have subcapsular or trabecular sinuses. Both the capsule and trabeculae in the spleen are thicker than in the lymph nodes and contain some smooth muscle cells.

PLATE 45 (Fig. 2)

SPLEEN: RED AND WHITE PULP

The figure illustrates a small area of red and white pulp and their structural associations.

The lymphatic (splenic) nodule represents the white pulp. Each nodule consists of a peripheral zone, the periarterial lymphatic sheath, densely packed small lymphocytes (8), a germinal center (9), which may not always be present, and an eccentric central artery (10). The cells in the periarterial lymphatic sheath are mainly T-lymphocytes. In a more lightly stained germinal center are found the B-lymphocytes (9), mainly medium-sized lymphocytes, some small lymphocytes, and lymphoblasts.

In the red pulp are found the splenic cords (6) (of Billroth) and venous sinuses (2, 7) which course between the cords. The splenic cords (6) are thin aggregations of lymphatic tissue containing small lymphocytes, associated cells and various blood cells. Venous sinuses (2, 7) are dilated vessels lined with modified endothelium whose elongated cells appear cuboidal in transverse sections.

Also present in the red pulp are pulp arteries (11) which are the branches of the central artery as it leaves the lymphatic nodule. Branches of these sheathed arteries are not illustrated; however, one vessel is seen in Figure 1:13. Capillaries and pulp veins (venules) are also present.

Trabeculae (1, 4) with trabecular arteries (1) and veins (4, 5) are also illustrated. These vessels have an intima and media but no apparent adventitia; connective tissue of the trabeculae surrounds the media.

PLATE 45 (Fig. 3)

SPLEEN: DEVELOPMENT OF LYMPHOCYTES AND RELATED CELLS

The illustrated cells may be found in lymph nodes, spleen, thymus, and other lymphatic tissues.

The large, phagocytic macrophage (1), ranging from 25 to 35 μm in diameter, exhibits an eccentric nucleus, cytoplasmic vacuoles (due to dissolved lipid inclusions), fragments of ingested nuclei, and a larger, unidentified inclusion.

The lymphoblast (2), about 15 to 20 μm in diameter, has intensely basophilic cytoplasm, a round nucleus with dilated chromatin filaments, and two or more nucleoli. In the medium-sized lymphocytes (prolymphocytes, 12 to 15 μm in diameter) (3), the cytoplasm is less basophilic, the nuclear chromatin is condensing, and the nucleoli are indistinct or absent. In small lymphocytes (6 to 12 μm in diameter) (4), the cytoplasm is reduced to a small rim. The cytoplasm is slightly basophilic and may contain azurophilic granules. Nuclear chromatin is in small clusters and deeply stained.

In a plasmablast (16 to 20 μm in diameter) (5), the nuclear chromatin forms a heavier reticulum than in the lymphoblast. In a proplasmacyte (12 to 18 μm in diameter) (6), the cytoplasm is more basophilic than in a prolymphocyte, the nucleus is eccentric, and the chromatin clumps are heavier. The plasma cell (mature plasmacyte) (7) is oval and exhibits an abundance of basophilic cytoplasm except for a pale area near the small, eccentric nucleus. The "cartwheel" arrangement of chromatin is a distinctive feature of plasma cells.

A monoblast (18 to 20 μm) (8) resembles a lymphoblast. The monocyte (15 to 18 μm) (9) has a bean-shaped or indented nucleus with chromatin in filaments and strands. The abundant cytoplasm may contain fine azurophilic granules (10).

PLATE 45

SPLEEN

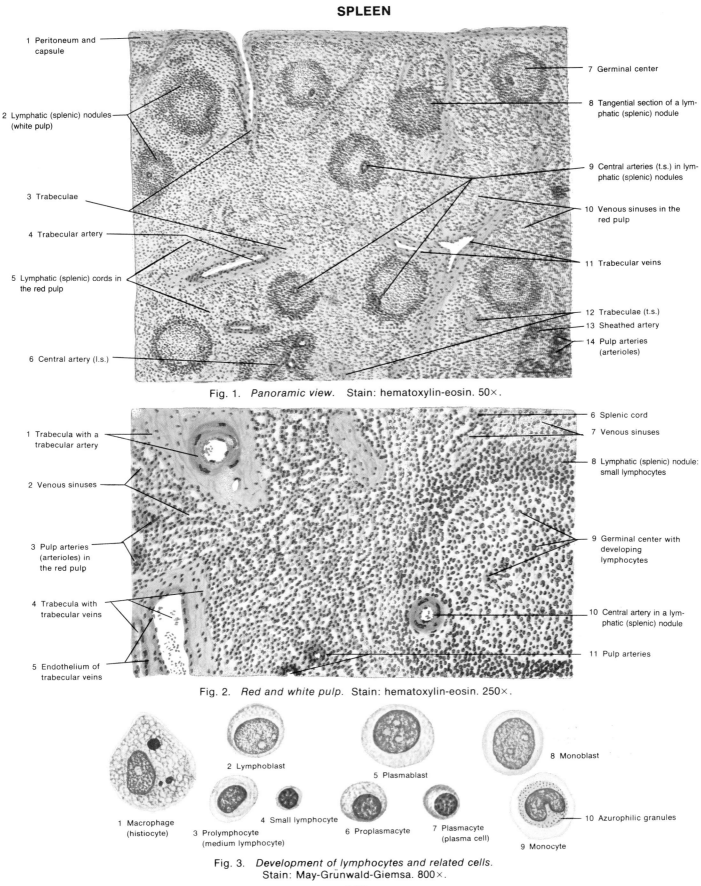

1 Peritoneum and capsule

2 Lymphatic (splenic) nodules (white pulp)

3 Trabeculae

4 Trabecular artery

5 Lymphatic (splenic) cords in the red pulp

6 Central artery (l.s.)

7 Germinal center

8 Tangential section of a lymphatic (splenic) nodule

9 Central arteries (t.s.) in lymphatic (splenic) nodules

10 Venous sinuses in the red pulp

11 Trabecular veins

12 Trabeculae (t.s.)

13 Sheathed artery

14 Pulp arteries (arterioles)

Fig. 1. *Panoramic view.* Stain: hematoxylin-eosin. 50×.

1 Trabecula with a trabecular artery

2 Venous sinuses

3 Pulp arteries (arterioles) in the red pulp

4 Trabecula with trabecular veins

5 Endothelium of trabecular veins

6 Splenic cord

7 Venous sinuses

8 Lymphatic (splenic) nodule: small lymphocytes

9 Germinal center with developing lymphocytes

10 Central artery in a lymphatic (splenic) nodule

11 Pulp arteries

Fig. 2. *Red and white pulp.* Stain: hematoxylin-eosin. 250×.

1 Macrophage (histiocyte)

2 Lymphoblast

3 Prolymphocyte (medium lymphocyte)

4 Small lymphocyte

5 Plasmablast

6 Proplasmacyte

7 Plasmacyte (plasma cell)

8 Monoblast

9 Monocyte

10 Azurophilic granules

Fig. 3. *Development of lymphocytes and related cells.* Stain: May-Grünwald-Giemsa. 800×.

PLATE 46 (Fig. 1)

INTEGUMENT: THIN SKIN
(CAJAL'S TRICHROME STAIN)

The skin is composed of two principal layers: epidermis and dermis. This illustration depicts a section of skin from the general body surface where wear and tear are minimal. In this type of skin, the epidermis (1) consists of stratified squamous epithelium and is thin in comparison to thick skin. The single layer of low columnar cells at the base of the epidermis is the stratum basale or germinativum (7). Directly above this layer are a few rows of polygonal cells, the stratum spinosum (6). Above these cells are usually one or two layers of granular cells which blend with the elongated, cornified cells of the stratum corneum (5). The narrow zone of dense irregular connective tissue below the epidermis is the papillary layer (2) of the dermis. Its projections into the base of the epidermis form the dermal papillae (8). The reticular layer (3) consists of dense, irregular connective tissue and comprises the bulk of the dermis. A small portion of hypodermis, the superficial region of the underlying subcutaneous tissue (4), is also illustrated.

Most of the skin appendages are located in the dermis. Illustrated in the figure are scattered hair follicles and a sweat gland, whose structure is seen in more detail on Plate 47. The lower portion of the hair follicle in longitudinal section (13) exhibits the papilla and hair bulb at its base, which is located deep in the dermis. The upper portion of another hair follicle (9) exhibits the smooth muscle, arrector pili muscle (10), and a sebaceous gland (11). An oblique section of the hair follicle (14) is illustrated in the subcutaneous tissue.

The dermis contains numerous examples of the cross sections of a coiled portion of the sweat gland. The sections with light-staining epithelium (12a) are from the secretory portion of the gland, whereas the deeper-staining sections (12b) are from the duct portion.

Cajal's trichrome stain illustrates the variations in collagenous fiber density and distinguishes between the muscle and connective tissue. Aniline dyes stain the nuclei and cytoplasm. The nuclei are stained bright red by basic fuchsin. Indigo carmine in picric acid solution is used to stain cytoplasm orange. Collagenous fibers stain deep blue.

PLATE 46 (Fig. 2)

THICK SKIN, PALM, SUPERFICIAL LAYERS

A section of palm skin is illustrated in which both the epidermis and dermis are much thicker than in the thin skin illustrated in Figure 1. The epidermis, in addition to being thicker, also has a more complex structure and five distinct cell layers. The outermost layer, the stratum corneum (1), is a wide layer of flattened, dead cells that are constantly desquamated or shed from the surface (10). Beneath this layer is a narrow, lightly stained stratum lucidum (2). At higher magnification are occasionally seen outlines of flattened cells and eleidin droplets. Located under the stratum lucidum is the stratum granulosum (3), whose cells contain dark-staining keratohyalin granules, better seen at a higher magnification (7).

Below this layer is the thick stratum spinosum (4), composed of several layers of polyhedral cells; and a basal layer, the stratum basale (5), consisting of columnar cells which rest on the basement membrane.

Cells of stratum spinosum (4) appear to be connected by spinous processes or intercellular bridges (8, 9), which represent the desmosomes (macula adherens). Mitotic activity (12) normally occurs in the deeper layers of stratum spinosum and stratum basale.

Ducts of sweat glands penetrate the epidermis in the area between two dermal papillae, lose their epithelial wall, and spiral through the epidermis (11) to the skin surface as channels with a thin cuticular lining.

Dermal papillae (6) are prominent in thick skin. Some of these papillae contain tactile corpuscles (Meissner's corpuscles) (13), while others have loops of capillaries.

PLATE 46

INTEGUMENT

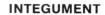
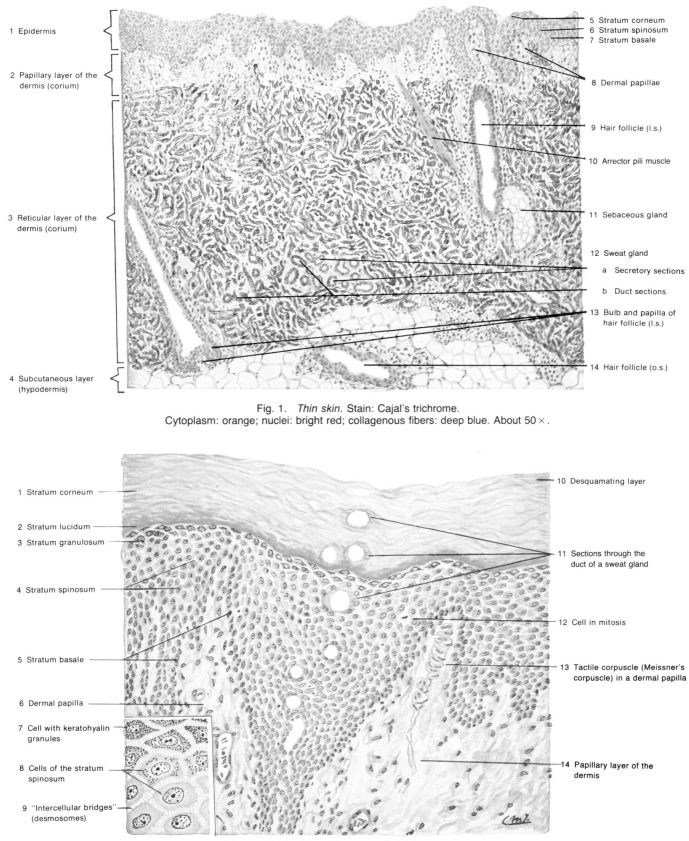

1 Epidermis

2 Papillary layer of the dermis (corium)

3 Reticular layer of the dermis (corium)

4 Subcutaneous layer (hypodermis)

5 Stratum corneum
6 Stratum spinosum
7 Stratum basale

8 Dermal papillae

9 Hair follicle (l.s.)

10 Arrector pili muscle

11 Sebaceous gland

12 Sweat gland

   a Secretory sections

   b Duct sections

13 Bulb and papilla of hair follicle (l.s.)

14 Hair follicle (o.s.)

Fig. 1. *Thin skin.* Stain: Cajal's trichrome.
Cytoplasm: orange; nuclei: bright red; collagenous fibers: deep blue. About 50×.

1 Stratum corneum

2 Stratum lucidum
3 Stratum granulosum

4 Stratum spinosum

5 Stratum basale

6 Dermal papilla

7 Cell with keratohyalin granules

8 Cells of the stratum spinosum

9 "Intercellular bridges" (desmosomes)

10 Desquamating layer

11 Sections through the duct of a sweat gland

12 Cell in mitosis

13 Tactile corpuscle (Meissner's corpuscle) in a dermal papilla

14 Papillary layer of the dermis

Fig. 2. *Thick skin, palm: superficial layers.*
Stain: hematoxylin-eosin. 200×.

PLATE 47

INTEGUMENT: SWEAT GLAND (DIAGRAM)

This plate illustrates a coiled tubular sweat gland. The coiled portion (B) is embedded either deep in the dermis or in the hypodermis. This section of the sweat gland comprises the secretory portion and stains light pink. The thinner, more proximal portion represents the excretory duct, which stains darker pink.

As the excretory duct passes through the dermis (7), it straightens out, penetrates the epidermis, loses its epithelial wall, and pursues a spiral course (6) through the epidermis.

Areas A, B, and C show the histologic appearance of different parts of the gland when the plane of section passes along lines a-a', b-b' and c-c', respectively. The secretory portions of the sweat gland are lined with large, light-staining columnar cells (3, 5, 8). Between the base of the secretory cells and the basal lamina are found myoepithelial cells; they are not illustrated in the figure. The excretory ducts are smaller in diameter and are lined with two rows of small, deep-staining cuboidal cells (4, 9). The duct cells increase somewhat in size as the duct approaches the epidermis (2); in the epidermis (1), the duct wall is gradually lost.

PLATE 47

INTEGUMENT

SWEAT GLAND (DIAGRAM)

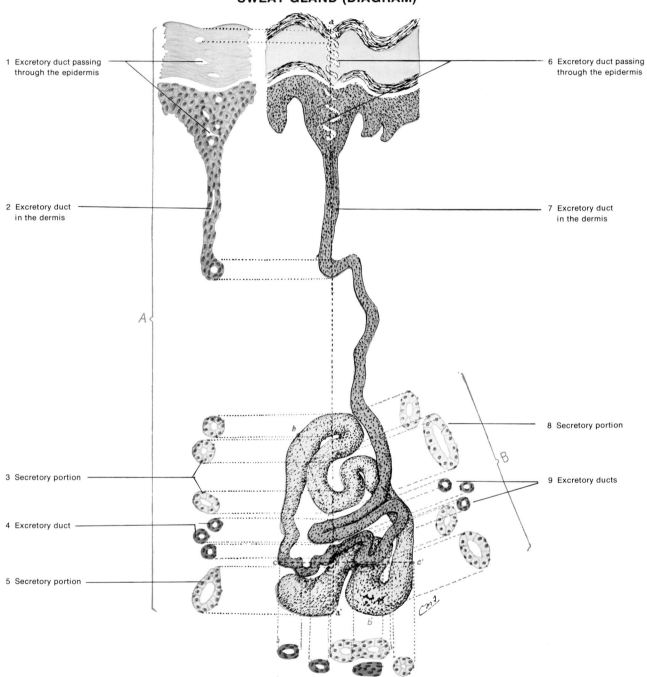

1 Excretory duct passing
through the epidermis

2 Excretory duct
in the dermis

3 Secretory portion

4 Excretory duct

5 Secretory portion

6 Excretory duct passing
through the epidermis

7 Excretory duct
in the dermis

8 Secretory portion

9 Excretory ducts

PLATE 48 (Fig. 1)

INTEGUMENT: SKIN (SCALP)

This section of skin illustrates stratum corneum (1) with cornified superficial cells, the stratum spinosum (2), and stratum basale.

Typical dermal papillae indenting the epidermis are clearly illustrated (3). The thin papillary layer of the dermis is not apparent at this magnification. The thick reticular layer (4) extends from just below the epidermis to the subcutaneous layer which contains increased adipose tissue (23). Beneath this layer is found the skeletal muscle (13).

Hair follicles in the scalp skin are numerous, close together, and placed at an angle to the surface of the skin. A complete hair follicle in longitudinal section (17) is illustrated in the center of the plate. Parts of other follicles, sectioned in different planes, are also illustrated (5, 8, 18, 20). The hair follicles consist of the following structures: cuticle, internal root sheath (18), external root sheath (20), connective tissue sheath (19), hair bulb (10), and a connective tissue papilla (11). The hair passes upward through the follicle (17, 21) to the surface of the skin.

Sebaceous glands (6, 15) are aggregated clusters of clear cells connected to a duct that opens into the hair follicles (see Fig. 2).

The arrector pili muscles (7) are smooth muscles that are aligned at an oblique angle, bind to the papillary layer of the dermis, and insert into the connective tissue sheath (19) of the hair follicle. Their contraction moves the hair shaft to a more vertical position.

The basal portions of the sweat glands lie deep in the dermis or in the subcutaneous layer (see also Plate 47). Sections of the gland with lightly stained columnar epithelium (12) represent the secretory portion of the gland and are distinct from sections of the duct (9) that exhibit two layers of smaller, darker-stained epithelial cells (stratified cuboidal). Each duct is coiled in the deep dermis (9), straightens out in the upper dermis (16), and follows a spiral course through the epidermis (14).

Pacinian corpuscles (22), located in the subcutaneous tissue, are the receptors for pressure and possibly vibration. (See also Plate 49, Fig. 2.)

PLATE 48 (Fig. 2)

SEBACEOUS GLAND AND ADJACENT HAIR FOLLICLE

This figure illustrates a sebaceous gland sectioned through the middle. The potential lumen is filled with secretory cells undergoing cytolysis (3) (holocrine secretion), a process whereby the entire cell breaks down to become the secretory product of the gland, an oily secretion called sebum. The gland is lined with a stratified epithelium that has continuity with the external root sheath (1) of the hair follicle. Its epithelium is modified, and along the base of the gland is a single row of columnar or cuboidal cells (5), the basal cells, whose nuclei may be flattened. These cells rest on a basement membrane which is surrounded by the connective tissue of the dermis. The basal cells exhibit mitotic activity and fill the alveolus with larger, polyhedral cells which enlarge, accumulate secretory material, and become round (4, 6). The cells in the interior of the alveolus undergo cytolysis (3) and, together with the secretory product sebum, pass through the short duct (2) of the gland into the lumen of the hair follicle.

The sebaceous glands lie in dermal connective tissue and in the angle between the hair follicles and the arrector pili muscles (11).

The various layers of the hair follicle at the level of the sebaceous gland may be identified. The follicle is surrounded by a connective tissue sheath (7) of the dermis. The external root sheath (8), composed of several cell layers, is continuous with stratum spinosum of the dermis. The internal root sheath (9) is composed of a thin, pale epithelial stratum (Henle's layer) and a thin, granular epithelial stratum (Huxley's layer) (9). The latter is in direct contact with the cortex of the hair (10), illustrated as a pale yellow layer with cells.

PLATE 48 (Fig. 3)

BULB OF HAIR FOLLICLE AND ADJACENT SWEAT GLAND

This figure illustrates the bulb of the hair follicle and its various layers. A sheath of fibrous connective tissue (7) surrounds the bulb. The external root sheath (1) at this level is a single layer of cells which are columnar above the bulb and flat at the base of the bulb, where they cannot be distinguished from matrix cells of the follicle. Above the bulb can be seen the internal root sheath, composed at this higher level of thin, pale epithelial stratum (Henle's layer) (2), and a thin granular stratum (Huxley's layer) (3). These layers become indistinguishable as their cells merge with those of the bulb. Internal to these layers are the cuticles (4), cortex (5), and medulla (6) of the hair. In the bulb, these layers merge into undifferentiated cells of the hair matrix (12) which cap the connective tissue papilla (11) of the hair follicle. Mitosis (10) is seen in the matrix cells.

In the dermal connective tissue and adjacent to the hair follicle are sections through the basal portion of a coiled sweat gland. The secretory cells (9) are tall columnar and stain light. Along their bases may be seen the flattened nuclei of myoepithelial cells (14). The excretory duct sections (8) are smaller in diameter than the secretory tubule, are lined with a stratified cuboidal epithelium, and stain darker.

PLATE 48

INTEGUMENT

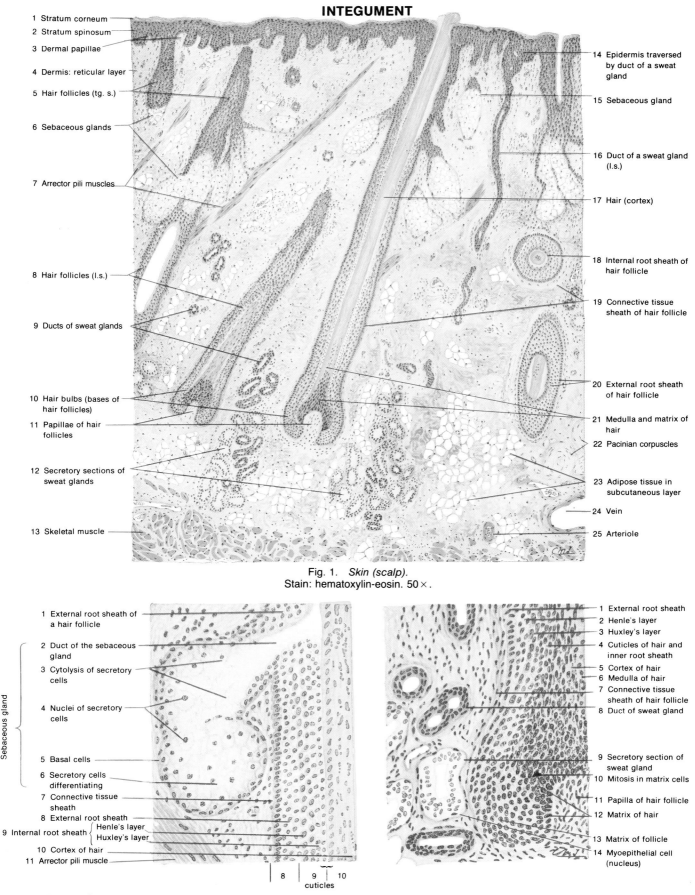

1 Stratum corneum
2 Stratum spinosum
3 Dermal papillae
4 Dermis: reticular layer
5 Hair follicles (tg. s.)
6 Sebaceous glands
7 Arrector pili muscles
8 Hair follicles (l.s.)
9 Ducts of sweat glands
10 Hair bulbs (bases of hair follicles)
11 Papillae of hair follicles
12 Secretory sections of sweat glands
13 Skeletal muscle

14 Epidermis traversed by duct of a sweat gland
15 Sebaceous gland
16 Duct of a sweat gland (l.s.)
17 Hair (cortex)
18 Internal root sheath of hair follicle
19 Connective tissue sheath of hair follicle
20 External root sheath of hair follicle
21 Medulla and matrix of hair
22 Pacinian corpuscles
23 Adipose tissue in subcutaneous layer
24 Vein
25 Arteriole

Fig. 1. *Skin (scalp).*
Stain: hematoxylin-eosin. 50×.

1 External root sheath of a hair follicle
Sebaceous gland
2 Duct of the sebaceous gland
3 Cytolysis of secretory cells
4 Nuclei of secretory cells
5 Basal cells
6 Secretory cells differentiating
7 Connective tissue sheath
8 External root sheath
9 Internal root sheath { Henle's layer
Huxley's layer
10 Cortex of hair
11 Arrector pili muscle

8   9   10
cuticles

Fig. 2. *Sebaceous gland and adjacent hair follicle.*

1 External root sheath
2 Henle's layer
3 Huxley's layer
4 Cuticles of hair and inner root sheath
5 Cortex of hair
6 Medulla of hair
7 Connective tissue sheath of hair follicle
8 Duct of sweat gland
9 Secretory section of sweat gland
10 Mitosis in matrix cells
11 Papilla of hair follicle
12 Matrix of hair
13 Matrix of follicle
14 Myoepithelial cell (nucleus)

Fig. 3. *Bulb of hair follicle and adjacent sweat gland.*

Stain: hematoxylin-eosin. 200×.

PLATE 49 (Fig. 1)

INTEGUMENT: GLOMUS IN THE DERMIS OF THICK SKIN

Arteriovenous anastomoses are numerous in the thick skin of fingers and toes. Some anastomoses are direct connections; in others, the arterial section of the anastomosis forms a specialized thick-walled structure, the glomus (2). The vessel is coiled and, as a result, more than one lumen may be seen in a transverse section. The smooth muscle cells in tunica media have hypertrophied and the specialized muscle cells with the epithelioid-like appearance are now called the epithelioid cells (5). The media wall, however, becomes thin again before the arteriole empties into a venule. The small artery (3, middle leader) may represent the terminal part of the glomus.

Small nerves and capillaries are present in the glomus and a connective tissue sheath (6) encloses the entire structure.

Present in the dermis that surrounds the glomus are blood vessels (3), nerves (4), and ducts of sweat glands (1, 7). The PAS and hematoxylin (PASH) stains demonstrate the basement membrane of these ducts.

PLATE 49 (Fig. 2)

PACINIAN CORPUSCLES IN THE DEEP DERMIS OF THICK SKIN

Pacinian corpuscles in thick skin are located deep in the dermis and subcutaneous tissue. They are receptors for pressure and possibly vibration. One corpuscle is illustrated in a transverse section (1) and another in an oblique section (6).

The corpuscles are ovoid structures when seen in longitudinal or oblique sections (6) and contain an elongated central core, the inner bulb (8). This area is usually empty in the sections, but in life, the corpuscle contains a terminal myelinated nerve fiber. Surrounding the inner bulb are concentric lamellae of compact collagenous fibers (10), which become denser peripherally (inner and outer lamellae). Between the lamellae is a small amount of loose connective tissue with flat fibroblasts (6). A thin dense connective tissue capsule (9) encloses the corpuscle.

In a transverse section of the corpuscle (1), the layers of lamellae surrounding the inner bulb resemble a sliced onion.

In the dense irregular connective tissue of the dermis (3) surrounding the corpuscle are adipose tissue (5), blood vessels (7), nerves (2, 11), and a sweat gland (4).

PLATE 49

INTEGUMENT

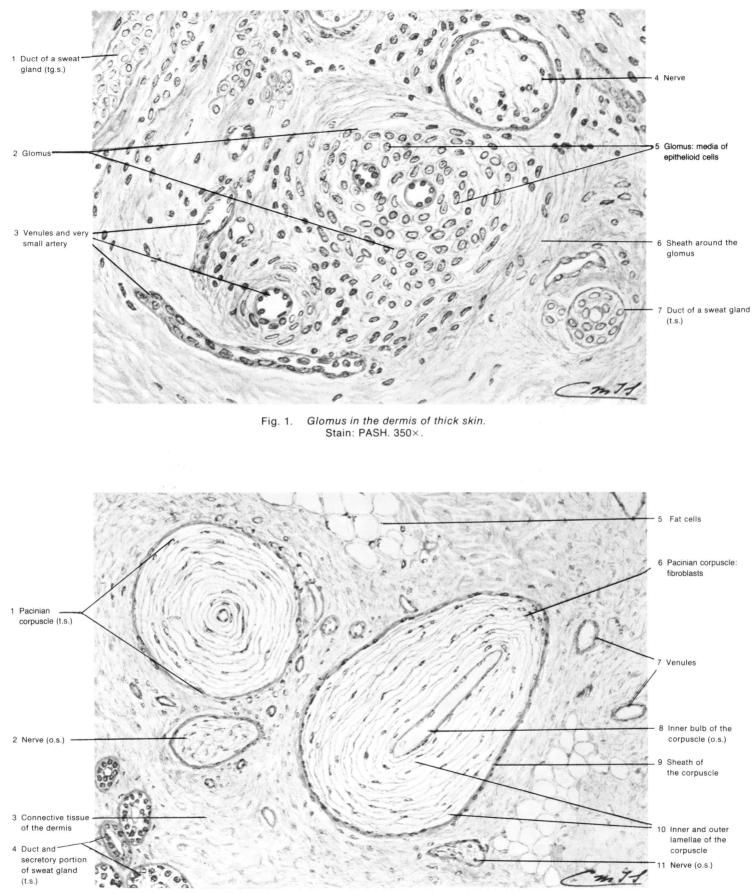

1 Duct of a sweat gland (tg.s.)

2 Glomus

3 Venules and very small artery

4 Nerve

5 Glomus: media of epithelioid cells

6 Sheath around the glomus

7 Duct of a sweat gland (t.s.)

Fig. 1.   *Glomus in the dermis of thick skin.*
Stain: PASH. 350×.

1 Pacinian corpuscle (t.s.)

2 Nerve (o.s.)

3 Connective tissue of the dermis

4 Duct and secretory portion of sweat gland (t.s.)

5 Fat cells

6 Pacinian corpuscle: fibroblasts

7 Venules

8 Inner bulb of the corpuscle (o.s.)

9 Sheath of the corpuscle

10 Inner and outer lamellae of the corpuscle

11 Nerve (o.s.)

Fig. 2.   *Pacinian corpuscles in the deep dermis of thick skin.*
Stain: PASH. 350×.

PLATE 50

LIP (LONGITUDINAL SECTION)

The core of the lip contains striated fibers of the orbicularis oris muscle (8). Special stains would reveal the presence of intermixed dense fibroelastic connective tissue in the core. The right side of the figure illustrates the skin of the lip and the left, the mucosal lining of the mouth.

The outer layer of the skin is lined with an epidermis (9) composed of stratified squamous, keratinized epithelium. Beneath the epidermis is the dermis (10) with sebaceous glands (11), hair follicles (12), and sweat glands (14), all of which are derivatives of the epidermis. Also found in the dermis are the arrector pili muscles (13, 15) and a neurovascular bundle on the lip periphery (7).

The mucosa is lined with a stratified squamous, nonkeratinized epithelium (1). The surface cells, without becoming cornified, slough off in the fluids of the mouth (see Plate 1, Fig. 1). Underlying the mucosal epithelium is the lamina propria (2), the counterpart of the dermis as related to the epidermis. In the submucosa are found tubuloalveolar labial glands (4), which are predominantly mucous with occasional serous demilunes. Their secretion moistens the oral mucosa and their small ducts (4, lower leader) open into the oral cavity.

Transition of the skin epidermis to epithelium of oral mucosa illustrates a muco-cutaneous junction. The "red line" or vermilion border of the lip is illustrated (6). Epithelium of the lip and oral mucosa is relatively smoother than that of the epidermis. The underlying papillae of the lip and oral mucosa are high, numerous, and abundantly supplied with capillaries. The color of the blood shows through the overlying cells, giving the lips a characteristic red color. The epithelium of the labial mucosa (1) is thicker than the epidermis of the skin (9).

PLATE 50

LIP (LONGITUDINAL SECTION)

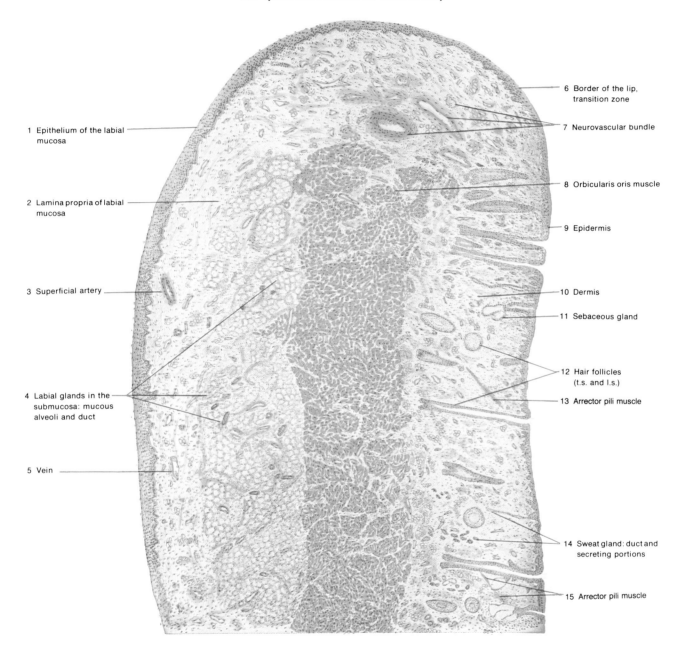

1 Epithelium of the labial
mucosa

2 Lamina propria of labial
mucosa

3 Superficial artery

4 Labial glands in the
submucosa: mucous
alveoli and duct

5 Vein

6 Border of the lip,
transition zone

7 Neurovascular bundle

8 Orbicularis oris muscle

9 Epidermis

10 Dermis

11 Sebaceous gland

12 Hair follicles
(t.s. and l.s.)

13 Arrector pili muscle

14 Sweat gland: duct and
secreting portions

15 Arrector pili muscle

Stain: hematoxylin-eosin. 20×.

PLATE 51

TONGUE: APEX (LONGITUDINAL SECTION, PANORAMIC VIEW)

The mucosa of the tongue consists of a stratified squamous epithelium and a thin papillated lamina propria (1), which may contain diffuse lymphatic tissue. The dorsal surface of the tongue is characterized by mucosal projections called papillae. Most numerous are the slender filiform papillae with cornified tips (6). Less numerous are the fungiform papillae (4, 7), which are characterized by a broad, round surface of noncornified epithelium and a prominent core of lamina propria (4). The papillae are found on the dorsal surface of the tongue but are absent on the entire ventral (lower) surface (18), where the mucosa is smooth.

Compact masses of skeletal muscle occupy the interior of the tongue. The muscle is typically seen as groups of fibers sectioned in longitudinal, transverse, or oblique planes. In the interfascicular connective tissue, which is continuous with the lamina propria, may be seen numerous blood vessels (9, 10, 15, 16) and nerves (8, 17).

In the lower half of the tongue near the apex and embedded in the muscle is illustrated a portion of the anterior lingual gland. This gland is of a mixed type and contains serous (11), mucous (13), and mixed alveoli with serous demilunes (not illustrated). Interlobular ducts (12) pass into the excretory ducts (14), which then open into the oral cavity on the ventral surface of the tongue.

PLATE 51

TONGUE: APEX (LONGITUDINAL SECTION, PANORAMIC VIEW)

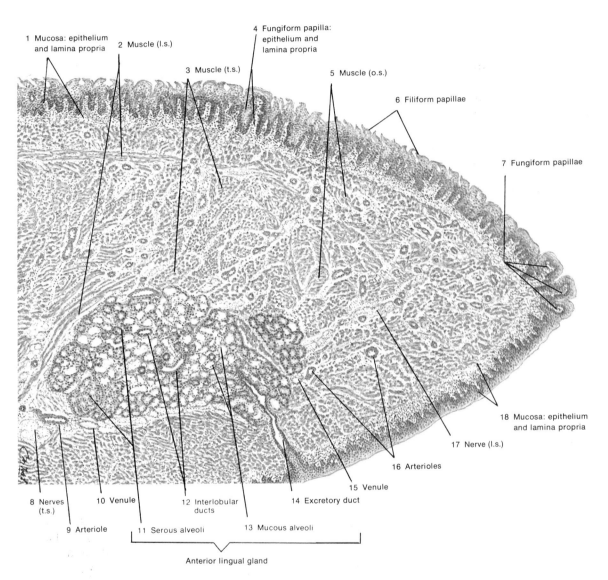

1 Mucosa: epithelium and lamina propria

2 Muscle (l.s.)

3 Muscle (t.s.)

4 Fungiform papilla: epithelium and lamina propria

5 Muscle (o.s.)

6 Filiform papillae

7 Fungiform papillae

18 Mucosa: epithelium and lamina propria

17 Nerve (l.s.)

16 Arterioles

15 Venule

14 Excretory duct

13 Mucous alveoli

12 Interlobular ducts

11 Serous alveoli

10 Venule

9 Arteriole

8 Nerves (t.s.)

Anterior lingual gland

Stain: hematoxylin-eosin. 25×.

PLATE 52 (Fig. 1)

TONGUE: CIRCUMVALLATE PAPILLA
(VERTICAL SECTION)

A vertical section through a circumvallate papilla is illustrated in Figure 1. The lamina propria of the papilla exhibits numerous, secondary papillae (3) which project into the overlying stratified squamous epithelium (8). Blood vessels (4) in the connective tissue stroma are abundant. The upper part of the circumvallate papilla usually does not project above the level of the adjacent lingual epithelium (1). A deep trench (9) or furrow encircles the papilla.

The barrel-shaped taste buds (5, 11) are located in the epithelium of the lateral surfaces of the papilla; some may also be present in the epithelium of the outer wall of the furrow.

Numerous serous alveoli of the tubuloalveolar glands (of von Ebner) (12) are located in the lamina propria and among the skeletal muscle fibers (6, 14). Ducts of the serous glands (7, 13) open at the bottom of the circular trench.

PLATE 52 (Fig. 2)

TASTE BUDS

Two taste buds are illustrated at a high magnification. They are embedded within the stratified epithelium of the lingual mucosa (1); however, they are distinguished from the surrounding epithelium by their oval shape and elongated cells (modified columnar) arranged perpendicularly to the surface.

Two of the several types of cells present in the buds are identified. Type I cells (6) are elongated with darker cytoplasm and slender, dark nucleus. Type II cells (5) have a lighter cytoplasm and a more oval, lighter nuclei. It is possible that these cells (Type II) are the neuroepithelial taste cells and Type I the supportive cells; however, it is difficult to assign a specific functional role to either type of cell with any degree of certainty. A third type of cell, the basal cell (not illustrated), is located at the periphery of the taste bud near the basement membrane. It is believed that this cell gives rise to the other two cell types. Large microvilli are present on both Type I and II cells. The taste hairs (2) represent clusters of microvilli that protrude through the taste pore (4) into the furrow surrounding the circumvallate papilla.

PLATE 52

TONGUE

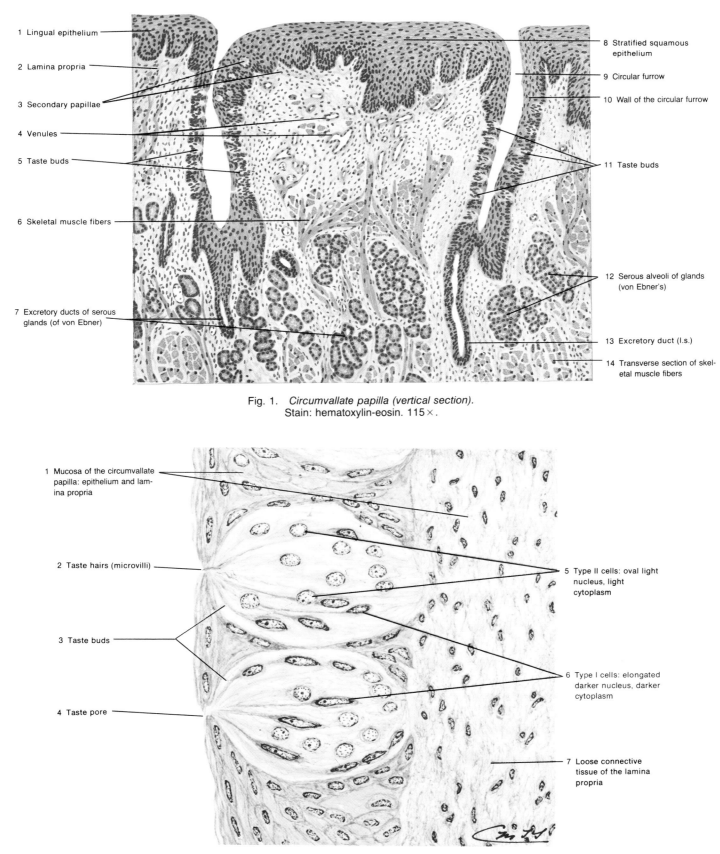

1 Lingual epithelium

2 Lamina propria

3 Secondary papillae

4 Venules

5 Taste buds

6 Skeletal muscle fibers

7 Excretory ducts of serous glands (of von Ebner)

8 Stratified squamous epithelium

9 Circular furrow

10 Wall of the circular furrow

11 Taste buds

12 Serous alveoli of glands (von Ebner's)

13 Excretory duct (l.s.)

14 Transverse section of skeletal muscle fibers

Fig. 1. *Circumvallate papilla (vertical section).*
Stain: hematoxylin-eosin. 115×.

1 Mucosa of the circumvallate papilla: epithelium and lamina propria

2 Taste hairs (microvilli)

3 Taste buds

4 Taste pore

5 Type II cells: oval light nucleus, light cytoplasm

6 Type I cells: elongated darker nucleus, darker cytoplasm

7 Loose connective tissue of the lamina propria

Fig. 2. *Taste buds.*
Stain: hematoxylin-eosin 900×.

PLATE 53 (Fig. 1)

POSTERIOR TONGUE NEAR CIRCUMVALLATE PAPILLA
(LONGITUDINAL SECTION)

This figure illustrates the posterior portion of the tongue, about 2 cm behind the circum-vallate papillae and near the lingual tonsils. The dorsal surface of the posterior tongue typically shows large mucosal ridges (1) and round elevations (6) or folds that resemble large fungiform papillae. Lymphatic nodules of the lingual tonsils can be seen in such elevations; typical filiform and fungiform papillae are absent in this region of the tongue.

The lamina propria of the mucosa is wider but similar to that in the anterior two thirds of the tongue. Under the epithelium are seen diffuse lymphatic tissue (2), adipose cells (3), blood vessels, and nerves. A large nerve is seen coursing along the vertical axis of the mucosal fold (9).

Numerous alveoli of the posterior lingual mucosal glands (4) lie deep in the lamina propria and in connective tissue trabeculae between the skeletal muscle fibers (5, 10) that extend deep into the muscles. The excretory ducts (7) open onto the dorsal surface of the tongue, usually between bases of the mucosal ridges and folds; however, in this figure, the duct appears to open at the apex of a ridge. Anteriorly, these glands come in contact with the serous glands (von Ebner's) of the circumvallate papilla; posteriorly, the glands extend through the root of the tongue.

PLATE 53 (Fig. 2)

LINGUAL TONSILS (TRANSVERSE SECTION)

This figure represents a transverse section of the posterior tongue and lingual tonsils.

The lymphatic nodules (2) are located in the lamina propria below the surface epithelium. The tonsilar crypts (3, 8) are deep invaginations of the surface and are lined with stratified squamous epithelium (9). The crypts may extend deep into the lamina propria.

Deep in the lamina propria and in the vicinity of the adipose tissue are mucous alveoli (5) of the posterior lingual glands. Small ducts (4, lower leader) unite to form larger excretory ducts, most of which open into the crypts, although some open on the lingual surface (4, upper leader). Skeletal muscles, not shown here, lie below the glands.

The lingual tonsils are an aggregation of small, individual tonsils, each with its own crypt and situated in the lamina propria at the root of the tongue. This arrangement may not be apparent in a small section of the tissue. The lingual tonsils are not a single encapsulated mass of lymphatic nodules as are the palatine tonsils.

PLATE 53

TONGUE AND TONSILS

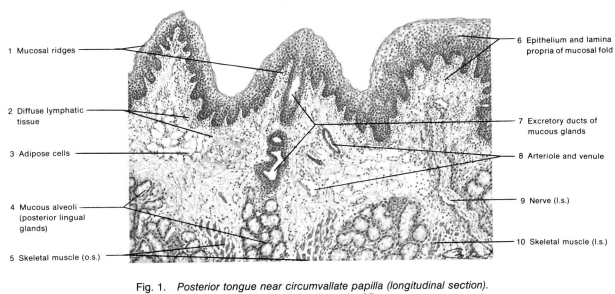

1 Mucosal ridges

2 Diffuse lymphatic tissue

3 Adipose cells

4 Mucous alveoli (posterior lingual glands)

5 Skeletal muscle (o.s.)

6 Epithelium and lamina propria of mucosal fold

7 Excretory ducts of mucous glands

8 Arteriole and venule

9 Nerve (l.s.)

10 Skeletal muscle (l.s.)

Fig. 1. *Posterior tongue near circumvallate papilla (longitudinal section).*
Stain: hematoxylin-eosin. 85×.

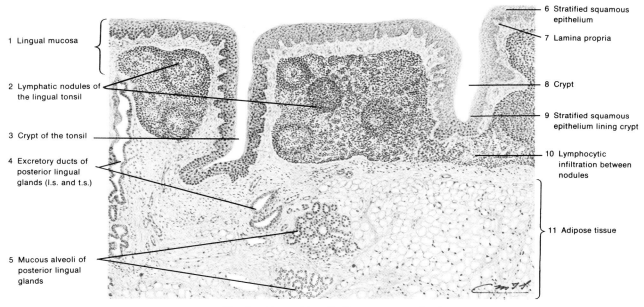

1 Lingual mucosa

2 Lymphatic nodules of the lingual tonsil

3 Crypt of the tonsil

4 Excretory ducts of posterior lingual glands (l.s. and t.s.)

5 Mucous alveoli of posterior lingual glands

6 Stratified squamous epithelium

7 Lamina propria

8 Crypt

9 Stratified squamous epithelium lining crypt

10 Lymphocytic infiltration between nodules

11 Adipose tissue

Fig. 2. *Lingual tonsils (transverse section).*
Stain: hematoxylin-eosin. 60×.

PLATE 54 (Fig. 1)

DRIED TOOTH: PANORAMIC VIEW, LONGITUDINAL SECTION

Dentin (3, 5) surrounds the pulp cavity (4) and its extension, the root canal (6). In life, the pulp cavity and root canal are filled with fine connective tissue which contains fibroblasts, histiocytes, odontoblasts, blood vessels, and nerves. Dentin (3) exhibits wavy, parallel dentinal tubules. The earlier or primary dentin is located at the periphery of the tooth (3); the later or secondary dentin lies along the pulp cavity (5), where it is formed throughout life by odontoblasts. In the crown of a dried tooth and at the periphery of dentin near its junction with enamel are numerous irregular, empty, air-filled spaces which appear black in the section. These are the interglobular spaces (12) which, in life, are filled with incompletely calcified dentin (interglobular dentin). Similar areas, but smaller and closer together, are present in the root, close to the dentinal-cementum junction, where they form the granular layer (of Tomes) (13).

The dentin in the crown is covered with a thick layer of enamel (1), composed of enamel rods or prisms held together by a small amount of interprismatic cementing substance. With adequate lighting, it is possible to see the incremental growth lines of Retzius (8), which represent variations in the rate of enamel deposition and the lighter bands of Schreger (9). Light rays passing through dried sections of tooth are refracted by twists that occur in the enamel rods as they course toward the surface of the tooth. These refracted rays are the light bands of Schreger (9). At the dentinoenamel junction may be seen enamel spindles (10) and enamel tufts (11), which are illustrated at a higher magnification in Figure 2.

Cementum (7) covers the dentin of the root. In life, cementum contains lacunae with cementocytes and canaliculi (14).

PLATE 54 (Fig. 2)

DRIED TOOTH: LAYERS OF THE CROWN

A section of enamel and dentin are illustrated at a high magnification. The enamel consists of elongated enamel rods or prisms (1). In the enamel near the dentinal junction are seen enamel spindles (2), which are pointed or spindle-shaped processes of dentin that penetrate the enamel for a short distance. Enamel tufts (3), which extend from the dentinoenamel junction (4) into the enamel, are groups of poorly calcified, twisted enamel rods. Dentin with its dentinal tubules (6) and black, air-filled interglobular spaces (5) is clearly visible.

PLATE 54 (Fig. 3)

DRIED TOOTH: LAYERS OF THE ROOT

Dentin (1) and cementum (4) are illustrated at a high magnification. Near the dentinoenamel junction is seen the granular layer (of Tomes) (2). Internal to this layer are the large, irregular interglobular (3) spaces which are commonly seen in the crown of the tooth but may also be present in the root. Cementum (4) contains lacunae (5) with their canaliculi.

PLATE 54

DRIED TOOTH

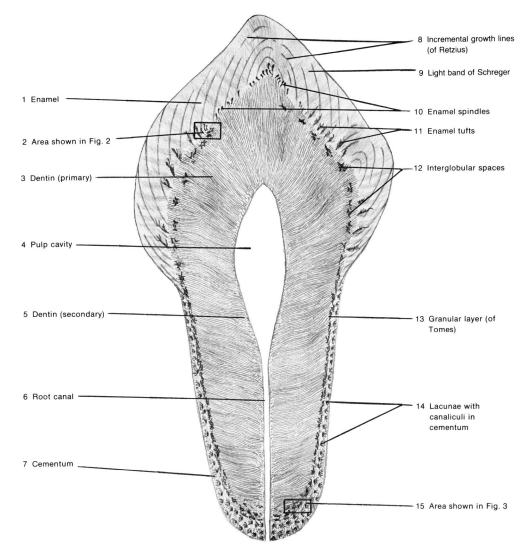

1 Enamel

2 Area shown in Fig. 2

3 Dentin (primary)

4 Pulp cavity

5 Dentin (secondary)

6 Root canal

7 Cementum

8 Incremental growth lines (of Retzius)

9 Light band of Schreger

10 Enamel spindles

11 Enamel tufts

12 Interglobular spaces

13 Granular layer (of Tomes)

14 Lacunae with canaliculi in cementum

15 Area shown in Fig. 3

Fig. 1.   *Panoramic view, longitudinal section.*

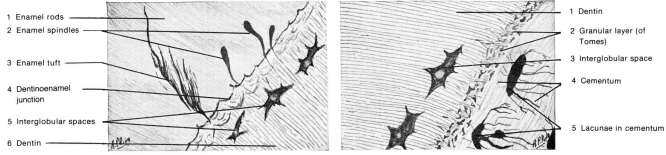

1 Enamel rods

2 Enamel spindles

3 Enamel tuft

4 Dentinoenamel junction

5 Interglobular spaces

6 Dentin

Fig. 2.   *Layers of the crown. Area corresponding to (2) in Fig. 1.* 160×.

1 Dentin

2 Granular layer (of Tomes)

3 Interglobular space

4 Cementum

5 Lacunae in cementum

Fig. 3.   *Layers of the root. Area corresponding to (15) in Fig. 1.* 160×.

PLATE 55 (Fig. 1)

DEVELOPING TOOTH: PANORAMIC VIEW

A developing deciduous tooth is shown embedded in a socket, the dental alveolus, in the bone of the jaw (4, 22). Connective tissue (3) surrounds the developing tooth and forms a compact layer immediately around the tooth, the dental sac (5). Enclosed within the sac is the enamel organ, composed of the external enamel epithelium (18), the stellate reticulum of enamel pulp (6, 19), the intermediate stratum (20), and the ameloblasts or inner enamel epithelium (7). All of these structures differentiate from the downgrowth of the gum epithelium. The ameloblasts secrete enamel around the dentin. The enamel (8, 15) is illustrated as a narrow band of deep-staining pink material.

The dental pulp (21) of primitive connective tissue forms the core of the developing tooth. Blood vessels and nerves innervate the dental pulp from below. The mesenchyme cells in the dental papilla differentiate into odontoblasts (11), which then produce the outer margin of the pulp. Odontoblasts secrete predentin (10, 17) which is an uncalcified dentin. As predentin calcifies, it forms a layer of dentin (9, 16) adjacent to enamel.

The oral mucosa (1, 13) covers the developing tooth. An epithelial downgrowth from the oral epithelium indicates the germ of a permanent tooth (2).

At the base of the tooth, the outer and inner enamel epithelium form the epithelial root sheath (of Hertwig) (12).

PLATE 55 (Fig. 2)

DEVELOPING TOOTH: SECTIONAL VIEW

The left side of the figure illustrates a small area of dental pulp with the fibroblasts (1) and the fine fibers. Odontoblasts (2) are at the margin of the pulp and secrete the uncalcified predentin (3), which later calcifies to become dentin (4). Processes of odontoblasts remain in the predentin and dentin as the odontoblast processes (of Tomes) (3).

On the right side of the figure is a small area of stellate reticulum (7) of enamel showing the nuclei, the processes of its modified epithelial cells, the intermediate stratum (8), a transition region, and the tall columnar ameloblasts (6) which secrete the enamel (5, 10) in the form of enamel rods or prisms. In the process of enamel formation, the apical end of each ameloblast becomes transformed into a terminal process of Tomes. These processes then appear collectively, in advanced enamel formation, as a separate layer of enamel processes (of Tomes) (9).

PLATE 55

DEVELOPING TOOTH

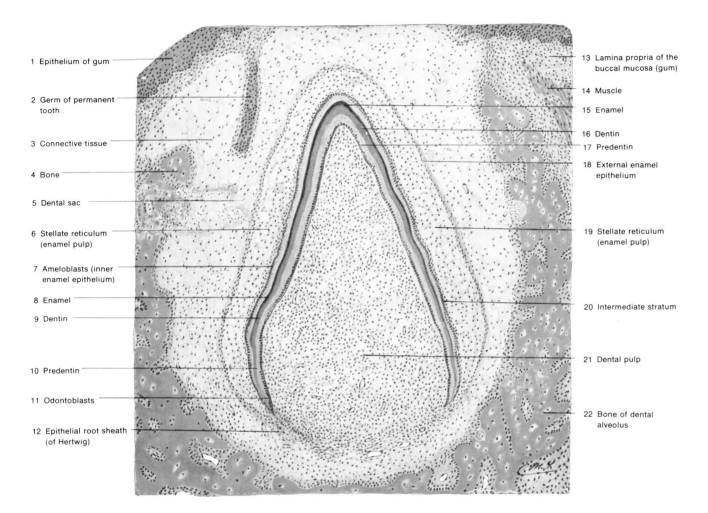

1 Epithelium of gum

2 Germ of permanent tooth

3 Connective tissue

4 Bone

5 Dental sac

6 Stellate reticulum (enamel pulp)

7 Ameloblasts (inner enamel epithelium)

8 Enamel

9 Dentin

10 Predentin

11 Odontoblasts

12 Epithelial root sheath (of Hertwig)

13 Lamina propria of the buccal mucosa (gum)

14 Muscle

15 Enamel

16 Dentin

17 Predentin

18 External enamel epithelium

19 Stellate reticulum (enamel pulp)

20 Intermediate stratum

21 Dental pulp

22 Bone of dental alveolus

Fig. 1. *Panoramic view.*
Stain: hematoxylin-eosin. 50×.

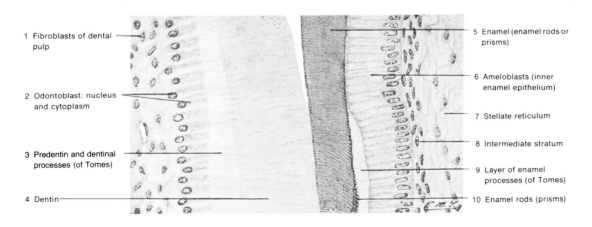

1 Fibroblasts of dental pulp

2 Odontoblast: nucleus and cytoplasm

3 Predentin and dentinal processes (of Tomes)

4 Dentin

5 Enamel (enamel rods or prisms)

6 Ameloblasts (inner enamel epithelium)

7 Stellate reticulum

8 Intermediate stratum

9 Layer of enamel processes (of Tomes)

10 Enamel rods (prisms)

Fig. 2. *Sectional view.*
Stain: hematoxylin-eosin. 300×.

PLATE 56

SALIVARY GLAND: PAROTID

The parotid salivary gland is classified as a compound tubuloalveolar gland (see Plate 6).

The parotid gland is a purely serous gland with well developed capsule and septa which subdivide the gland into lobes and lobules. Parts of several lobules are illustrated in the figure.

Each lobule consists of masses of serous alveoli (1, 15) supported by thin connective tissue partitions. Each alveolus consists of pyramid-shaped cells arranged around a small, barely visible lumen (1); in certain sections, the lumen is not visible in all alveoli. The serous cells have a small, round nucleus located at the base of deeply basophilic cytoplasm. At the apices, the cytoplasm is lighter-staining (15). At higher magnification, basal striations (I) are often visible at the base of the cells (22) and small acidophilic secretory granules (zymogen granules) (21) at the cell apices; the number of secretory granules varies with the state of activity of the cell or gland. Myoepithelial cells (basket cells) (23) lie between the basement membrane and the epithelial cells; usually, only the nucleus is visible.

Distributed within the lobules and among the alveoli are small blood vessels (18), adipose cells (2, 19), striated ducts (5, 7), and intercalated ducts (8, 17, 25). The intercalated ducts drain the alveoli (17), have small diameters and lumina, and are lined with low cuboidal cells (II). Striated ducts (5, 7) have larger lumina and are lined with columnar epithelium that exhibit basal striations (III, 24). In all duct cells, the nucleus has a central location in the cytoplasm.

Striated ducts drain into the interlobular excretory ducts (6, 9, 12, 14), which are found in the connective tissue septa (11, 13, 16). The lumina become progressively wider as the ducts increase in size. The ductal epithelium varies from low columnar (6, IV) to pseudostratified or stratified columnar in large excretory ducts (9, 12)

The interlobular connective tissue contains blood vessels (3, 4, 10) of various sizes, nerves, and occasionally, parasympathetic ganglia (20).

PLATE 56

SALIVARY GLAND: PAROTID

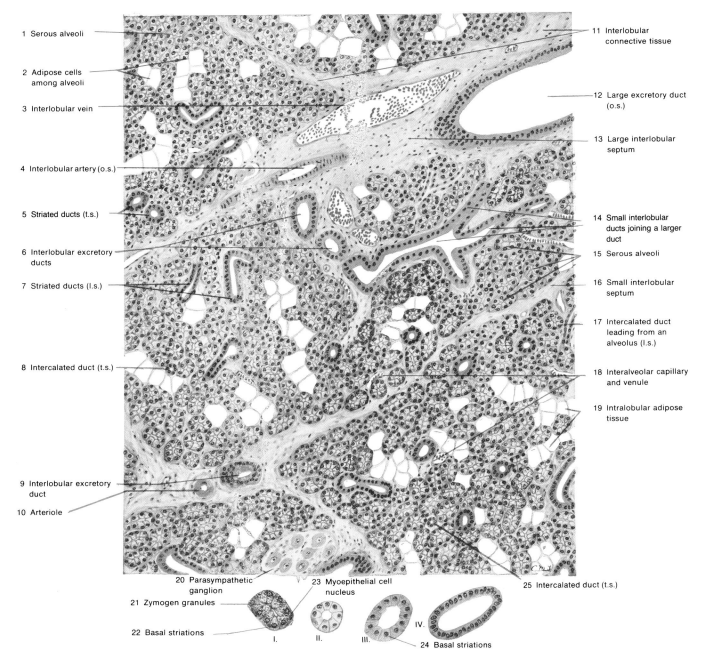

1 Serous alveoli

2 Adipose cells among alveoli

3 Interlobular vein

4 Interlobular artery (o.s.)

5 Striated ducts (t.s.)

6 Interlobular excretory ducts

7 Striated ducts (l.s.)

8 Intercalated duct (t.s.)

9 Interlobular excretory duct

10 Arteriole

11 Interlobular connective tissue

12 Large excretory duct (o.s.)

13 Large interlobular septum

14 Small interlobular ducts joining a larger duct

15 Serous alveoli

16 Small interlobular septum

17 Intercalated duct leading from an alveolus (l.s.)

18 Interalveolar capillary and venule

19 Intralobular adipose tissue

20 Parasympathetic ganglion

21 Zymogen granules

22 Basal striations

23 Myoepithelial cell nucleus

24 Basal striations

25 Intercalated duct (t.s.)

I. II. III. IV.

I. serous alveolus; II. intercalated duct; III. striated duct; IV. interlobular excretory duct.

Stain: hematoxylin-eosin. 120×.

PLATE 57

SALIVARY GLAND: SUBMANDIBULAR

This plate illustrates parts of several lobules of the submandibular gland, which is a compound tubuloalveolar gland.

The submandibular gland is a mixed type, but is composed predominantly of serous alveoli. Intermixed with serous alveoli are a few mucous alveoli. The presence of mixed alveoli distinguishes the submandibular gland from the parotid gland, which is a purely serous gland.

The serous alveoli (3, 10, II), similar to those in the parotid gland, are recognized by their smaller size, intensely stained pyramidal cells with deep basophilic cytoplasm, round nucleus, light-stained apical area, and narrow lumina (3, II). The mucous alveoli (4, 9, IV) are larger and more variable in size and shape. The mucous cells are more columnar, are pale or almost colorless after staining, and have flat, basal nuclei; the alveoli exhibit somewhat larger and more apparent lumina.

Mixed alveoli (8, V) are normally mucous alveoli surrounded by one or more groups of serous cells, the serous demilunes (14, 15). Myoepithelial cells (basket cells) (16) are disposed around serous, mucous, and intercalated duct cells.

The duct system is similar to that seen in the parotid gland. Intralobular intercalated ducts (I, 12) with small lumina and striated ducts (7, III, 13) are present in the gland. A longitudinal section (IV) shows an alveolus opening into an intercalated duct (12), which then opens into a striated duct (13). Interlobular excretory ducts (1, 5) course in the interlobular connective tissue septa. Adipose cells (11) are scattered among the alveoli; however, they are less numerous than in the parotid gland.

PLATE 57

SALIVARY GLAND: SUBMANDIBULAR

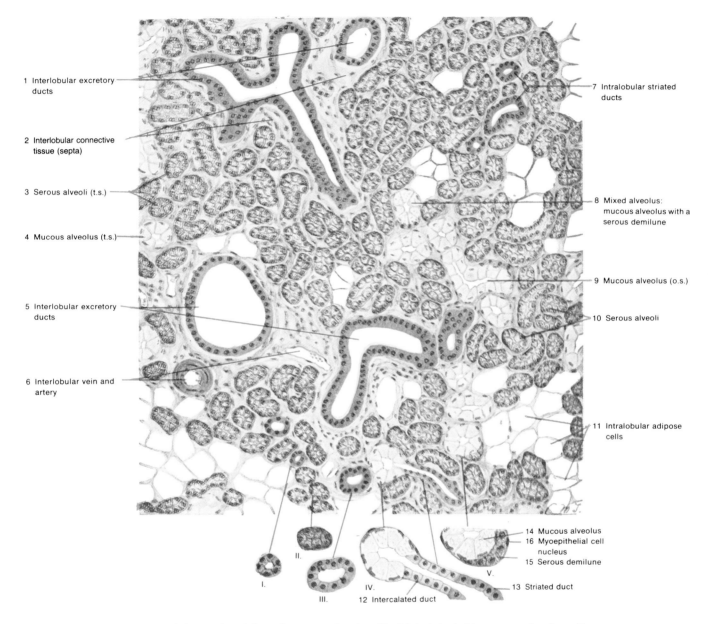

1 Interlobular excretory ducts

2 Interlobular connective tissue (septa)

3 Serous alveoli (t.s.)

4 Mucous alveolus (t.s.)

5 Interlobular excretory ducts

6 Interlobular vein and artery

7 Intralobular striated ducts

8 Mixed alveolus: mucous alveolus with a serous demilune

9 Mucous alveolus (o.s.)

10 Serous alveoli

11 Intralobular adipose cells

II.

I.

III.

IV.

12 Intercalated duct

V.

14 Mucous alveolus

16 Myoepithelial cell nucleus

15 Serous demilune

13 Striated duct

I. intercalated duct; II. serous alveolus; III. striated duct; IV. mucous alveolus with intercalated and striated ducts (l.s.); V. mixed alveolus.

Stain: hematoxylin-eosin. 170×.

PLATE 58

SALIVARY GLAND: SUBLINGUAL

The sublingual gland is also a mixed gland, but is composed predominantly of mucous alveoli (4, 6, I) and mucous alveoli with serous demilunes (2, 7, II). Purely serous alveoli are scarce; however, the composition of the gland is variable. In this figure, serous alveoli are comparatively numerous (3), whereas in other sections of the gland, these alveoli may be absent. Myoepithelial cells may be seen around alveoli, normally situated between the basement membrane and the base of the epithelial cell.

Typical intercalated ducts (8, IV) are infrequent or absent and the striated ducts are seen only occasionally. Poorly developed striated or non-striated intralobular ducts are more prevalent (1, 9, V).

The interlobular connective tissue (13) is characteristically more abundant in the sublingual than in the parotid and submandibular glands. Epithelial lining of interlobular excretory ducts varies from low columnar in the smaller ducts to pseudostratified or stratified columnar in the larger ducts (15, VI), as seen in the parotid and submandibular glands. Blood vessels (5, 11, 12), nerves (10), and parasympathetic ganglia (14) are seen in the interlobular connective tissue.

PLATE 58

SALIVARY GLAND: SUBLINGUAL

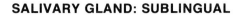

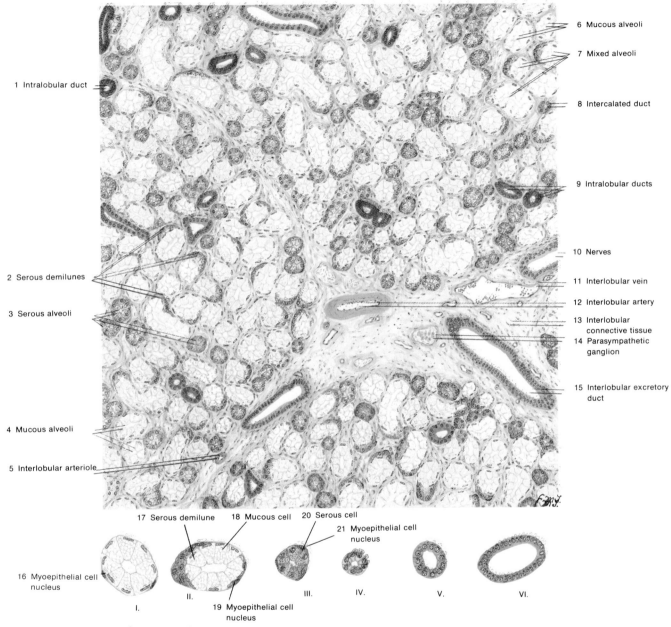

1 Intralobular duct

2 Serous demilunes

3 Serous alveoli

4 Mucous alveoli

5 Interlobular arteriole

6 Mucous alveoli

7 Mixed alveoli

8 Intercalated duct

9 Intralobular ducts

10 Nerves

11 Interlobular vein

12 Interlobular artery

13 Interlobular connective tissue

14 Parasympathetic ganglion

15 Interlobular excretory duct

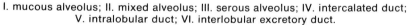

16 Myoepithelial cell nucleus

17 Serous demilune

18 Mucous cell

19 Myoepithelial cell nucleus

20 Serous cell

21 Myoepithelial cell nucleus

I.

II.

III.

IV.

V.

VI.

I. mucous alveolus; II. mixed alveolus; III. serous alveolus; IV. intercalated duct;
V. intralobular duct; VI. interlobular excretory duct.

Stain: hematoxylin-eosin. 85×.

PLATE 59

UPPER ESOPHAGUS: WALL (TRANSVERSE SECTION)

The esophagus is a tubular organ whose wall is composed of four distinct parts: the mucosa, submucosa, muscularis externa, and adventitia.

The mucosa consists of an inner lining of nonkeratinized stratified squamous epithelium (1); an underlying thin layer of fine connective tissue, the lamina propria (2); and a layer of longitudinal smooth muscle fibers, the muscularis mucosae (3). Connective tissue papillae in the lamina propria indent the epithelium. Present in the lamina propria are small blood vessels, diffuse lymphatic tissue, and a small lymphatic nodule (9). The muscularis mucosae (3) is composed of longitudinal smooth muscle fibers, illustrated in either cross or oblique sections.

The submucosa (4) is a wide layer of moderately dense irregular connective tissue which often contains adipose cells (14). Tubuloalveolar mucous glands, the esophageal glands proper (11), are present in the submucosa and occur at intervals throughout the length of the esophagus. Ducts (12) arising from the alveoli of the esophageal glands pass through the muscularis mucosae (10) and the lamina propria and open into the lumen of the esophagus; their epithelium merges with stratified squamous surface epithelium of the esophagus (see Plate 60). Large blood vessels (13) course in the submucosa.

Located beneath the submucosa is the muscularis externa, composed of two well-defined muscle layers. The inner muscle layer (5) is circular and, in this transverse section of the esophagus, sectioned longitudinally; the outer muscle layer is longitudinal (7), and in it the muscle fibers are seen mainly in transverse sections. A thin layer of connective tissue lies between the two muscle layers (6). Although highly variable in different species of animals, in humans the muscularis externa in the upper third of the esophagus consists primarily of striated skeletal muscle fibers. In the middle third, both layers exhibit an increasing mixture of smooth muscle, and in the lower third of the esophagus, only smooth muscle is found. The peripheral location of the nuclei in the striated muscle fibers is best seen in the fibers cut transversely (7).

The adventitia (8) of the esophagus consists of a loose connective tissue layer which blends with the adventitia of the trachea and the surrounding structures. Adipose tissue (16) is frequently present in this layer. Adventitia also contains large blood vessels (17, 18) and nerves (19) forming neuro-vascular bundles as well as smaller divisions of the bundle.

PLATE 59

UPPER ESOPHAGUS: WALL (TRANSVERSE SECTION)

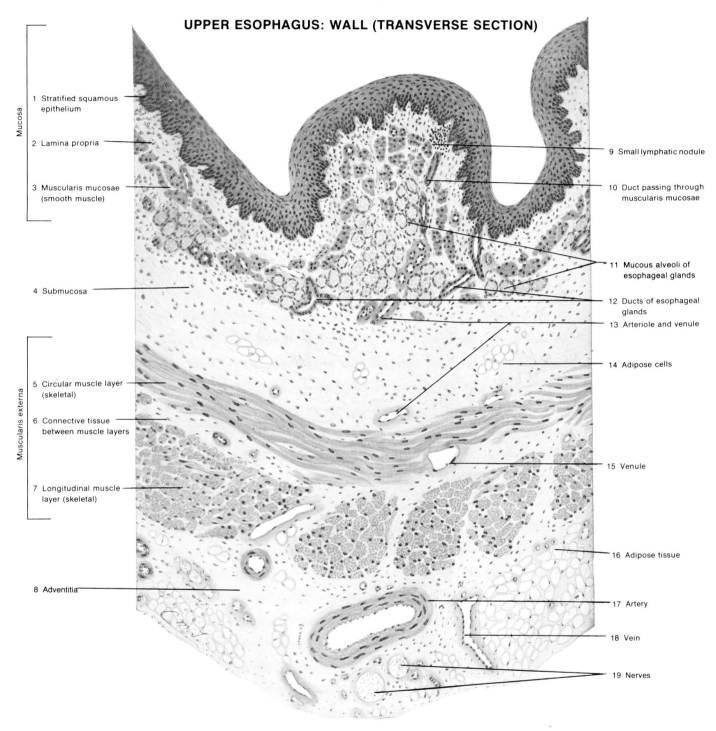

Mucosa

1 Stratified squamous epithelium

2 Lamina propria

3 Muscularis mucosae (smooth muscle)

4 Submucosa

Muscularis externa

5 Circular muscle layer (skeletal)

6 Connective tissue between muscle layers

7 Longitudinal muscle layer (skeletal)

8 Adventitia

9 Small lymphatic nodule

10 Duct passing through muscularis mucosae

11 Mucous alveoli of esophageal glands

12 Ducts of esophageal glands

13 Arteriole and venule

14 Adipose cells

15 Venule

16 Adipose tissue

17 Artery

18 Vein

19 Nerves

Stain: hematoxylin-eosin. 50×.

PLATE 60

UPPER ESOPHAGUS: MUCOSA AND SUBMUCOSA
(TRANSVERSE SECTION)

Higher magnification of the upper esophageal wall illustrates the mucosa (1, 2, 3) and the submucosa (4). The surface stratified squamous epithelium (1) exhibits typical cell layers normally seen in this type of epithelium: squamous cells (6) forming the outer layers, numerous polyhedral cells (7) of the intermediate layers, and low columnar cells (9) in the basal layer. Mitotic activity is usually observed in the deeper layers of the epithelium (8).

In the lamina propria (2, 10) are the blood vessels (11) and scattered or aggregated lymphocytes (12). The muscularis mucosae (which is always smooth muscle) is illustrated as small bundles of muscle fibers sectioned in a transverse plane (13).

In the submucosa are found mucous alveoli (filled with mucigen) of the esophageal glands proper (15). Small ducts from these glands (16, lower leaders) lined with simple epithelium join the larger excretory ducts (16, upper leader) that are lined with stratified epithelium. A large duct is sectioned tangentially (14), revealing that its epithelium becomes continuous with the stratified squamous epithelium of the esophageal lumen.

In the submucosa (4) are seen blood vessels (17, 18), nerves (19), and adipose cells (20). A small section of skeletal muscle fibers from the inner circular layer of the muscularis externa (5) is illustrated in the lower left corner.

PLATE 60

UPPER ESOPHAGUS: MUCOSA AND SUBMUCOSA
(TRANSVERSE SECTION)

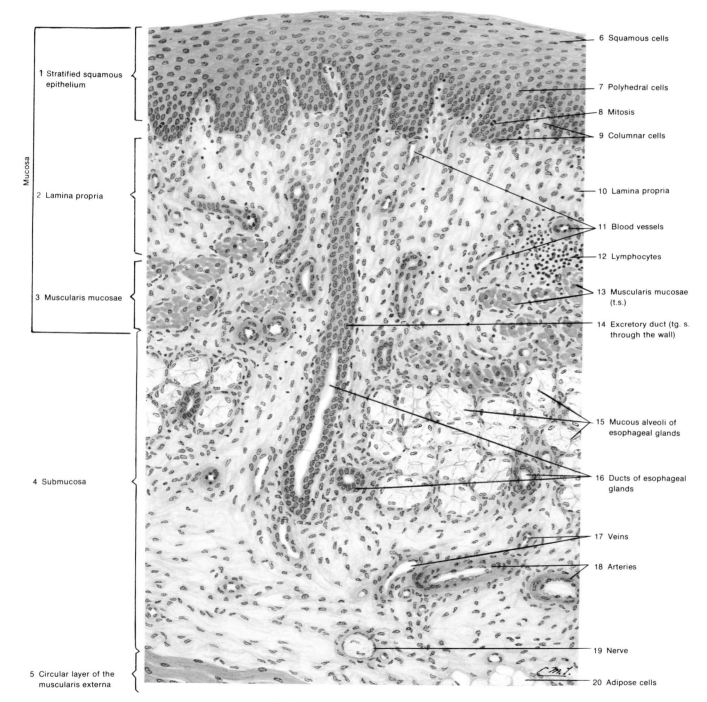

Mucosa

1 Stratified squamous epithelium

2 Lamina propria

3 Muscularis mucosae

4 Submucosa

5 Circular layer of the muscularis externa

6 Squamous cells

7 Polyhedral cells

8 Mitosis

9 Columnar cells

10 Lamina propria

11 Blood vessels

12 Lymphocytes

13 Muscularis mucosae (t.s.)

14 Excretory duct (tg. s. through the wall)

15 Mucous alveoli of esophageal glands

16 Ducts of esophageal glands

17 Veins

18 Arteries

19 Nerve

20 Adipose cells

Stain: hematoxylin-eosin. 250×.

PLATE 61 (Fig. 1)

UPPER ESOPHAGUS (TRANSVERSE SECTION)

This section of upper esophagus is similar to that illustrated in Plate 59; however, it is stained with Heidenhain's modification of Mallory's trichrome (Mallory-azan). Azocarmine stains the nuclei an intense red. A mixture of aniline blue and orange G then selectively stains other tissue components. Collagenous fibers stain bright blue (1, 4, 5, 7, 9), whereas cytoplasm of epithelial and muscle cells stains orange to red (2, 3, 6, 8).·

The layers of the esophagus are easily distinguishable. Because this section is from the upper esophagus (as in Plate 60), the outermost layer is the adventitia (1) and the muscularis externa is composed of skeletal muscle (2, 3). Aniline blue stains not only the large amounts of connective tissue in the submucosa (9) and adventitia (1) but also the smaller amounts between (4) and within (5) muscle layers. The connective tissue of the lamina propria (7) is distinct from the smooth muscle of the muscularis mucosae (8).

PLATE 61 (Fig. 2)

LOWER ESOPHAGUS (TRANSVERSE SECTION)

This section of the terminal portion of the esophagus (in the peritoneal cavity near the stomach) is stained with Van Gieson's trichrome, which employs iron hematoxylin (Weigert's or Heidenhain's) as a nuclear stain and picrofuchsin to stain other components. As a result, cellular details are not well defined; the stain is useful for differentiating between connective tissue and muscle. Nuclei are stained dark brown. Collagenous fibers are stained red with acid fuchsin (3, 5, 7), whereas muscle (and other tissues) are stained yellow with picric acid (2, 4, 6, 8, 9).

Except for regional differences, the layers in the wall of the lower esophagus are generally similar to those in the upper region. The outermost layer of the esophagus in the peritoneal cavity is the serosa (visceral peritoneum) (1) in contrast to adventitia in the thoracic cavity. The muscularis externa layers are entirely smooth muscle (2, 4), although this is not apparent with this stain and at this magnification. Distribution of the mucous glands in the submucosa is variable, and in some regions they may be absent; however, some are illustrated in this section (9).

In addition to the abundant collagenous fibers in the submucosa (5), distribution of finer fibers in lesser amounts may be seen between and around bundles of smooth muscle fibers (3, 8), in serosa (1) and in the lamina propria (7).

PLATE 61

ESOPHAGUS (TRANSVERSE SECTIONS)

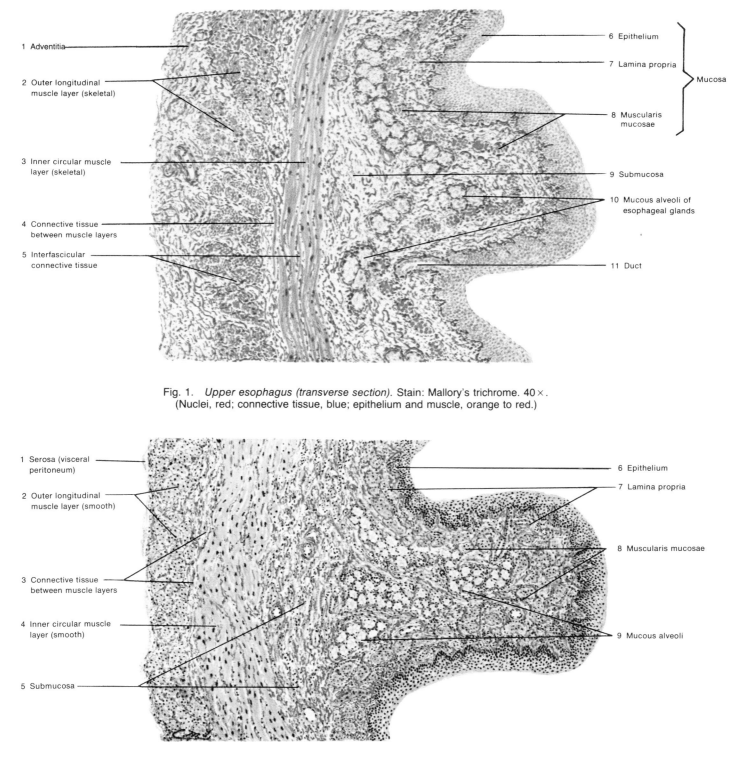

1 Adventitia

2 Outer longitudinal muscle layer (skeletal)

3 Inner circular muscle layer (skeletal)

4 Connective tissue between muscle layers

5 Interfascicular connective tissue

6 Epithelium

7 Lamina propria

8 Muscularis mucosae

Mucosa

9 Submucosa

10 Mucous alveoli of esophageal glands

11 Duct

Fig. 1. *Upper esophagus (transverse section).* Stain: Mallory's trichrome. 40×.
(Nuclei, red; connective tissue, blue; epithelium and muscle, orange to red.)

1 Serosa (visceral peritoneum)

2 Outer longitudinal muscle layer (smooth)

3 Connective tissue between muscle layers

4 Inner circular muscle layer (smooth)

5 Submucosa

6 Epithelium

7 Lamina propria

8 Muscularis mucosae

9 Mucous alveoli

Fig. 2. *Lower esophagus (transverse section).* Stain: Van Gieson's trichrome. 40×.
(Nuclei, dark brown; connective tissue, red; epithelium and muscle, yellow.)

PLATE 62

CARDIA (LONGITUDINAL SECTION)

At the terminal end of the esophagus, the esophageal glands proper that are normally located in the submucosa may still be present (11). Ducts (13) from these glands penetrate the muscularis mucosae, course through the lamina propria (15) and empty into the lumen of the esophagus. The lamina propria (14) may contain few cardiac glands (12).

At the cardia or the esophageal-stomach junction, stratified squamous epithelium of the esophagus changes abruptly to simple columnar, mucus-secreting epithelium of the stomach. As a result, the boundary between these two organs is sharply defined.

The lamina propria of the stomach (16) is continuous with that of the esophagus and becomes a wide layer containing diffuse lymphatic tissue and glands. The lamina propria is penetrated by a multitude of shallow gastric pits (19) into which the mucosal glands empty (17).

In the upper region of the stomach are two types of glands. The simple tubular cardiac glands (17) are primarily limited to the transition region, the cardia of the stomach. They are lined with a single type of cell, the mucus-secreting columnar cell. Below the cardia of the stomach, the glands are replaced by simple tubular gastric glands (20), which may exhibit basal branching. The gastric glands are composed of four different cell types: the chief or zymogenic cells (21), parietal cells (23), mucous neck cells (22), and several different types of endocrine cells (not illustrated), collectively called enteroendocrine cells (see Plate 69). The mucous neck cells (22) are located at the distal end of the of the gastric glands before they open into the gastric pits.

The muscularis mucosae (8) is continuous from esophagus to the stomach. In the esophagus, muscularis mucosae is usually a single layer of longitudinal fibers. In the stomach, a second layer of smooth muscle is added, the inner circular layer (8).

The submucosa (7) and muscularis externa (6) layers are continuous. Numerous blood vessels course through the length of submucosa (1, 2, 3, 4, 5, 9). The larger vessels distribute smaller vessels to other regions of the esophagus.

PLATE 62

CARDIA (LONGITUDINAL SECTION)

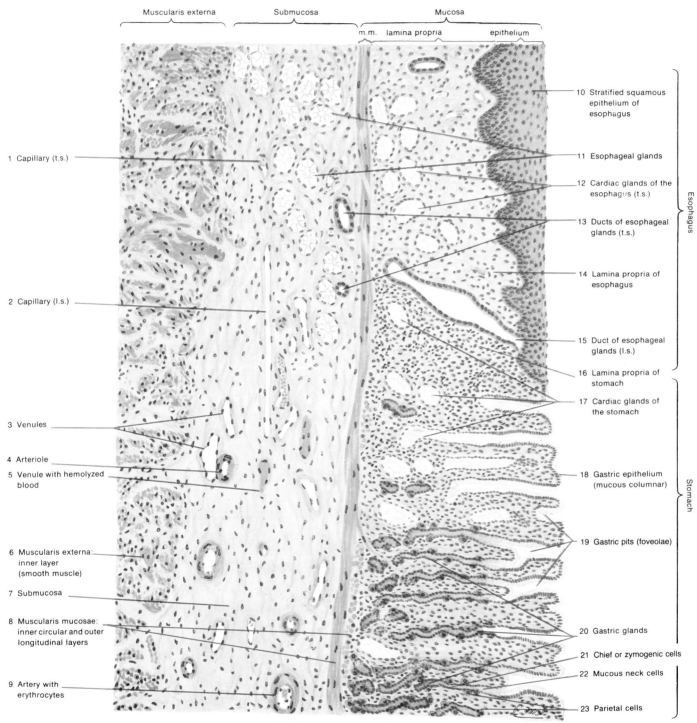

Muscularis externa — Submucosa — Mucosa

m.m. lamina propria epithelium

1 Capillary (t.s.)

2 Capillary (l.s.)

3 Venules

4 Arteriole

5 Venule with hemolyzed blood

6 Muscularis externa: inner layer (smooth muscle)

7 Submucosa

8 Muscularis mucosae: inner circular and outer longitudinal layers

9 Artery with erythrocytes

10 Stratified squamous epithelium of esophagus

11 Esophageal glands

12 Cardiac glands of the esophagus (t.s.)

13 Ducts of esophageal glands (t.s.)

14 Lamina propria of esophagus

15 Duct of esophageal glands (l.s.)

16 Lamina propria of stomach

17 Cardiac glands of the stomach

18 Gastric epithelium (mucous columnar)

19 Gastric pits (foveolae)

20 Gastric glands

21 Chief or zymogenic cells

22 Mucous neck cells

23 Parietal cells

Esophagus

Stomach

Stain: hematoxylin-eosin. 70×.

PLATE 63

THE STOMACH: FUNDUS OR BODY
(TRANSVERSE SECTION)

The human stomach is divided into three distinct histological areas: the cardia, fundus or body, and pylorus. The fundus or body is the most extensive region in the stomach.

This low-magnification figure illustrates a transverse section of the fundic stomach. The stomach wall exhibits four general regions that are characteristic of the entire digestive tract: the mucosa (1, 2, 3), submucosa (4), muscularis externa (5, 6, 7), and serosa (8).

Mucosa (1, 2, 3): the mucosa of the stomach consists of three layers: the epithelium, lamina propria, and muscularis mucosae. The luminal surface of the mucosa is lined with a layer of simple columnar epithelium (1, 11). This epithelium also extends into and lines the gastric pits (10), which are tubular infoldings of the surface epithelium. In the fundic region of the stomach, the gastric pits are not deep and extend into the mucosa about one-fourth of its thickness. Beneath the surface epithelium is a layer of loose connective tissue, the lamina propria (2, 12), which fills the narrow spaces between the gastric glands. The outer layer of mucosa is lined by a thin band of smooth muscle, the muscularis mucosae (3, 15), consisting of an inner circular layer and an outer longitudinal layer. Thin slips of muscle from the muscularis mucosae (3, 15) extend into lamina propria (2, 12) between the gastric glands (13, 14) toward the surface epithelium (1, 11) (see Plate 64:8).

The gastric glands (13, 14) are tightly packed in the lamina propria and occupy the entire thickness of the mucosa (1, 2, 3). These glands open in small groups into the bottom of the gastric pits (10). The surface epithelium of the entire gastrc mucosa contains the same cell type, from the cardiac to the pyloric region; however, there are distinct regional differences in the types of cells that comprise the gastric glands. At lower magnification, two distinct types of cells can be identified in the gastric glands of the fundic stomach. The acidophilic parietal cells (13) are seen in the upper portions of the glands; the more basophilic chief (zymogenic) (14) cells occupy the lower regions. The subglandular regions of the lamina propria may contain small accumulations of lymphatic tissue or nodules (16).

The mucosa of an empty stomach exhibits numerous folds called the rugae (9). These folds are temporary and are formed from the contractions of the smooth muscle layer, the muscularis mucosae (3, 15). As the stomach fills with solid or liquid material, the rugae disappear and the mucosa appears smooth.

Submucosa (4): The prominent layer directly beneath the muscularis mucosae (3, 15) is the submucosa (4). In an empty stomach, this layer can extend into the folds or the rugae (9). The submucosa contains denser irregular connective tissue and more collagenous fibers (17) than the lamina propria. In addition to the normal complement of connective tissue cells, the submucosa also contains numerous lymph vessels, capillaries (22), large arterioles (18), and venules (19). Isolated or small clusters of the parasympathetic ganglia of the submucosal (Meissner's) nerve plexus (21) are also seen in the deeper regions of the submucosa.

Muscularis Externa (5, 6, 7): In the stomach, the muscularis externa (5, 6, 7) consists of three layers of smooth muscle, each oriented in a different plane: an inner oblique layer (5), a middle circular layer (6) and an outer longitudinal layer (7). The oblique layer is not complete and, as a result, is not always seen in sections of stomach wall. In this illustration, the circular layer has been sectioned longitudinally and the longitudinal layer transversely. Located between the circular and longitudinal smooth muscle layers is a prominent myenteric (Auerbach's) nerve plexus (23) of parasympathetic ganglia and nerve fibers.

Serosa (8): The outermost layer of the stomach wall is the serosa (8). This is a thin layer of connective tissue that overlies the muscularis externa (5, 6, 7). Externally, this layer is covered by a simple squamous mesothelium of the visceral peritoneum (8). The connective tissue covered by the visceral peritoneum can contain numerous adipose cells (24).

PLATE 63

STOMACH: FUNDUS OR BODY (TRANSVERSE SECTION)

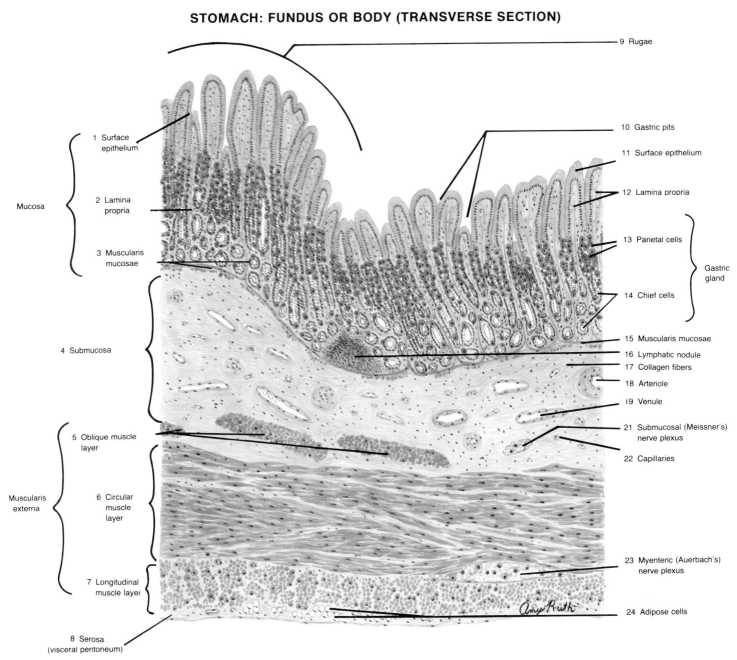

9 Rugae

1 Surface epithelium

Mucosa

2 Lamina propria

3 Muscularis mucosae

10 Gastric pits

11 Surface epithelium

12 Lamina propria

13 Parietal cells

Gastric gland

14 Chief cells

4 Submucosa

15 Muscularis mucosae

16 Lymphatic nodule

17 Collagen fibers

18 Arteriole

19 Venule

21 Submucosal (Meissner's) nerve plexus

22 Capillaries

5 Oblique muscle layer

Muscularis externa

6 Circular muscle layer

7 Longitudinal muscle layer

23 Myenteric (Auerbach's) nerve plexus

24 Adipose cells

8 Serosa (visceral peritoneum)

Stain: hematoxylin-eosin. 57×.

PLATE 64

STOMACH: MUCOSA OF THE FUNDUS OR BODY
(TRANSVERSE SECTION)

The mucosa and the adjacent submucosa of the fundic stomach are illustrated at a higher magnification. The extension of the simple columnar surface epithelium (1, 13) into the gastric pits (11) and the opening of the tubular gastric glands (5) into these pits are clearly seen. The loose irregular connective tissue of the lamina propria (6) fills the narrow spaces between the tightly packed gastric glands and extends from the surface epithelium (1) to the muscularis mucosae (9).

The lamina propria (6) is better seen in the mucosal ridges (2); it consists primarily of fine reticular and collagenous fibers. Scattered throughout this connective tissue are the oval nuclei of the fibroblasts. Also seen in the lamina propria are accumulations of lymphoid tissue in the form of a lymphatic nodule (17), in addition to individual lymphocytes and other cell types normally encountered in the loose connective tissue.

The gastric glands (5) extend the entire length of the mucosa. In the deeper regions of the mucosa, the gastric glands may branch, as seen by the numerous transverse and oblique sections. Each gastric gland generally consists of three regions. At the junction of the gastric pit with the gastric gland is the isthmus (14), containing the surface epithelial cells (1, 13) and parietal cells (4). Lower in the gland is the neck (15), composed primarily of mucous neck cells (3) and also parietal cells (4). The base or the fundus (16) is the deep portion of the gland and is composed predominantly of chief (zymogenic) cells (7) with a few scattered parietal cells (4). In addition to these cells, the fundic glands also contain undifferentiated cells and a variety of enteroendocrine cells that belong to the APUD group. (The characteristics of the APUD cells are discussed in greater detail with Plate 69.)

In the hematoxylin–eosin preparations, three types of cells can be easily identified in the fundic gastric glands. In this illustration, the parietal cells stain intensely and uniformly acidophilic (4). This staining characteristic distinguishes the parietal cells from other cells in the fundic glands. In contrast, the chief cells (zymogenic) (7) are distinctly basophilic and readily distinguishable from the acidophilic parietal cells. The mucous neck cells (3) are located just below the gastric pits and are interspersed between the parietal cells in the neck region of the glands.

The muscularis mucosae (9) is well illustrated in this stomach section. It is composed of two thin strips of smooth muscle, the inner circular (9a) and outer longitudinal layer (9b). In this illustration, the circular layer is sectioned longitudinally while the outer layer is sectioned transversely. Extending into the lamina propria (6) from the muscularis mucosae (9) toward the surface epithelium (1, 13) are strands of smooth muscle (8, 12).

Directly below the muscularis mucosae is a prominent layer of denser connective tissue, the submucosa (10). In this section, abundant collagen fibers (18) and the nuclei of numerous fibroblasts (19) are readily seen. The submucosa layer also contains numerous vessels, including arterioles (20), venules (21), lymphatics, and capillaries. Some adipose cells may be seen in this layer.

PLATE 64

STOMACH: MUCOSA OF THE FUNDUS OR BODY
(TRANSVERSE SECTION)

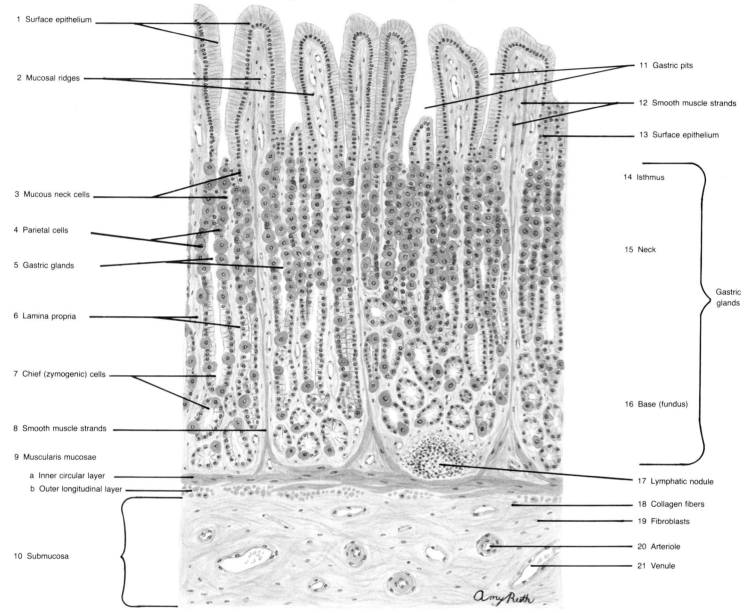

1 Surface epithelium

2 Mucosal ridges

3 Mucous neck cells

4 Parietal cells

5 Gastric glands

6 Lamina propria

7 Chief (zymogenic) cells

8 Smooth muscle strands

9 Muscularis mucosae
  a Inner circular layer
  b Outer longitudinal layer

10 Submucosa

11 Gastric pits

12 Smooth muscle strands

13 Surface epithelium

14 Isthmus

15 Neck

Gastric glands

16 Base (fundus)

17 Lymphatic nodule

18 Collagen fibers

19 Fibroblasts

20 Arteriole

21 Venule

Stain: hematoxylin-eosin. 180×.

PLATE 65 (Fig. 1)

STOMACH: FUNDUS OR BODY, SUPERFICIAL
REGION OF THE GASTRIC MUCOSA

Higher magnification of the stomach wall illustrates the characteristic features of various cells that compose the superficial region of the gastric mucosa of the fundus or body.

The tall columnar surface epithelium (1) is lightly stained due to mucigen droplets, has basal oval nuclei, and exhibits a thin but distinct basement membrane (2). The surface epithelium extends into the gastric pits (4). The underlying lamina propria (3) is a fibroreticular connective tissue.

Gastric glands lie in the lamina propria (11) below the gastric pits. The neck region of the gastric glands (5) is lined with low columnar mucous neck cells (6) with round, basal nuclei. The constricted necks of the gastric glands (10) open by a short transition region (9) into the bottom of the gastric pit (8).

Parietal cells (7) are interspersed among the mucous neck cells; their free surfaces are on the border of the glandular lumen. The parietal cells are the most conspicuous cells in the gastric mucosa and are primarily found in the upper half of the gland. The cells are large and pyramidal in shape with a round nucleus and highly acidophilic cytoplasm; some pyramidal cells may be binucleate.

Deeper in the gastric gland, toward the lower half or third of the gland, the mucous cells are replaced by basophilic chief or zymogenic cells (13), which border on the lumen of the gland. Parietal cells are also seen here; however, they are displaced peripherally and lie against the basement membrane without reaching the lumen.

PLATE 65 (Fig. 2)

DEEP REGION OF THE MUCOSA

Gastric glands are branched tubular glands; the branching occurs at the base of the glands. A section through the deep region of the mucosa illustrates basal portions of the glands sectioned in various planes (1, 10).

As in the higher regions of the gland, the chief or zymogenic cells border the glandular lumen (4, 9, 12). Parietal cells are wedged against the basement membrane (3, 8, 11) and are not in direct contact with the lumen. This is well demonstrated in several transverse sections of the glands (3, lower leader).

Also illustrated are the lamina propria between glands (2) and a narrow zone of subglandular lamina propria (5), which is not always distinguishable.

The two layers of the muscularis mucosae are seen (13, 14).

PLATE 65

STOMACH: FUNDUS OR BODY

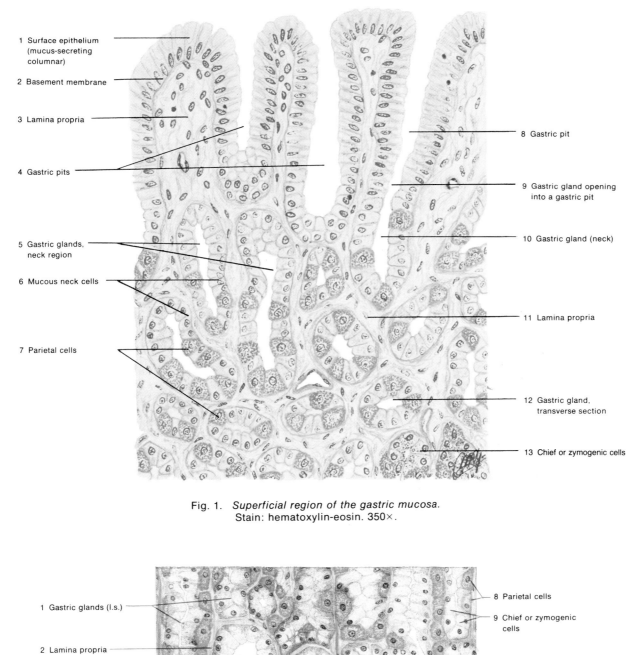

1 Surface epithelium (mucus-secreting columnar)

2 Basement membrane

3 Lamina propria

4 Gastric pits

5 Gastric glands, neck region

6 Mucous neck cells

7 Parietal cells

8 Gastric pit

9 Gastric gland opening into a gastric pit

10 Gastric gland (neck)

11 Lamina propria

12 Gastric gland, transverse section

13 Chief or zymogenic cells

Fig. 1. *Superficial region of the gastric mucosa.*
Stain: hematoxylin-eosin. 350×.

1 Gastric glands (l.s.)

2 Lamina propria

3 Parietal cells

4 Chief or zymogenic cells

5 Subglandular region of the lamina propria

6 Venule

7 Submucosa

8 Parietal cells

9 Chief or zymogenic cells

10 Gastric glands (t.s.) (basal coiled portions)

11 Parietal cell

12 Chief or zymogenic cells

13 Muscularis mucosae (circular layer)

14 Muscularis mucosae (longitudinal layer)

Fig. 2. *Deep region of the gastric mucosa.*
Stain: hematoxylin-eosin. 350×.

PLATE 66

STOMACH: MUCOSA OF THE PYLORIC REGION

In the mucosa of the pyloric region, the gastric pits (4, 12) are deeper than those in the fundus or body of the stomach and extend into the mucosa to about one half or more of its thickness. The simple columnar mucous epithelium (10) that lines the surface of the stomach also lines the gastric pits.

The gastric glands that are observed in the body and fundus of the stomach are replaced by pyloric glands in the pyloric region of the stomach (5, 6, 14). These are either branched or coiled tubular mucous glands. Typically, one type of cell is identified in these glands, a tall columnar cell, with slightly granular cytoplasm, lightly stained due to mucigen content, and a flattened or oval nucleus at the base. The pyloric glands open into the bottom of the gastric pits (4, lower leader). Enteroendocrine cells are also present in this region of the stomach and can be demonstrated with special staining techniques.

The remaining structures in this region are similar to those seen in the upper stomach. The lamina propria contains diffuse lymphatic tissue (13) and an occasional lymphatic nodule (16) in its deepest part. These nodules may increase in size and penetrate through the muscularis mucosae into the submucosa. Smooth muscle fibers from the circular layer of the muscularis mucosae pass into the lamina propria (7) between the pyloric glands and into mucosal ridges (2, 3).

PLATE 66

STOMACH: MUCOSA OF THE PYLORIC REGION

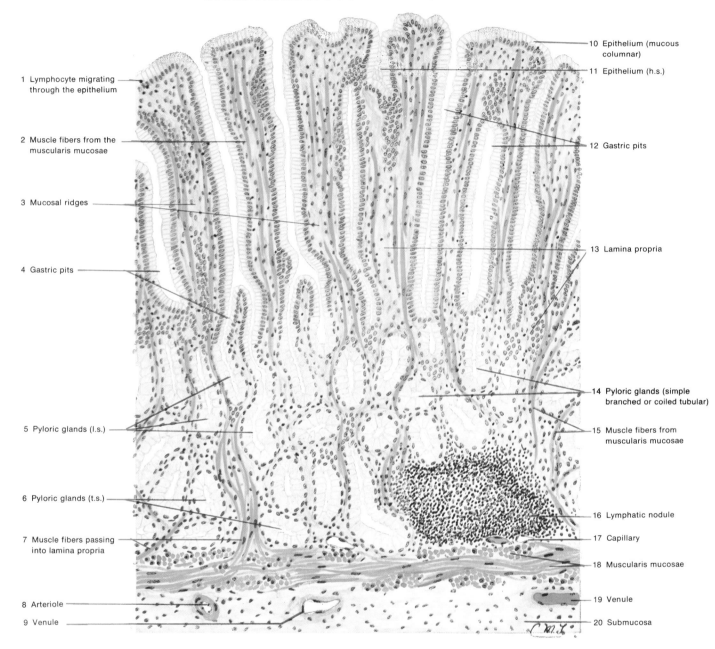

1 Lymphocyte migrating through the epithelium

2 Muscle fibers from the muscularis mucosae

3 Mucosal ridges

4 Gastric pits

5 Pyloric glands (l.s.)

6 Pyloric glands (t.s.)

7 Muscle fibers passing into lamina propria

8 Arteriole

9 Venule

10 Epithelium (mucous columnar)

11 Epithelium (h.s.)

12 Gastric pits

13 Lamina propria

14 Pyloric glands (simple branched or coiled tubular)

15 Muscle fibers from muscularis mucosae

16 Lymphatic nodule

17 Capillary

18 Muscularis mucosae

19 Venule

20 Submucosa

Stain: hematoxylin-eosin. 100×.

PLATE 67

PYLORIC-DUODENAL JUNCTION (LONGITUDINAL SECTION)

Located in the pyloric region of the stomach (1), just before its junction with the duodenum (2), is the pyloric sphincter (7). This sphincter is formed by thickening of the circular layer of the muscularis externa. Several features in this region differentiate the pyloric stomach from the duodenum.

As the pylorus joins the duodenum, the mucosal ridges (5), which surround the gastric pits (6), become broader and more irregular in outline, and as a result, become highly variable in sectioned material. Coiled tubular pyloric (mucous) glands (4) are present in the lamina propria and open into the bottom of gastric pits (6). Lymphatic nodules (10) are frequently seen at the transition region.

The duodenal surface (2) exhibits surface modification in the form of villi (13). Each villus is a leaf-shaped surface projection (13) with a pointed end. Between individual villi are intervillous spaces (16) which represent the continuation of the intestinal lumen. The mucus-secreting epithelium of the stomach (3) exhibits an abrupt transition (11) to intestinal epithelium. This epithelium contains goblet and columnar cells with striated borders (microvilli), which are present throughout the length of the small intestine.

Short simple tubular intestinal glands (crypts of Lieberkühn) (12) are now seen in the lamina propria. These glands are also lined with goblet cells and cells with striated borders (microvilli) from the surface epithelium. One or more intestinal glands open into spaces between the villi (17).

Duodenal glands (Brunner's glands) (14) occupy most of the submucosa in the upper duodenum and frequently extend through the muscularis mucosae into the deep mucosa. In this region, the muscularis mucosae is disrupted (15) and strands of its muscle may be dispersed among the mucous tubules of the glands. Except for the esophageal (submucosal) glands proper, the duodenal glands are the only submucosal glands in the digestive tract.

Plate 67

PYLORIC-DUODENAL JUNCTION (LONGITUDINAL SECTION)

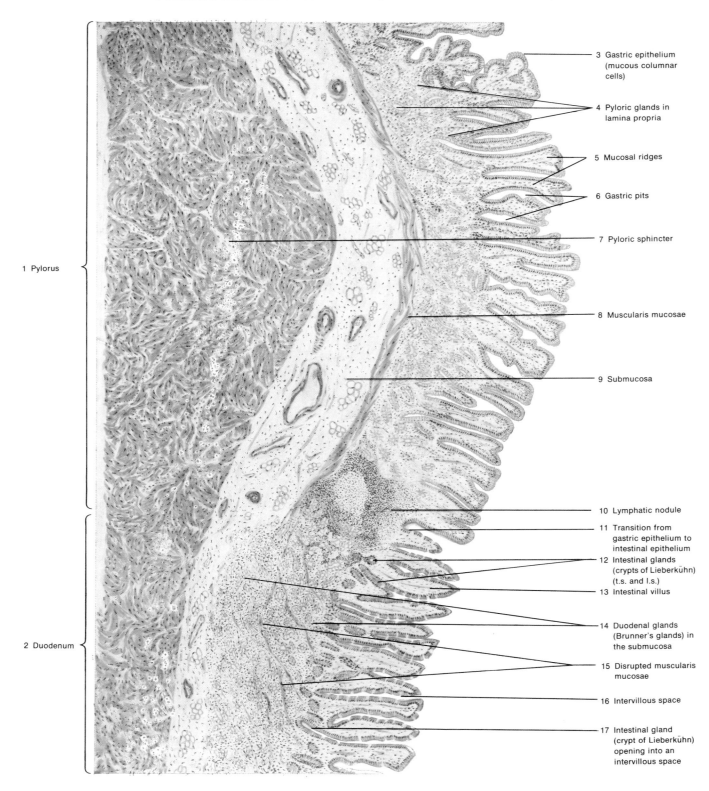

1 Pylorus

2 Duodenum

3 Gastric epithelium (mucous columnar cells)

4 Pyloric glands in lamina propria

5 Mucosal ridges

6 Gastric pits

7 Pyloric sphincter

8 Muscularis mucosae

9 Submucosa

10 Lymphatic nodule

11 Transition from gastric epithelium to intestinal epithelium

12 Intestinal glands (crypts of Lieberkühn) (t.s. and l.s.)

13 Intestinal villus

14 Duodenal glands (Brunner's glands) in the submucosa

15 Disrupted muscularis mucosae

16 Intervillous space

17 Intestinal gland (crypt of Lieberkühn) opening into an intervillous space

Stain: hematoxylin-eosin. 25×.

PLATE 68

SMALL INTESTINE: DUODENUM (LONGITUDINAL SECTION)

The wall of the duodenum consists of four layers: mucosa (13, 14, 15), submucosa (17), muscularis externa (18) and serosa (visceral peritoneum) (19). These layers are continuous with those in the stomach and those in the small and large intestines.

Distinctive features of the small intestine are the villi (3, 13), a surface epithelium of columnar cells with striated borders, the goblet cells (1), and short tubular intestinal glands (crypts of Lieberkühn) (5, 6, 7) in the lamina propria. The presence of mucous duodenal glands (Brunner's glands) (17) in the submucosa is a characteristic feature of the upper duodenum. These submucosal glands are absent elsewhere in the small or large intestine.

The villi (3, 13) are mucosal surface modifications with intervillous spaces (2). The lining epithelium (1) covers the villi, lines the spaces, and continues into the intestinal glands (5). Each villus has a core of lamina propria (3, 13), some smooth muscle fibers (4) that extend from the muscularis mucosae (15), and a central lacteal (not illustrated). (See Plate 70, Fig. 2, for detailed structure of a villus.)

The lamina propria (14) contains intestinal glands (crypts of Lieberkühn) (6, 7) which open into the intervillous spaces (5). In certain sections, extensions of submucosal duodenal glands (Brunner's glands) are seen in the lamina propria (8, upper leader, and 16). The lamina propria contains fine connective tissue with reticular cells, diffuse lymphatic tissue, or lymphatic nodules that may be seen in the deep lamina propria.

The submucosa (17) is almost completely filled with highly branched tubular duodenal glands (Brunner's glands) (8, 17). The muscularis mucosae may be disrupted if these glands penetrate into the mucosal lamina propria, and strands of smooth muscle may be observed in the glandular area (9). The duodenal glands open into the bottom of the intestinal glands.

The muscularis externa (18) consists of an inner circular and outer longitudinal layer of smooth muscle. Parasympathetic ganglia cells of the myenteric nerve plexus (Auerbach's plexus) (12) are seen in the thin layer of connective tissue between the two muscle layers; this nerve plexus is found between these muscle layers throughout the small and large intestine. Similar but smaller ganglion cells are likewise found in the submucosa throughout the small and large intestine (submucosal or Meissner's plexus).

Serosa (visceral peritoneum) (19) forms the outermost layer.

PLATE 68

SMALL INTESTINE: DUODENUM (LONGITUDINAL SECTION)

1 Lining epithelium: columnar cells with striated borders and goblet cells

2 Intervillous spaces

3 Intestinal villus (l.s.)

4 Muscle fibers in a villus

5 Intestinal glands (crypts of Lieberkühn) opening into intervillous spaces

6 Intestinal glands (l.s.)

7 Intestinal glands (t.s.)

8 Duodenal glands (Brunner's glands)

9 Displaced fibers of the muscularis mucosae

10 Arteriole

11 Venule

12 Parasympathetic ganglion of the myenteric plexus (Auerbach's plexus)

13 Villi with core of lamina propria and muscle fibers

14 Lamina propria proper

15 Muscularis mucosae

16 Duodenal glands extending into the mucosa

17 Submucosa with duodenal glands

18 Muscularis externa; inner circular and outer longitudinal layers

19 Serosa (visceral peritoneum)

Mucosa

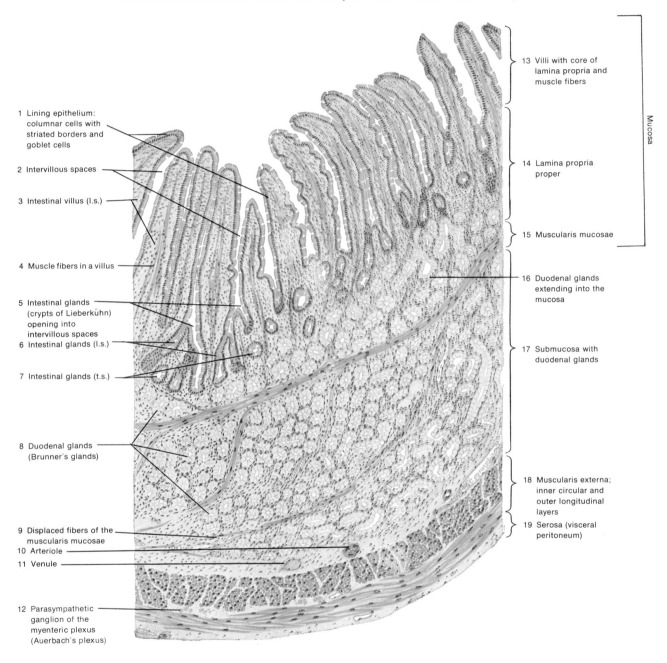

Stain: hematoxylin-eosin. 50×.

Plate 69 (Fig. 1)

SMALL INTESTINE: JEJUNUM-ILEUM
(TRANSVERSE SECTION)

Histologic structure of the lower duodenum, jejunum, and ileum remains similar to that of the upper duodenum illustrated on Plate 68. The only exceptions are the duodenal glands, which are usually limited to the upper part of the duodenum. The villi differ somewhat in shape and length in different regions, but this is not usually apparent in histological sections. Aggregated lymphatic nodules (Peyer's patches) occur at different intervals in the ileum (see Plate 70, Fig. 1).

This figure illustrates villi that have been sectioned in longitudinal (1), oblique (13), and transverse (12, 16) planes. A contracted villus (14) appears shorter and broader than other villi. Each villus exhibits a typical structure: a surface epithelium with striated border and goblet cells (11), a core of lamina propria with diffuse lymphatic tissue, and groups of smooth muscle fibers (15). (The central lacteal and small blood vessels in the villus are illustrated on Plate 70, Fig. 2.)

Intestinal glands (crypts of Lieberkühn) (3, 17) in the lamina propria are close together and open into the intervillous spaces (3, middle leader).

A lymphatic nodule (21) located in the submucosa originated initially in the mucosa and then extended through the muscularis mucosae into the submucosa.

Muscularis mucosae (6), submucosa (7), muscularis externa (8, 9), and serosa (10) are typical, although adipose tissue (19) is not always present in the serosa. Ganglion cells of the myenteric nerve plexus (18) are seen in the connective tissue between the muscle layers. Ganglion cells of the submucosal nerve plexuses are also present but not illustrated.

Plate 69 (Fig. 2)

INTESTINAL GLANDS WITH PANETH CELLS

At the base of the jejunal mucosa and adjacent to the muscularis mucosae (4) are several intestinal glands. The characteristic goblet cells (1) and cells with striated borders (2) are present in the glands. In addition, at the base of each gland is found a group of pyramid-shaped cells with large, acidophilic granules. These are the Paneth cells (3). The coarse granules, which stain reddish-orange in this preparation, fill most of the cytoplasm and displace the nucleus toward the base of the cell.

The exact function of the Paneth cell has not been clarified; however, lysozyme that possesses antibacterial activity has been detected in the eosinophilic granules, which may have a role in regulating the intestinal flora.

Paneth cells are found throughout the small intestine and occasionally in the large intestine.

Plate 69 (Fig. 3)

INTESTINAL GLANDS WITH ENTEROENDOCRINE CELLS

This section was prepared from an operative section of ileum. Transverse and oblique sections of intestinal glands are illustrated. The cytoplasm and nuclei of the goblet cells and striated epithelium are stained with Darrow red, as are the nuclei of fibroblasts in the stroma.

Special silver technique demonstrates fine argyrophilic granules in the basal portions of some cells; in these cells the nuclei lie above the granules. These are the enteroendocrine cells (2), which appear similar under the light microscope; however, numerous types of cells with varied endocrine functions are presently recognized. Most of the enteroendocrine cell types can take up and decarboxylate precursors of biogenic monoamines and are therefore considered a part of a larger group of diffuse endocrine cells designated as the amine precursor uptake and decarboxylation (APUD) cell series. The APUD cell types are found in epithelia of the gastrointestinal (stomach, small and large intestine) and respiratory tracts and in the pancreas and thyroid gland. The former terms used to describe these cells, argentaffin or enterochromaffin cells, implied more limited functions.

The silver staining technique also reveals argyrophilic reticular fibers (1) in the connective tissue of the lamina propria.

PLATE 69

SMALL INTESTINE

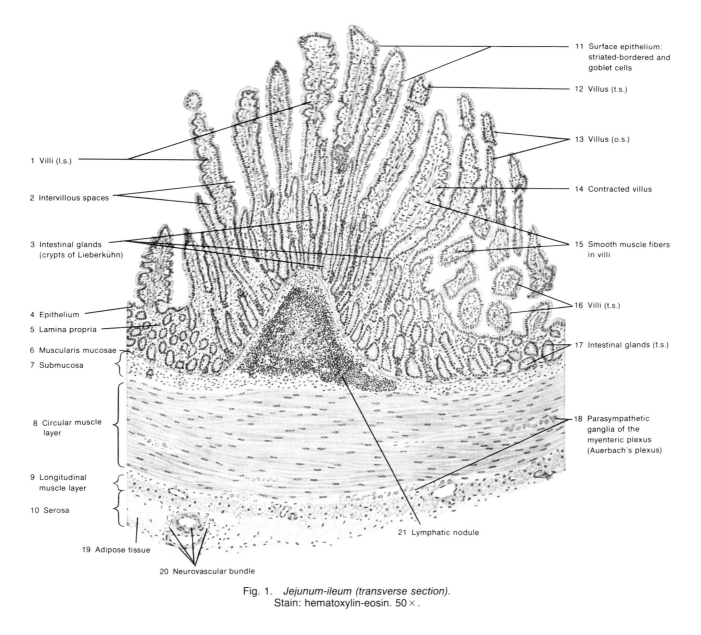

11 Surface epithelium:
striated-bordered and
goblet cells

12 Villus (t.s.)

13 Villus (o.s.)

1 Villi (l.s.)

14 Contracted villus

2 Intervillous spaces

3 Intestinal glands
(crypts of Lieberkühn)

15 Smooth muscle fibers
in villi

4 Epithelium

5 Lamina propria

16 Villi (t.s.)

6 Muscularis mucosae

7 Submucosa

17 Intestinal glands (t.s.)

8 Circular muscle
layer

18 Parasympathetic
ganglia of the
myenteric plexus
(Auerbach's plexus)

9 Longitudinal
muscle layer

10 Serosa

21 Lymphatic nodule

19 Adipose tissue

20 Neurovascular bundle

Fig. 1. *Jejunum-ileum (transverse section).*
Stain: hematoxylin-eosin. 50×.

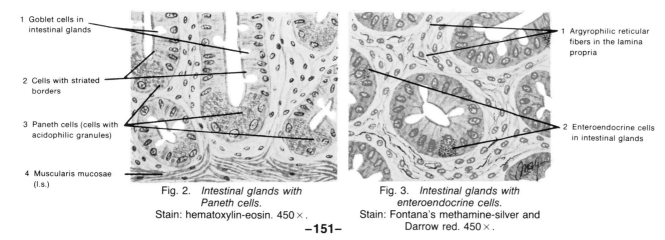

1 Goblet cells in
intestinal glands

2 Cells with striated
borders

3 Paneth cells (cells with
acidophilic granules)

4 Muscularis mucosae
(l.s.)

1 Argyrophilic reticular
fibers in the lamina
propria

2 Enteroendocrine cells
in intestinal glands

Fig. 2. *Intestinal glands with
Paneth cells.*
Stain: hematoxylin-eosin. 450×.

Fig. 3. *Intestinal glands with
enteroendocrine cells.*
Stain: Fontana's methamine-silver and
Darrow red. 450×.

PLATE 70 (Fig. 1)

SMALL INTESTINE: ILEUM WITH AGGREGATED NODULES (PEYER'S PATCH, TRANSVERSE SECTION)

In this figure, four coats of the intestinal wall are illustrated (9 through 16 inclusive). The villi are seen in various planes of section (1, 2, 9) and the intestinal glands (crypts of Lieberkühn) (3, 10) are present in the lamina propria; two of these glands are illustrated opening into an intervillous space (upper 3, upper 10).

A characteristic feature of the ileum are the aggregated lymphatic nodules (Peyer's patches); each patch is an aggregation of 10 or more lymphatic nodules. The patches are located in the wall of the ileum opposite the attachment of the mesentery. The portion of the Peyer's patch illustrated in this figure shows nine lymphatic nodules (4, 5, and others), most of which exhibit germinal centers (5). The nodules coalesce and the boundaries between them are not usually discernible.

The nodules originate in the diffuse lymphatic tissue of the lamina propria. Villi are absent in the area where the nodules reach the surface of the mucosa (4). Typically, the nodules extend into the submucosa (7), disrupt the muscularis mucosae (6), and spread out in the loose connective tissue of the submucosa.

PLATE 70 (Fig. 2)

SMALL INTESTINE: VILLI

The distal parts of three villi are illustrated at a higher magnification; two villi are sectioned longitudinally (left and right). The central villus was bent and sectioned in two parts: the apex has been sectioned transversely (1) and the lower portion tangentially (7) and longitudinally (8).

The surface epithelium (2) contains goblet cells (9, 10, 13) and columnar cells with striated borders (14, 15). The thin basement membrane is visible in different areas (5) of the villi. In the core of lamina propria (12) are seen reticular cells of the stroma, lymphocytes, and smooth muscle fibers (4, 16). Present in each villus (but not always seen in sections) is a central lacteal, a small, dilated lymphatic vessel lined with endothelium (3, 17). Blood vessels in a villus consist of an arteriole, one or more venules, and numerous capillaries (11).

PLATE 70

SMALL INTESTINE

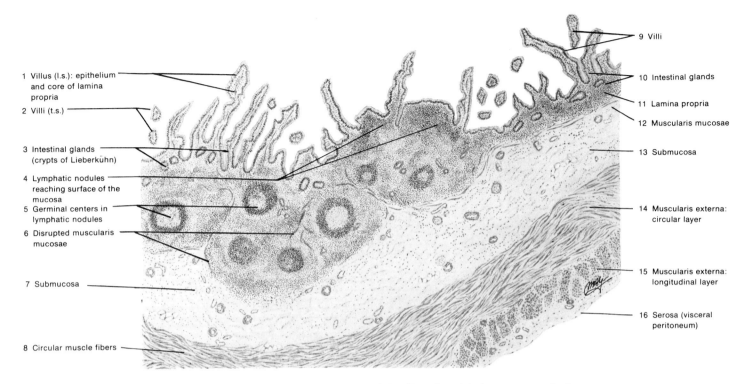

1 Villus (l.s.): epithelium and core of lamina propria

2 Villi (t.s.)

3 Intestinal glands (crypts of Lieberkühn)

4 Lymphatic nodules reaching surface of the mucosa

5 Germinal centers in lymphatic nodules

6 Disrupted muscularis mucosae

7 Submucosa

8 Circular muscle fibers

9 Villi

10 Intestinal glands

11 Lamina propria

12 Muscularis mucosae

13 Submucosa

14 Muscularis externa: circular layer

15 Muscularis externa: longitudinal layer

16 Serosa (visceral peritoneum)

Fig. 1. *Ileum with aggregated nodules (Peyer's patch, transverse section).*
Stain: hematoxylin-eosin. 25×.

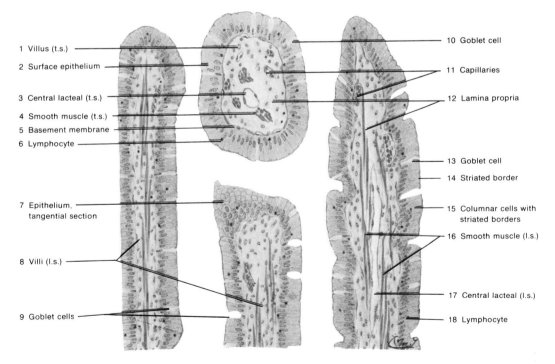

1 Villus (t.s.)

2 Surface epithelium

3 Central lacteal (t.s.)

4 Smooth muscle (t.s.)

5 Basement membrane

6 Lymphocyte

7 Epithelium, tangential section

8 Villi (l.s.)

9 Goblet cells

10 Goblet cell

11 Capillaries

12 Lamina propria

13 Goblet cell

14 Striated border

15 Columnar cells with striated borders

16 Smooth muscle (l.s.)

17 Central lacteal (l.s.)

18 Lymphocyte

Fig. 2. *Small intestine: villi.*
Stain: hematoxylin-eosin. 200×.

PLATE 71

LARGE INTESTINE: COLON (PANORAMIC VIEW, TRANSVERSE SECTION) AND MESENTERY

In the colon, the layers of the wall remain the same as in the small intestine: the mucosa (5, 6), submucosa (4), muscularis externa with two layers of muscle (1, 15, 16), and serosa (2) (in the region of the transverse and sigmoid colon). Plate 72 shows the detailed structure of one of these regions.

There are, however, several modifications that distinguish the colon from other regions of the digestive tract. The villi are absent and the luminal surface of the mucosa is smooth. Plicae circularis are absent, but temporary folds (7) of submucosa and mucosa are present in the undistended colon. The outer longitudinal layer of the muscularis externa is condensed into three broad, longitudinal bands of muscle called taeniae coli (3, 12, 19). In the rest of the colon wall, a very thin muscle layer is found between the bands of taeniae coli (1, upper leader, 15); this muscle layer is often discontinuous. Between the two muscle layers are found the ganglion cells of the myenteric (Auerbach's) nerve plexus (18).

Attached to the transverse and sigmoid colon, as well as to the small intestine, is the mesentery. The serosa (2) extends from the colon and over the mesentery (8) as the outermost layer. The mesentery contains loose connective tissue, adipose tissue, blood vessels, and nerves (10).

PLATE 71

LARGE INTESTINE: COLON
(PANORAMIC VIEW, TRANSVERSE SECTION) AND MESENTERY

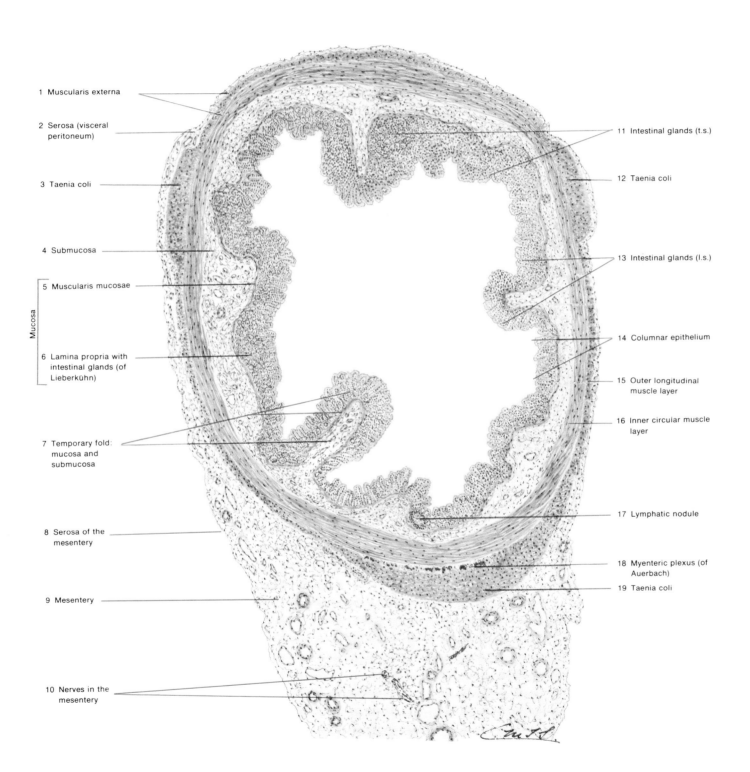

1 Muscularis externa

2 Serosa (visceral peritoneum)

3 Taenia coli

4 Submucosa

5 Muscularis mucosae

Mucosa

6 Lamina propria with intestinal glands (of Lieberkühn)

7 Temporary fold: mucosa and submucosa

8 Serosa of the mesentery

9 Mesentery

10 Nerves in the mesentery

11 Intestinal glands (t.s.)

12 Taenia coli

13 Intestinal glands (l.s.)

14 Columnar epithelium

15 Outer longitudinal muscle layer

16 Inner circular muscle layer

17 Lymphatic nodule

18 Myenteric plexus (of Auerbach)

19 Taenia coli

Stain: hematoxylin-eosin. 20×.

PLATE 72

LARGE INTESTINE: COLON (WALL, TRANSVERSE SECTION)

A section of the colon wall is illustrated in detail. The four representative layers are indicated: mucosa (27), submucosa (26), muscularis externa (25), and serosa (24). All layers are continuous with those of the small intestine.

Because the villi are absent in the colon, the mucosal surface appears smooth. It is indented at close intervals by long tubular intestinal glands (crypts of Lieberkühn) (20), which extend through the lamina propria to the muscularis mucosae.

The surface epithelium is primarily columnar, with thin striated borders (14) and goblet cells. This epithelium continues into the intestinal glands (16, 20), where the goblet cells are in great abundance and are the principal cells. Parts of the glands may be seen sectioned longitudinally (20), transversely (21), or tangentially (16).

The lamina propria (19), similar to that in the small intestine, contains abundant diffuse lymphatic tissue. Lymphatic nodules (17, 23) are located deep in the lamina propria and may extend through the muscularis mucosae into the submucosa.

The structures of the muscularis mucosae (10), submucosa (9), and serosa (1) are typical. In this section, muscularis externa (5, 6) appears typical; however, in other parts of the colon, the longitudinal layer of the muscularis externa is arranged into bands of taeniae coli.

Serosa (1) covers the entire transverse and sigmoid colon; the ascending and descending colon are retroperitoneal, and the outer layer of its posterior surface is adventitia.

PLATE 72

LARGE INTESTINE: COLON (WALL, TRANSVERSE SECTION)

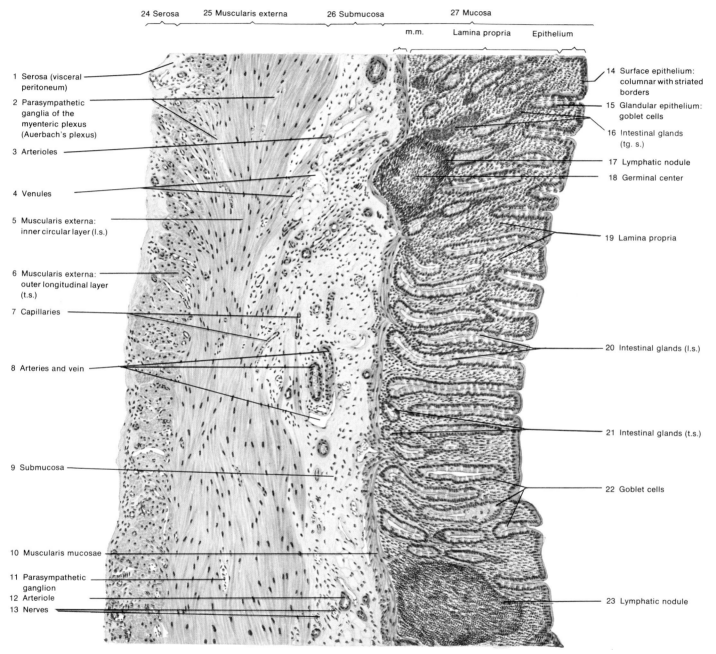

24 Serosa   25 Muscularis externa   26 Submucosa   27 Mucosa

m.m.   Lamina propria   Epithelium

1 Serosa (visceral peritoneum)

2 Parasympathetic ganglia of the myenteric plexus (Auerbach's plexus)

3 Arterioles

4 Venules

5 Muscularis externa: inner circular layer (l.s.)

6 Muscularis externa: outer longitudinal layer (t.s.)

7 Capillaries

8 Arteries and vein

9 Submucosa

10 Muscularis mucosae

11 Parasympathetic ganglion

12 Arteriole

13 Nerves

14 Surface epithelium: columnar with striated borders

15 Glandular epithelium: goblet cells

16 Intestinal glands (tg. s.)

17 Lymphatic nodule

18 Germinal center

19 Lamina propria

20 Intestinal glands (l.s.)

21 Intestinal glands (t.s.)

22 Goblet cells

23 Lymphatic nodule

Colon: a sector of the wall. Stain: hematoxylin-eosin. 53×.

PLATE 73

APPENDIX (PANORAMIC VIEW, TRANSVERSE SECTION)

This figure represents a panoramic view of a cross section of the vermiform appendix. Its structure is similar to that of the colon except for several modifications that are characteristic features of the appendix.

The component parts of the mucosa are similar to those of the colon: a similar surface epithelium (9), lamina propria (5, 11) with intestinal glands (crypts of Lieberkühn) (6, 10), and the muscularis mucosae (12). The intestinal glands (6, 10) are less well developed, shorter, and often farther apart than in the colon. Diffuse lymphatic tissue in the lamina propria is abundant and is often observed in the adjacent submucosa.

Lymphatic nodules (1, 7, 19) are numerous in the appendix and often exhibit large germinal centers (7). These nodules originate in the lamina propria (19) and because of their size, may extend to the surface epithelium (19, lower leader). Characteristically, the lymphatic nodules also extend into the submucosa and disrupt the muscularis mucosae (16) as their size increases.

The submucosa is highly vascular (8). The muscularis externa (14) has the characteristic inner circular and outer longitudinal layers of smooth muscle (17, 18) which may vary in thickness. Serosa (15) is the outermost layer and covers the muscularis externa.

PLATE 73

APPENDIX (PANORAMIC VIEW, TRANSVERSE SECTION)

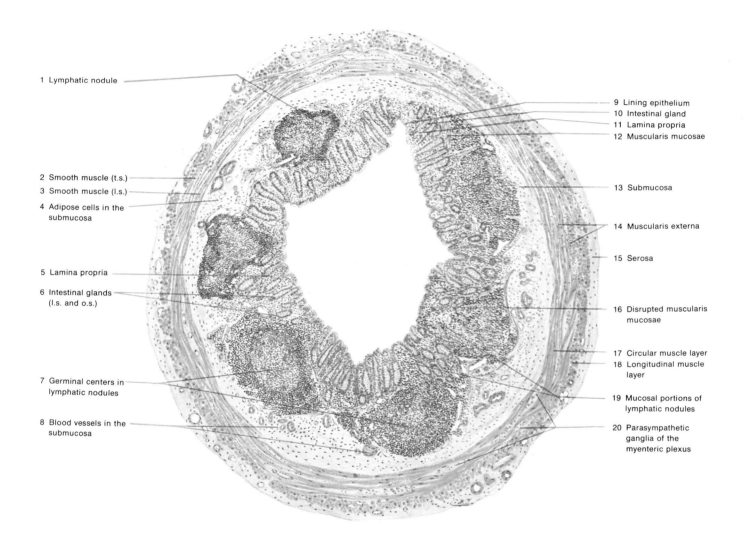

1 Lymphatic nodule

2 Smooth muscle (t.s.)

3 Smooth muscle (l.s.)

4 Adipose cells in the
submucosa

5 Lamina propria

6 Intestinal glands
(l.s. and o.s.)

7 Germinal centers in
lymphatic nodules

8 Blood vessels in the
submucosa

9 Lining epithelium
10 Intestinal gland
11 Lamina propria
12 Muscularis mucosae

13 Submucosa

14 Muscularis externa

15 Serosa

16 Disrupted muscularis
mucosae

17 Circular muscle layer
18 Longitudinal muscle
layer

19 Mucosal portions of
lymphatic nodules

20 Parasympathetic
ganglia of the
myenteric plexus

Stain: hematoxylin-eosin. 25×.

PLATE 74

RECTUM: PANORAMIC VIEW, TRANSVERSE SECTION

This illustration represents a transverse section through the upper rectum. The histologic structure of the rectum is generally similar to that of the colon; the same layers are present in the wall (3, 9, 12–15), and the same components are found in each layer. Except for the difference in the longitudinal muscle layer, this figure could be a histologic section of the colon.

Surface epithelium (8) is lined by columnar cells with striated borders and goblet cells. Intestinal glands (10, 11) in the wide lamina propria are similar to those in the colon; however, the glands are longer and closer together, and contain more goblet cells. In fact, almost all cells in the intestinal glands are goblet cells.

Temporary longitudinal folds (4) may be present in the upper rectum and in the colon. These folds have a core of submucosa and are covered by mucosa (4). Permanent transverse folds of the rectum, if present in a section, would contain smooth muscle fibers from the circular layers of the muscularis externa.

Permanent longitudinal folds (rectal columns) appear in the lower rectum, the anal canal.

Taeniae coli of the colon continue into the rectum where the muscularis externa (13, 14) again acquires the typical inner circular and outer longitudinal muscle layers.

Adventitia (15) covers part of the rectum and serosa the remainder.

PLATE 74

RECTUM (PANORAMIC VIEW, TRANSVERSE SECTION)

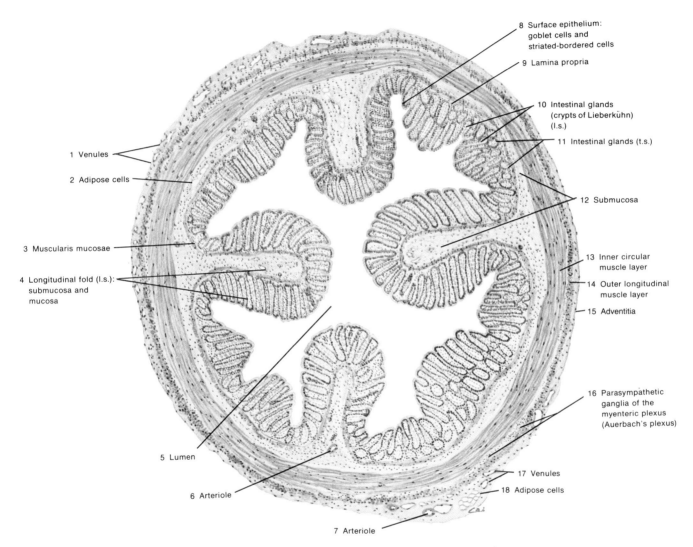

1 Venules

2 Adipose cells

3 Muscularis mucosae

4 Longitudinal fold (l.s.):
submucosa and
mucosa

5 Lumen

6 Arteriole

7 Arteriole

8 Surface epithelium:
goblet cells and
striated-bordered cells

9 Lamina propria

10 Intestinal glands
(crypts of Lieberkühn)
(l.s.)

11 Intestinal glands (t.s.)

12 Submucosa

13 Inner circular
muscle layer

14 Outer longitudinal
muscle layer

15 Adventitia

16 Parasympathetic
ganglia of the
myenteric plexus
(Auerbach's plexus)

17 Venules

18 Adipose cells

Stain: hematoxylin-eosin. 40×.

PLATE 75

ANAL CANAL (LONGITUDINAL SECTION)

The upper portion of the anal canal (A), above the anal valves (11), represents the lowermost part of the rectum. The lower part of the anal canal (B), below the anal valves (11), is the transition area between the simple columnar epithelium and the stratified squamous epithelium of the skin. The change from rectal mucosa to anal mucosa takes place at the apex of the anal valves (10), and is called the anorectal line.

The rectal mucosa (4–8) is typical in structure to that of the colon; however, the intestinal glands (7) are shorter and farther apart. As a result, more of the lamina propria is seen (8) between intestinal glands, diffuse lymphatic tissue is more abundant, and the solitary lymphatic nodules (6) are numerous. The muscularis mucosae (5) terminates in the vicinity of the anal valve (12).

At the apex of the anal valve, the columnar epithelium of the rectum is abruptly replaced by noncornified stratified squamous epithelium (10) of the anal canal. Intestinal glands also terminate at this region. The lamina propria of the rectum is replaced by dense irregular connective tissue of lamina propria of the anal canal (13, lower leader). The submucosa of the rectum (9) merges with the lamina propria of the anal canal.

In this region of the anal canal, the submucosa and lamina propria are highly vascular. The internal hemorrhoidal plexus of veins (15) lies in the mucosa of the anal canal. Blood vessels from this region continue into the submucosa of the rectum. Internal hemorrhoids result from chronic dilation of these vessels. External hemorrhoids develop from vessels of the external venous plexus (not illustrated in this figure) of the anus.

The circular muscle layer of the muscularis externa (1) increases greatly in thickness in the upper region of the anal canal and forms the internal anal sphincter (1, 14). In the lower region of the anal canal, this sphincter is replaced by skeletal muscles, the external anal sphincter (16). External to this sphincter is the levator ani muscle (skeletal), a portion of which is illustrated in the figure (3). The longitudinal muscle layer of the muscularis externa (2) becomes thin and disappears in the connective tissue around the external anal sphincter.

PLATE 75

ANAL CANAL (LONGITUDINAL SECTION)

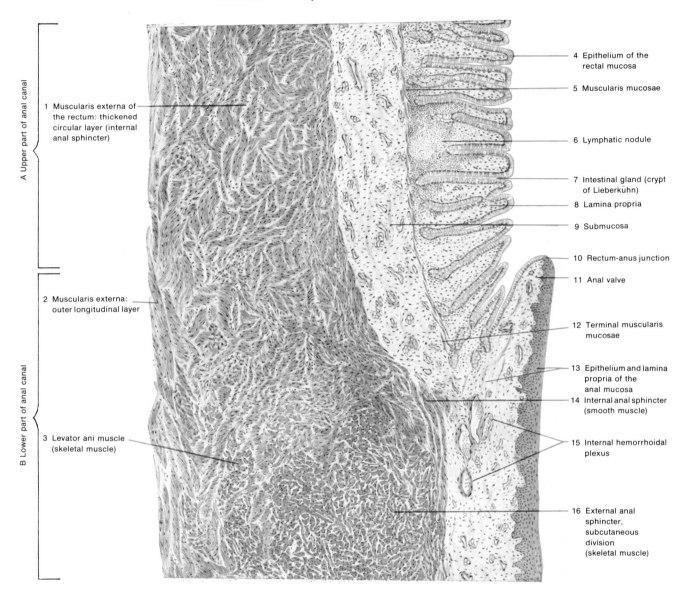

A Upper part of anal canal

B Lower part of anal canal

1 Muscularis externa of the rectum: thickened circular layer (internal anal sphincter)

2 Muscularis externa: outer longitudinal layer

3 Levator ani muscle (skeletal muscle)

4 Epithelium of the rectal mucosa

5 Muscularis mucosae

6 Lymphatic nodule

7 Intestinal gland (crypt of Lieberkühn)

8 Lamina propria

9 Submucosa

10 Rectum-anus junction

11 Anal valve

12 Terminal muscularis mucosae

13 Epithelium and lamina propria of the anal mucosa

14 Internal anal sphincter (smooth muscle)

15 Internal hemorrhoidal plexus

16 External anal sphincter, subcutaneous division (skeletal muscle)

Stain: hematoxylin-eosin. 25×.

PLATE 76

LIVER LOBULE (PANORAMIC VIEW, TRANSVERSE SECTION)

The connective tissue in the liver hilus extends between the liver lobes as the interlobular septa (2) that partially outline the small hepatic (liver) lobules (1). These septa that contain the interlobular branches of the portal vein, hepatic artery, and bile ducts can be collectively considered portal canals or area. Also, in the interlobular septa are found small lymphatic vessels and nerves.

This figure illustrates, in transverse section, one complete hepatic lobule in the center and parts of several adjacent lobules (1 and others). The boundaries between lobules are conspicuous where three lobules join at the interlobular septa (portal canal or area). In transverse sections, the septum at these corners appears triangular (7, 18) and forms the portal canals, consisting of the following structures: the interlobular branches of the portal vein, hepatic artery, and bile duct (4, 5, 6, 16, 17, 19; and others). In the human liver, the well-defined connective tissue partitions between lobules are not conspicuous and the liver sinusoids are continuous from one lobule to the next (10).

In the center of each hepatic lobule is the central vein (9, 13). Around the periphery of each lobule are several portal canals and the interlobular connective tissue. The hepatic lobule in the center of the figure exhibits portal areas and partial connective tissue boundaries (4–7, 11–12, 16–19). Any one portal area forms a partial boundary for more than one lobule.

Within the lobule are plates of hepatic cells (14, 20) that radiate from the central vein toward the periphery. Located between the hepatic plates are the hepatic sinusoids (15, 21), which are formed from small distributing branches of the interlobular vein. Arterial and venous blood mixes in these sinusoids and flows toward the central vein. Bile is formed in the liver cells and drains through the bile canaliculi in the opposite direction into the interlobular bile ducts (Plate 77, Fig. 3).

Interlobular vessels and bile ducts exhibit numerous branches in the liver parenchyma. Thus, in a section of liver, it is possible to see more than one section of each of these structures within a portal area. In one such area and connective tissue (4–7) are illustrated five cross sections of bile ducts, three portal vein branches, and one artery. Conversely, all three structures may not be seen in any one portal area (11, 12) in which the hepatic artery is not seen in this plane of section. Lymphatics and nerves are small, inconspicuous, and seen only occasionally.

PLATE 76

LIVER LOBULE (PANORAMIC VIEW, TRANSVERSE SECTION)

1 Hepatic lobule

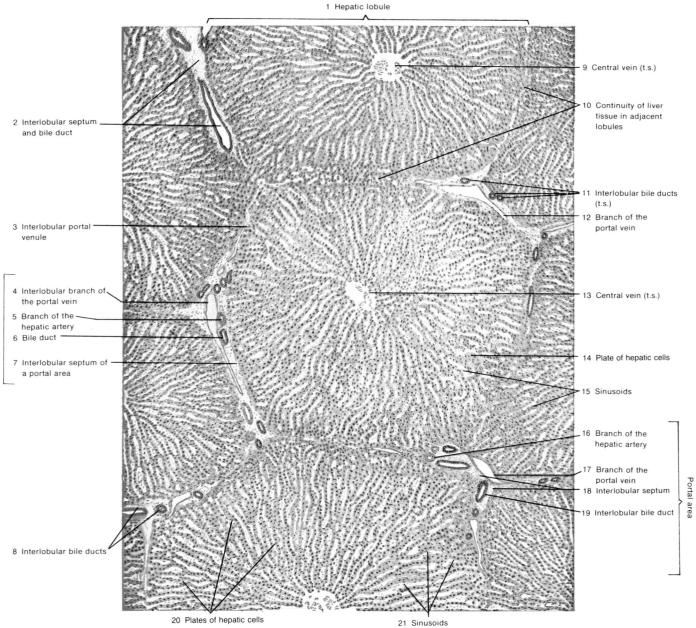

2 Interlobular septum and bile duct

3 Interlobular portal venule

Portal area

4 Interlobular branch of the portal vein

5 Branch of the hepatic artery

6 Bile duct

7 Interlobular septum of a portal area

8 Interlobular bile ducts

9 Central vein (t.s.)

10 Continuity of liver tissue in adjacent lobules

11 Interlobular bile ducts (t.s.)

12 Branch of the portal vein

13 Central vein (t.s.)

14 Plate of hepatic cells

15 Sinusoids

16 Branch of the hepatic artery

17 Branch of the portal vein

18 Interlobular septum

19 Interlobular bile duct

Portal area

20 Plates of hepatic cells

21 Sinusoids

Stain: hematoxylin-eosin. 45×.

PLATE 77 (Fig. 1)

LIVER LOBULE (SECTIONAL VIEW, TRANSVERSE SECTION)

Part of a hepatic lobule between the central vein (1) and the peripheral interlobular septum (9) is illustrated. This section illustrates, in more detail, the structures seen in Plate 76.

The central vein (1), a venule, is lined with endothelium. At the periphery of the lobule is the interlobular septum (9) with the portal area, which consists of a portal vein (8), two hepatic artery branches (6, 12), four sections of the bile duct (7, 14), and a lymphatic vessel (13).

The liver lobule consists of plates of hepatic cells (11) which branch and anastomose, except at the periphery of the lobule, where a solid plate of hepatic cells forms the limiting plate (10). This plate separates the hepatic plates and sinusoids from the interlobular connective tissue. Distributing portal venules and hepatic arterioles penetrate through the interlobular connective tissue to give rise to the sinusoids.

The hepatic cells (11) are polygonal, vary in size, contain a large, round vesicular nucleus, and may occasionally be binucleate. The cells have a granular acidophilic cytoplasm which varies with the functional state of the cells (see also Fig. 2).

The sinusoids (2, 5) are situated between the plates, and follow their branchings and anastomoses. The lumina of the sinusoids are incompletely lined with endothelial cells (3). Also present in the sinusoid wall are fixed macrophages, the Kupffer cells. The sinusoids, containing erythrocytes (4) and leukocytes, open into the central vein (1).

PLATE 77 (Fig. 2)

LIVER: KUPFFER CELLS (INDIA INK PREPARATION)

To demonstrate the phagocytic system, a rabbit liver was intravenously injected with India ink. A section of injected liver with hepatic plates (4) and sinusoids (2) is illustrated.

The phagocytic cells (Kupffer cells) (1, 5) are prominent in the sinusoids because of their phagocytosis of the carbon particles. Kupffer cells are large, with several processes, and exhibit an irregular or stellate outline. Because of increased phagocytosis, the nucleus is obscured by the accumulation of the carbon particles. Endothelial cells are also present in the sinusoids; these cells are smaller and usually only the nucleus is visible (3).

PLATE 77 (Fig. 3)

LIVER: BILE CANALICULI (OSMIC ACID PREPARATION)

A small block of liver was fixed in osmic acid; sections were prepared and stained with hematoxylin-eosin. Penetration of osmic acid into the liver tissue reveals bile canaliculi (2, 8), which are minute channels between individual hepatic cells within the plates (1, 6). The canaliculi follow an irregular course in the hepatic cells and branch freely within the hepatic plates. In this figure, some canaliculi are illustrated in transverse plane (8).

The sinusoids (4, 5) contain endothelial cells (7) with small nuclei and a Kupffer cell (9) with larger nucleus and branched cytoplasm.

Also illustrated is a sinusoid opening into the central vein (4, upper leader).

PLATE 77

LIVER

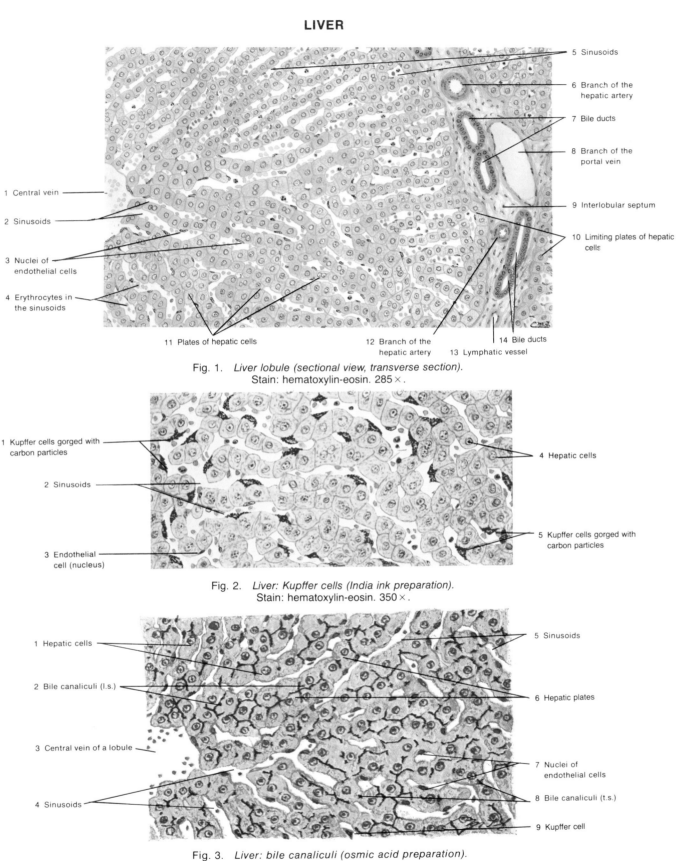

5 Sinusoids

6 Branch of the
hepatic artery

7 Bile ducts

8 Branch of the
portal vein

9 Interlobular septum

10 Limiting plates of hepatic
cells

1 Central vein

2 Sinusoids

3 Nuclei of
endothelial cells

4 Erythrocytes in
the sinusoids

11 Plates of hepatic cells

12 Branch of the
hepatic artery

13 Lymphatic vessel

14 Bile ducts

Fig. 1.   *Liver lobule (sectional view, transverse section).*
Stain: hematoxylin-eosin. 285×.

1 Kupffer cells gorged with
carbon particles

2 Sinusoids

3 Endothelial
cell (nucleus)

4 Hepatic cells

5 Kupffer cells gorged with
carbon particles

Fig. 2.   *Liver: Kupffer cells (India ink preparation).*
Stain: hematoxylin-eosin. 350×.

1 Hepatic cells

2 Bile canaliculi (l.s.)

3 Central vein of a lobule

4 Sinusoids

5 Sinusoids

6 Hepatic plates

7 Nuclei of
endothelial cells

8 Bile canaliculi (t.s.)

9 Kupffer cell

Fig. 3.   *Liver: bile canaliculi (osmic acid preparation).*
Stain: hematoxylin-eosin. 300×.

PLATE 78 (Fig. 1)

MITOCHONDRIA AND FAT DROPLETS IN LIVER CELLS
(ALTMANN'S STAIN)

The illustrated liver specimen was fixed in potassium bichromate and osmic acid, stained with acid fuchsin and picric acid. The mitochondria (2) stain red. The fat droplets (1) usually stain black after osmic acid fixation, but in this preparation stain blue.

PLATE 78 (Fig. 2)

GLYCOGEN IN LIVER CELLS (BEST'S CARMINE STAIN)

Liver sections stained with alcohol and ammonia solution of carmine demonstrate glycogen (1) as red granules that exhibit an irregular distribution within the cytoplasm. If the sections are previously stained with Meyer's hemalum, the nuclei appear violet.

PLATE 78 (Fig. 3)

RETICULAR FIBERS IN A HEPATIC LOBULE
(DEL RIO HORTEGA'S STAIN)

The use of Del Rio Hortega's modification of the ammonium silver carbonate method for silver impregnation demonstrates the fine fibrillar structure of the stroma. Reticular fibers are stained black and the liver cells a pale violet.

Reticular fibers form most of the supporting connective tissue of the liver. They line the liver sinusoids (1), disposed between the hepatocytes and the discontinuous endothelial cells, and form a dense network (3) around the central vein (2).

The collagenous fibers in the dense irregular connective tissue of the interlobular septa stain a dark brown (4); the reticular fibers merge with these fibers.

PLATE 78

LIVER

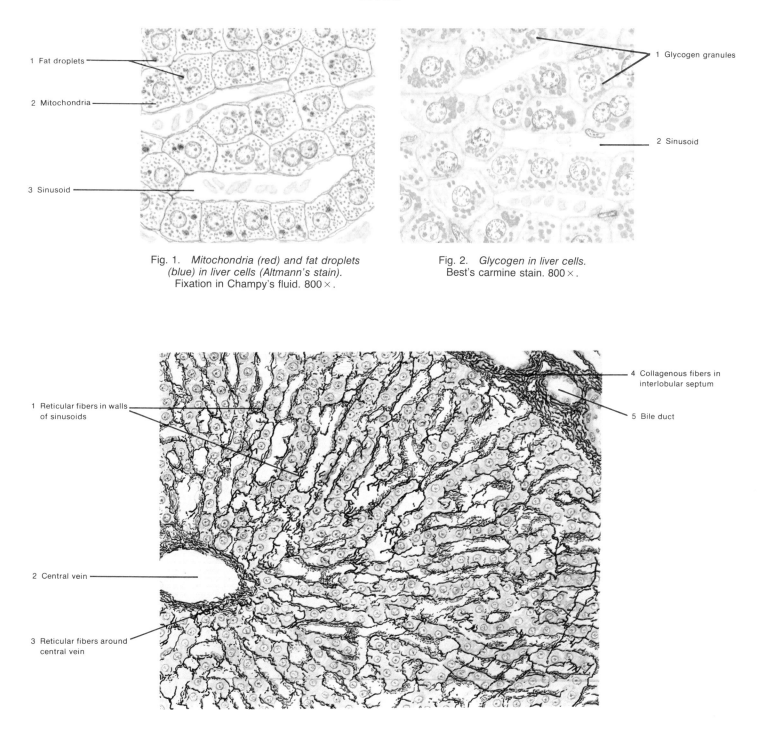

1 Fat droplets

2 Mitochondria

3 Sinusoid

1 Glycogen granules

2 Sinusoid

Fig. 1. *Mitochondria (red) and fat droplets (blue) in liver cells (Altmann's stain).* Fixation in Champy's fluid. 800×.

Fig. 2. *Glycogen in liver cells.* Best's carmine stain. 800×.

1 Reticular fibers in walls of sinusoids

4 Collagenous fibers in interlobular septum

5 Bile duct

2 Central vein

3 Reticular fibers around central vein

Fig. 3. *Reticular fibers in a hepatic lobule.* Stain: Del Rio Hortega. 300×.

PLATE 79

GALLBLADDER

The wall of the gallbladder consists of a mucosa (3, 4, 5), a fibromuscular layer (2), a perimuscular connective tissue layer (1, 10), and a serosa (6) on all of its surface except the hepatic, where an adventitia attaches it to the liver.

The mucosa is thrown into temporary folds (15) which disappear when the gallbladder is distended with bile. These folds resemble villi; however, they are different due to their variable size, shape, and irregular arrangement. The crypts or diverticula between the folds often form deep indentations (16) in the mucosa. In cross section, these diverticula in the lamina propria resemble tubular glands (18); however, there are no glands in the gallbladder proper (except in the neck region).

The lining epithelium (5, 14, 20) is simple tall columnar with lightly stained cytoplasm and basal nuclei. The lamina propria (4, 17) contains loose connective and some diffuse lymphatic tissue.

The smooth muscle fibers (7) in the fibromuscular layer (2) do not form a compact layer but are interspersed with layers of loose connective tissue rich in elastic fibers (8). In contrast to other organs where a serosa or adventitia covers the muscular layer, the gallbladder has a wide layer of perimuscular loose connective tissue (1, 10) which contains blood vessels (11, 13), lymphatics, and nerves (12); serosa is the outermost layer and covers all of these structures.

PLATE 79

GALLBLADDER

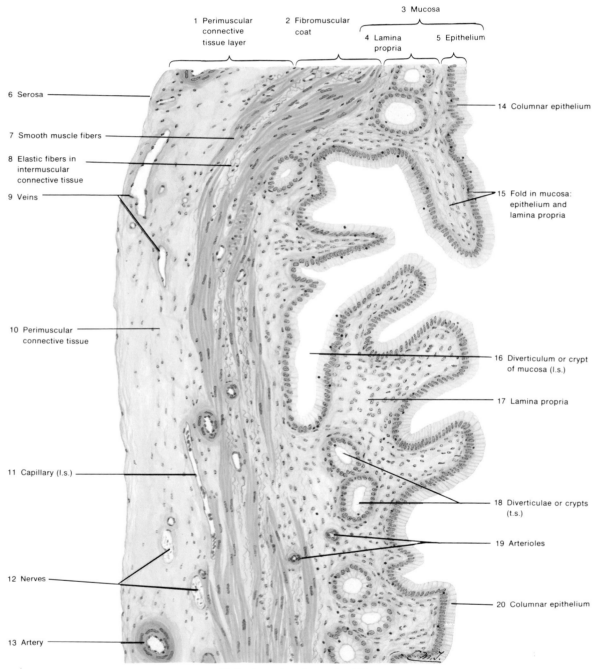

3 Mucosa

1 Perimuscular connective tissue layer

2 Fibromuscular coat

4 Lamina propria

5 Epithelium

6 Serosa

7 Smooth muscle fibers

8 Elastic fibers in intermuscular connective tissue

9 Veins

10 Perimuscular connective tissue

11 Capillary (l.s.)

12 Nerves

13 Artery

14 Columnar epithelium

15 Fold in mucosa: epithelium and lamina propria

16 Diverticulum or crypt of mucosa (l.s.)

17 Lamina propria

18 Diverticulae or crypts (t.s.)

19 Arterioles

20 Columnar epithelium

Stain: hematoxylin-eosin. 120×.

PLATE 80 (Fig. 1)

PANCREAS (SECTIONAL VIEW)

The pancreas is composed of masses of serous acini (2, 15) arranged into numerous small lobules surrounded by intralobular and interlobular connective tissue with their corresponding ducts (1, 5, 20; 10, 11). The pancreatic islets (of Langerhans) (4, 8, 9) are the characteristic features of the organ.

A pancreatic acinus (2, 15, I) consists of pyramidal secretory zymogenic cells (I, 21) and small centroacinar cells (22) within its lumen.

Individual acini are drained by long, narrow intercalated ducts (intralobular ducts) (1, 5, 20, II) that exhibit small lumina and are lined by low cuboidal cells (II). The ductal epithelium extends into each acinus and becomes visible as the pale-staining centroacinar cells (22).

Intercalated ducts drain into larger interlobular ducts (11, 19, III), which are lined with columnar epithelium and are found in the connective tissue septa (10, 11).

The pancreatic islets (of Langerhans) (4, 8, 9) are round masses of endocrine cells of varying size that are demarcated from the surrounding acinar tissue by a thin layer of reticular fibers; the islets are larger than the acini. Under higher magnification (IV), the islets are compact clusters of epithelial cells (23) permeated by a rich network of capillaries (24).

Located in the connective tissue septa are blood vessels (6, 7, 12, 13, 18), nerves (14, 17), occasional small ganglia, and Pacinian corpuscles (16).

PLATE 80 (Fig. 2)

PANCREATIC ACINI (SPECIAL PREPARATION)

A small portion of the pancreas illustrates cellular detail in acini after special staining with Gomori's chrome hematoxylin–phloxine. Zymogen granules stain red (1) and the basophilic (chromophilic) substance stains blue (2).

The upper triangle of the figure is comparable to Figure 1 (90×). The lower triangle has a higher magnification (450×) and illustrates the zymogen granules (1) filling the apical portion of the cells (storage phase).

In the basal portion of the cells, this stain illustrates the basophilic cytoplasm and its striations (2). The nucleus lies in this zone.

PLATE 80 (Fig. 3)

PANCREATIC ISLETS (SPECIAL PREPARATION)

This figure illustrates the pancreatic islet (of Langerhans), the surrounding connective tissue (4), and a few adjacent acini (5). The Gomori's chrome hematoxylin-phloxine stain distinguishes the alpha (A) and beta (B) cells of the islets. In addition, another cell type, the delta cell (D) (not illustrated) can be demonstrated with selective staining. Granules of A or alpha cells stain red (1), while the granules of B or beta cells stain blue (2). Cell membranes are usually more distinguishable in alpha cells. Alpha (A) cells are situated more peripherally in the islet and the beta (B) cells, in general, lie deeper. Also, the B cells are the predominant cell type that are distributed throughout the islets and constitute about 60% of their mass. The D cells are least abundant, have variable cell shape, and may occur anywhere in the pancreatic islets.

Capillaries (3) are clearly visible, demonstrating the rich vascularity of the islet.

PLATE 80

PANCREAS

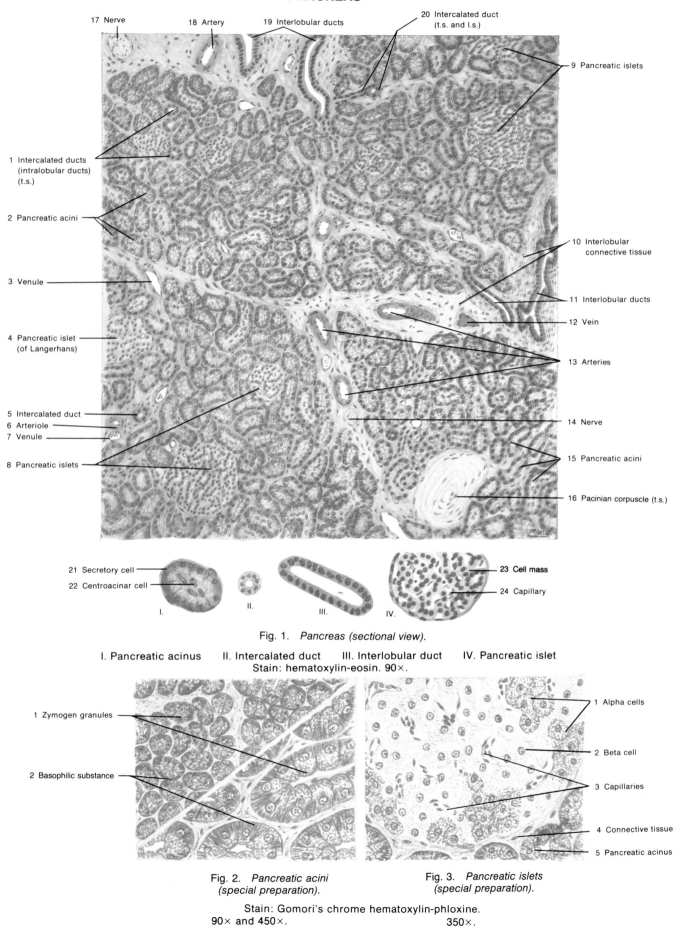

17 Nerve 18 Artery 19 Interlobular ducts 20 Intercalated duct (t.s. and l.s.)

9 Pancreatic islets

1 Intercalated ducts (intralobular ducts) (t.s.)

2 Pancreatic acini

3 Venule

4 Pancreatic islet (of Langerhans)

5 Intercalated duct
6 Arteriole
7 Venule

8 Pancreatic islets

10 Interlobular connective tissue

11 Interlobular ducts

12 Vein

13 Arteries

14 Nerve

15 Pancreatic acini

16 Pacinian corpuscle (t.s.)

21 Secretory cell
22 Centroacinar cell

23 Cell mass
24 Capillary

I. II. III. IV.

Fig. 1. *Pancreas (sectional view).*

I. Pancreatic acinus   II. Intercalated duct   III. Interlobular duct   IV. Pancreatic islet
Stain: hematoxylin-eosin. 90×.

1 Zymogen granules

2 Basophilic substance

1 Alpha cells

2 Beta cell

3 Capillaries

4 Connective tissue

5 Pancreatic acinus

Fig. 2. *Pancreatic acini (special preparation).*

Fig. 3. *Pancreatic islets (special preparation).*

Stain: Gomori's chrome hematoxylin-phloxine.
90× and 450×.   350×.

PLATE 81 (Fig. 1)

OLFACTORY MUCOSA AND SUPERIOR CONCHA, RHESUS MONKEY
(GENERAL VIEW)

In this figure, the olfactory mucosa (2) is illustrated on the surface of the superior concha (1).

The respiratory epithelium lining the nasal cavity is pseudostratified ciliated columnar with goblet cells. The olfactory epithelium is specialized for reception of smell (5 and Fig. 2) and differs from the respiratory epithelium; it is pseudostratified tall columnar epithelium that lacks goblet cells. The olfactory epithelium is found in the roof of each nasal cavity, on each side of the septum and the upper nasal conchae.

In the loose connective tissue of lamina propria are found branched tuboloalveolar olfactory glands of Bowman (3, 6). These glands produce a serous secretion, in contrast to mixed mucous and serous secretion produced by the glands in the nasal cavity. Numerous small nerves found in the lamina propria are the olfactory nerves or fila olfactoria (4, 7) which represent the aggregated axons of the olfactory cells. Small blood vessels and nerves are also present in the connective tissue. The lamina propria merges with the periosteum of the bone.

PLATE 81 (Fig. 2)

OLFACTORY MUCOSA: DETAIL OF A TRANSITION AREA

In the human nose, olfactory mucosa occupies a small area. It extends over the superior concha and for a short distance on each side of the nasal septum. This illustration depicts a transition area between the olfactory (1) and respiratory (9) epithelia. In this region, the histologic differences between these two important epithelia become obvious.

The olfactory epithelium is tall, pseudostratified columnar, composed of three different types of cells: the supporting, basal, and neuroepithelial olfactory cells. The individual cell outlines are difficult to distinguish in a routine histologic preparation; however, the location and shape of the nuclei allow some identification of different cell types that comprise the olfactory epithelium.

The supportive or sustentacular cells (3) are elongated with their oval nuclei situated more apically or superficially in the epithelium. Their broad apical surfaces contain slender microvilli that protrude into the overlying layer of surface mucus (2); basally, the cells are slender.

The olfactory cells are the sensory bipolar neurons (4). Their oval or round nuclei occupy a region in the epithelium that is somewhat between the nuclei of the supporting cells (3) and the basal cells (5). The apices of the olfactory cells are slender and pass to the epithelial surface. Radiating from these apices are long and nonmotile olfactory cilia that lie parallel to the epithelial surface in the overlying mucus (2); these cilia function as receptors for odor. Extending from the slender cell bases are axons that pass into the underlying connective tissue of lamina propria (6), where they aggregate into small bundles of unmyelinated olfactory nerves, the fila olfactoria (14). These nerves ultimately leave the nasal cavity and pass into the olfactory bulb of the brain.

The basal cells (5) are short, small cells located at the base of the epithelium and between the bases of the supportive and olfactory cells.

The transition from the olfactory (1) to the respiratory (9) epithelium is abrupt. In this illustration, the respiratory epithelium is pseudostratified columnar with distinct surface cilia (10) and an abundance of goblet cells (11); these cells are not present in the olfactory epithelium. Also, in the transitional region, the height of the respiratory epithelium appears similar to that of the olfactory; however, in other regions of the respiratory tract, the epithelial height is much reduced when compared to olfactory epithelium.

Beneath the olfactory epithelium is the lamina propria (6), containing a rich supply of capillaries, lymphatic vessels, arterioles (8) and venules (13). In addition to the olfactory nerves (14), the lamina propria also contains branched, tubuloalveolar olfactory glands (of Bowman) (7). These serous glands deliver their secretions through narrow ducts (12), which penetrate the olfactory epithelium and open onto the surface. The secretions from these glands moisten the olfactory mucosa and provide the necessary solvent for odoriferous substances.

PLATE 81

OLFACTORY MUCOSA

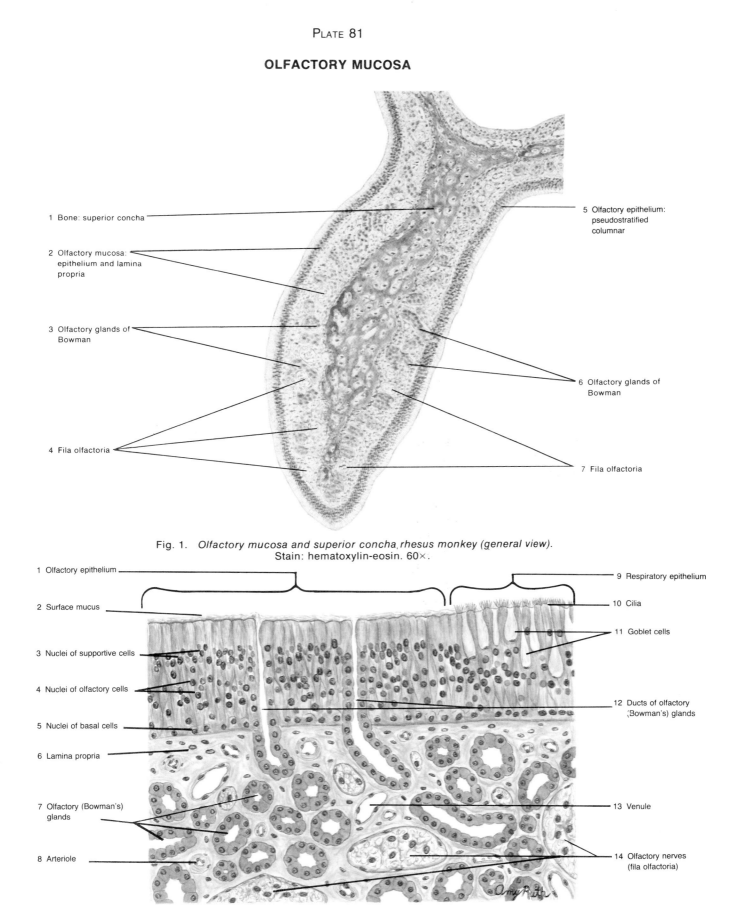

1 Bone: superior concha

2 Olfactory mucosa:
  epithelium and lamina
  propria

3 Olfactory glands of
  Bowman

4 Fila olfactoria

5 Olfactory epithelium:
  pseudostratified
  columnar

6 Olfactory glands of
  Bowman

7 Fila olfactoria

Fig. 1. *Olfactory mucosa and superior concha, rhesus monkey (general view).*
Stain: hematoxylin-eosin. 60×.

1 Olfactory epithelium

2 Surface mucus

3 Nuclei of supportive cells

4 Nuclei of olfactory cells

5 Nuclei of basal cells

6 Lamina propria

7 Olfactory (Bowman's)
  glands

8 Arteriole

9 Respiratory epithelium

10 Cilia

11 Goblet cells

12 Ducts of olfactory
  (Bowman's) glands

13 Venule

14 Olfactory nerves
  (fila olfactoria)

Fig. 2. *Olfactory mucosa: detail of a transition area.*
Stain: hematoxylin-eosin. 500×.

PLATE 82

EPIGLOTTIS (LONGITUDINAL SECTION)

The epiglottis is the uppermost part of the larynx, projecting upward from its anterior wall as a flat flap.

A central plate of elastic cartilage, the epiglottic cartilage (7), forms the framework for the epiglottis. Its anterior or lingual surface (6, 9) is covered with noncornified stratified squamous epithelium. The underlying lamina propria merges with the perichondrium of the epiglottic cartilage (8).

The anterior or lingual mucosa covers the apex of the epiglottis and more than half of the posterior or laryngeal surface (2, 3). The stratified squamous epithelium, however, becomes lower (3), connective tissue papillae disappear, and a transition is made to respiratory epithelium, which is pseudostratified ciliated columnar epithelium (5) with goblet cells.

Tubuloalveolar mucous, serous, or mixed glands are present in the lamina propria (4). Occasional taste buds (1) may be seen in the epithelium. Solitary lymphatic nodules may be present in the lingual or laryngeal mucosa.

PLATE 82

EPIGLOTTIS (LONGITUDINAL SECTION)

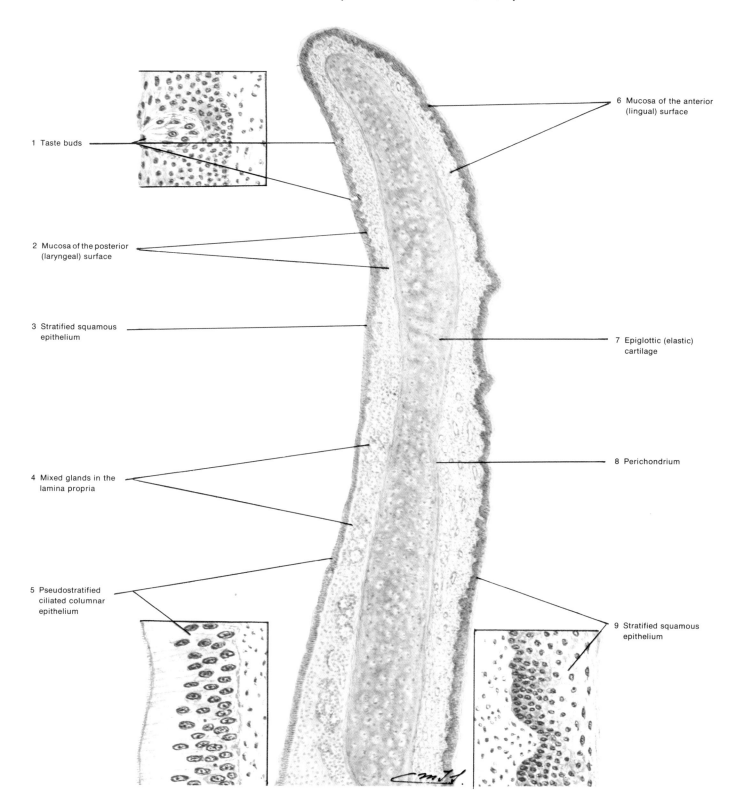

1 Taste buds

2 Mucosa of the posterior (laryngeal) surface

3 Stratified squamous epithelium

4 Mixed glands in the lamina propria

5 Pseudostratified ciliated columnar epithelium

6 Mucosa of the anterior (lingual) surface

7 Epiglottic (elastic) cartilage

8 Perichondrium

9 Stratified squamous epithelium

Stain: hematoxylin-eosin. 25× and 300×.

PLATE 83

LARYNX (FRONTAL SECTION)

The larynx has been sectioned vertically to show the two prominent folds (13, 18–20), the supporting cartilages (8, 11), and muscles (10, 20).

The superior or false vocal fold (13) is formed by the mucosa and is continuous with the posterior surface of the epiglottis (12). The covering epithelium is pseudostratified ciliated columnar (14) with goblet cells. Below the epithelium in the lamina propria are found mixed glands which are predominantly mucous (15). Excretory ducts (16), which open onto the epithelial surface, are seen among the glands (15). Lymphatic nodules (7) are located in the lamina propria on the ventricular side of the vocal fold.

The ventricle (17) is a deep indentation and recess separating the false vocal fold (13) from the true vocal fold (18–20). The mucosa in the lateral wall (3, 4, 5, 6) is similar to that of the false vocal fold. Lymphatic nodules are more numerous and are sometimes called the "laryngeal tonsils" (7). The lamina propria (3) blends with the perichondrium (9) of the thyroid cartilage (8); there is no distinct submucosa. The lower wall of the ventricle makes the transition to true vocal fold.

The mucosa of the true vocal fold consists of noncornified, stratified squamous epithelium (18) and a thin, dense lamina propria devoid of glands, lymphatic tissue, or blood vessels. At the apex of the true vocal fold is the vocal ligament (19), consisting of dense elastic fibers which spread out into the adjacent lamina propria and the vocalis muscle (20). The thyroarytenoid muscle (10) and the thyroid cartilage (8) comprise the remaining wall.

The epithelium in the lower larynx changes to pseudostratified ciliated columnar (21), and the underlying lamina propria contains mixed glands (22). The cricoid cartilage (11) is the lowermost cartilage of the larynx.

PLATE 83

LARYNX (FRONTAL SECTION)

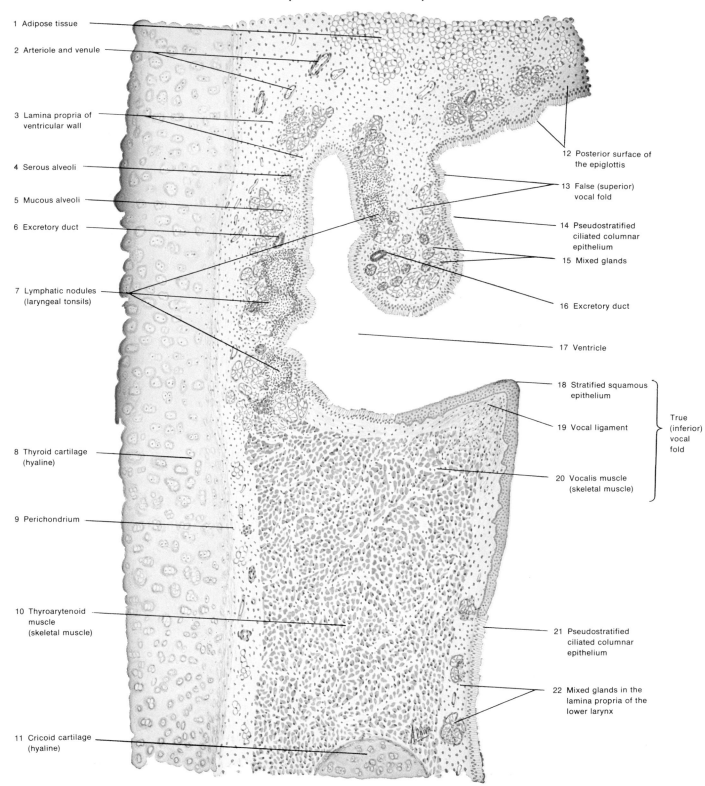

1 Adipose tissue

2 Arteriole and venule

3 Lamina propria of
   ventricular wall

4 Serous alveoli

5 Mucous alveoli

6 Excretory duct

7 Lymphatic nodules
   (laryngeal tonsils)

8 Thyroid cartilage
   (hyaline)

9 Perichondrium

10 Thyroarytenoid
   muscle
   (skeletal muscle)

11 Cricoid cartilage
   (hyaline)

12 Posterior surface of
   the epiglottis

13 False (superior)
   vocal fold

14 Pseudostratified
   ciliated columnar
   epithelium

15 Mixed glands

16 Excretory duct

17 Ventricle

18 Stratified squamous
   epithelium

19 Vocal ligament

20 Vocalis muscle
   (skeletal muscle)

True
(inferior)
vocal
fold

21 Pseudostratified
   ciliated columnar
   epithelium

22 Mixed glands in the
   lamina propria of the
   lower larynx

Stain: hematoxylin-eosin. 35×.

PLATE 84 (Fig. 1)

TRACHEA: PANORAMIC VIEW, TRANSVERSE SECTION

The wall of the trachea consists of a mucosa, submucosa, hyaline cartilage, and adventitia. The cartilage in the trachea is a series of C-shaped rings between whose ends lies the smooth trachealis muscle (9).

Approximately half of a transverse section of the trachea is illustrated in Figure 1. The mucosa consists of pseudostratified ciliated columnar epithelium with goblet cells (13) and a lamina propria (11, 14) of fine connective tissue. Present also are diffuse lymphatic tissue (14) and occasional solitary nodules. Deep in the lamina propria, the elastic fibers form a longitudinal elastic membrane (15). In the loose connective tissue of the submucosa are tubuloalveolar mixed glands (4, 5) whose ducts (10, 17) pass through the lamina propria to the tracheal lumen.

The hyaline cartilage (3) is surrounded by a perichondrium (2) of dense connective tissue which merges with the submucosa (16) on one side and the adventitia (1) on the other side. Numerous blood vessels and nerves (6) course in the adventitia and provide smaller branches to the outer layers.

The mucosa exhibits folds (12) along the posterior wall of the trachea where the cartilage is absent. The trachealis muscle (9) lies deep to the elastic membrane of the mucosa and is embedded in the fibroelastic tissue that occupies the area between the ends of the cartilage rings. Most of the muscle fibers insert into the perichondrium of the cartilage (2, upper leader). Mixed glands are present in the submucosa; these can intermingle with the muscle fibers and extend into the adventitia (8).

PLATE 84 (Fig. 2)

TRACHEA (SECTIONAL VIEW)

A small section of trachea, illustrated at a higher magnification and stained with hematoxylin–eosin, shows detailed structure of the wall. The pseudostratified surface epithelium contains ciliated (5) and goblet cells (10), the typical irregular disposition of nuclei, and the thickened basement membrane (6). A longitudinal elastic membrane (7) is visible in the deeper region of the lamina propria; in this illustration, the fibers are illustrated in transverse sections. A duct (8) and a group of mucous alveoli (9) indicate the tracheal glands. Located adjacent to the tracheal glands is the perichondrium (1) of the cartilage. The typical association of cartilage with perichondrium is seen; the larger lacunae and chondrocytes in the interior of the plate become progressively flatter (3) toward the perichondrium and the matrix, gradually blending with the connective tissue.

PLATE 84 (Fig. 3)

TRACHEA (SECTIONAL VIEW): ELASTIC FIBER STAIN

This section is similar to Figure 2 except that it has been stained with Gallego's method to demonstrate elastic fibers, which stain red with carbol–fuchsin. The elastic fibers of the elastic membrane (8) are prominent. Collagenous fibers stain blue with aniline blue and provide a contrast where these intermix with the elastic fibers. Collagenous fibers are also demonstrated in the perichondrium (1, lower leader), submucosa (3), and superficial lamina propria (9).

PLATE 84

TRACHEA

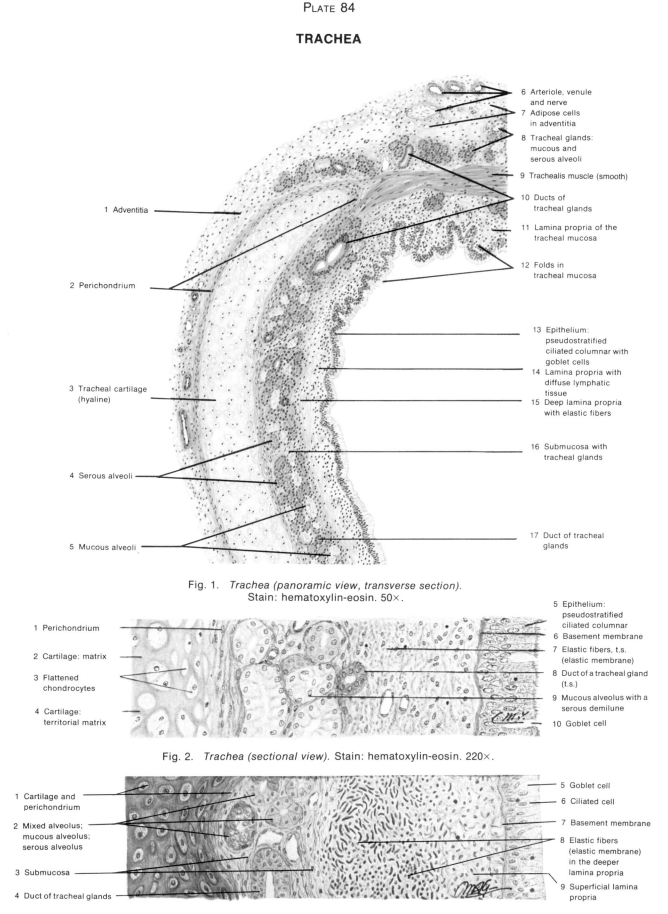

6 Arteriole, venule
and nerve

7 Adipose cells
in adventitia

8 Tracheal glands:
mucous and
serous alveoli

9 Trachealis muscle (smooth)

10 Ducts of
tracheal glands

11 Lamina propria of the
tracheal mucosa

12 Folds in
tracheal mucosa

13 Epithelium:
pseudostratified
ciliated columnar with
goblet cells

14 Lamina propria with
diffuse lymphatic
tissue

15 Deep lamina propria
with elastic fibers

16 Submucosa with
tracheal glands

17 Duct of tracheal
glands

1 Adventitia

2 Perichondrium

3 Tracheal cartilage
(hyaline)

4 Serous alveoli

5 Mucous alveoli

Fig. 1. *Trachea (panoramic view, transverse section).*
Stain: hematoxylin-eosin. 50×.

1 Perichondrium

2 Cartilage: matrix

3 Flattened
chondrocytes

4 Cartilage:
territorial matrix

5 Epithelium:
pseudostratified
ciliated columnar

6 Basement membrane

7 Elastic fibers, t.s.
(elastic membrane)

8 Duct of a tracheal gland
(t.s.)

9 Mucous alveolus with a
serous demilune

10 Goblet cell

Fig. 2. *Trachea (sectional view).* Stain: hematoxylin-eosin. 220×.

1 Cartilage and
perichondrium

2 Mixed alveolus;
mucous alveolus;
serous alveolus

3 Submucosa

4 Duct of tracheal glands

5 Goblet cell

6 Ciliated cell

7 Basement membrane

8 Elastic fibers
(elastic membrane)
in the deeper
lamina propria

9 Superficial lamina
propria

Fig. 3. *Trachea (sectional view).* Stain: Gallego's method for elastic fibers. 220×.

PLATE 85

LUNG (PANORAMIC VIEW)

The respiratory system consists of the lungs and the air passages. The passages of the respiratory tract are divided into the conducting portion and respiratory portion. The conducting portion consists of the nasal cavity, nasopharynx, larynx, trachea, bronchi, bronchioles, and terminal bronchioles. The respiratory portion consists of the respiratory bronchioles, alveolar ducts, alveolar sacs, and alveoli. The histologic characteristics of several of these divisions are shown in greater detail on Plate 86 and the distinguishing features of the lung are illustrated in this panoramic view. All cartilage in the lung is hyaline.

The histologic structure of the extrapulmonary bronchi is similar to that of the trachea. In the intrapulmonary bronchi, the C-shaped cartilage rings are replaced by cartilage plates that encircle individual bronchi. The smooth muscle spreads out from the trachealis muscle to form an incomplete layer around the lumen.

The intrapulmonary (33) bronchus is identified by several cartilage plates (30) located in close proximity to each other (33 and Plate 86, Fig. 1). The epithelium is pseudostratified columnar ciliated with goblet cells (32). The rest of the wall consists of a thin lamina propria, a narrow layer of smooth muscle (31), a submucosa with scattered bronchial glands, hyaline cartilage plates (30), and adventitia.

As the intrapulmonary bronchi divide into smaller bronchi, there is a decrease in the epithelial height and the amount of cartilage. Farther down the airway tube, only occasional small pieces of cartilage are seen. In bronchi that are about 1 mm in diameter, cartilage disappears completely.

In bronchioles (16), the epithelium is low, pseudostratified columnar ciliated with occasional goblet cells. The mucosa is typically folded and the smooth muscle is prominent. Adventitia surrounds these structures; glands and cartilage plates are no longer present (16).

Terminal bronchioles (6, 12) exhibit a wavy mucosal lining and ciliated columnar epithelum; goblet cells are lacking in these tubules. Still present, however, are a thin lamina propria, a layer of smooth muscle, and an adventitia.

The respiratory bronchioles (5, 8, 17, 23, 26, 27) are characterized by a direct connection with the alveolar ducts and alveoli. The epithelium is low columnar or cuboidal (5, 8) and may be ciliated in the proximal portion of the respiratory bronchioles. A minimal amount of connective tissue supports the band of intermixed smooth muscle, the elastic fibers of the lamina propria and the accompanying blood vessels. Individual alveoli appear in the wall of the respiratory bronchioles (5, 26, left side) as outpockets. Alveoli increase in number distally in the tubules. The epithelium and muscle in the distal respiratory bronchioles appear as small, intermittent areas between the openings of the numerous alveoli (5, upper leader; 17, 23, 24, 25).

Each distal respiratory bronchiole terminates by branching into several alveolar ducts; in histologic sections only one such alveolar duct may be seen (5 and 2, lower leader; 23, upper leader; and 22, middle leader). The walls of the alveolar ducts are formed by a series of alveoli situated adjacent to each other (2, 15, 22). A cluster of alveoli that opens into an alveolar duct is called an alveolar sac (14, 20).

The alveoli (4, 21, 25) form the parenchyma of the lung, giving it the appearance of fine lace (See Fig. 4, Plate 86 for details).

A plane of section shows a continuous passageway from the terminal bronchiole into the alveolar ducts (6, 5, lowest leader of 2; 23, 26, middle leader of 22).

The pulmonary artery branches repeatedly to accompany the divisions of the bronchial tree (7, 10, 28). Large pulmonary vein branches accompany the bronchi and bronchioles; numerous small branches of the vein are seen in the lung trabeculae (3).

Very small bronchial arteries supply the walls of various bronchi, bronchioles, and other areas. Small bronchial veins (29) may be seen in the walls of the larger bronchi.

The visceral pleura (1) is composed of a thin layer of connective tissue (19) and a layer of mesothelium (18).

PLATE 85

LUNG (PANORAMIC VIEW)

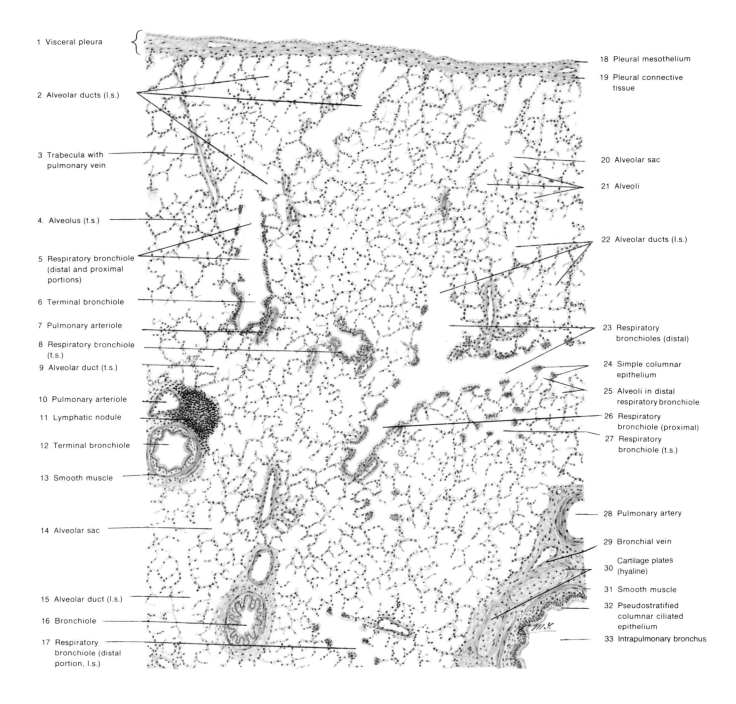

1 Visceral pleura

2 Alveolar ducts (l.s.)

3 Trabecula with pulmonary vein

4. Alveolus (t.s.)

5 Respiratory bronchiole (distal and proximal portions)

6 Terminal bronchiole

7 Pulmonary arteriole

8 Respiratory bronchiole (t.s.)

9 Alveolar duct (t.s.)

10 Pulmonary arteriole

11 Lymphatic nodule

12 Terminal bronchiole

13 Smooth muscle

14 Alveolar sac

15 Alveolar duct (l.s.)

16 Bronchiole

17 Respiratory bronchiole (distal portion, l.s.)

18 Pleural mesothelium

19 Pleural connective tissue

20 Alveolar sac

21 Alveoli

22 Alveolar ducts (l.s.)

23 Respiratory bronchioles (distal)

24 Simple columnar epithelium

25 Alveoli in distal respiratory bronchiole

26 Respiratory bronchiole (proximal)

27 Respiratory bronchiole (t.s.)

28 Pulmonary artery

29 Bronchial vein

30 Cartilage plates (hyaline)

31 Smooth muscle

32 Pseudostratified columnar ciliated epithelium

33 Intrapulmonary bronchus

Stain: hematoxylin-eosin. 30×.

PLATE 86 (Fig. 1)

LUNG: INTRAPULMONARY BRONCHUS

The primary or extrapulmonary bronchi divide further to give rise to a series of intrapulmonary bronchi. Such a bronchus is lined by pseudostratified columnar ciliated epithelium (12), a thin lamina propria (13) of fine connective tissue with many elastic fibers (not illustrated), and scanty lymphocytes. Ducts (2) from the submucosal glands pass through these layers to open into the bronchial lumen. A thin layer of smooth muscle (6) surrounds the lamina propria.

The submucosa contains glands that may consist of either serous (5, 8), mucous, or mucoserous alveoli (10). In addition, serous demilunes may be present.

The cartilage plates (4) are close together; they will become smaller and farther apart as the bronchi continue to divide and their size decreases. Between the plates, the submucosal connective tissue blends with the well-developed adventitia (3).

The accompanying branch of the pulmonary artery (15) is located either adjacent to it or in the outer adventitia. A small branch of the pulmonary artery (7) probably accompanies a small bronchus or bronchiole which is in another plane of section.

Bronchial vessels are seen in the connective tissue of a bronchus. These are an artery (16), a venule (11), and capillaries (9).

PLATE 86 (Fig. 2)

TERMINAL BRONCHIOLE

Bronchioles are of small diameter, about 1 mm or less. Mucosal folds are prominent and the epithelium is low pseudostratified columnar ciliated with few goblet cells. The epithelium becomes columnar ciliated in terminal bronchioles (5) and the goblet cells are absent. A well-developed smooth muscle layer (3) surrounds the thin lamina propria, which is, in turn, surrounded by the adventitia (2). Cartilage plates and the glands are absent, in addition to the goblet cells.

Adjacent to the bronchiole is a branch of the pulmonary artery (6); the bronchiole is surrounded by alveoli of the lung (7).

PLATE 86 (Fig. 3)

RESPIRATORY BRONCHIOLE

This figure illustrates a respiratory bronchiole and associated structures. The wall of the bronchiole is lined with cuboidal epithelium (4). Cilia may be present in the epithelium of the proximal but disappear in the distal portion of the respiratory bronchiole. Smooth muscle forms a layer close to the epithelium (3). A branch of the pulmonary artery (5) accompanies the respiratory bronchiole.

An alveolar duct (2) arises from the respiratory bronchiole and numerous alveoli (1) open into the alveolar duct.

PLATE 86 (Fig. 4)

ALVEOLAR WALLS (INTERALVEOLAR SEPTA)

The oval alveoli (5) are lined by a simple squamous epithelium, which is not very obvious at this magnification. Adjacent alveoli share a common interalveolar septum (4). Located in the thin septum are capillary plexi (1, 3) supported by fine connective tissue with fibroblasts and other cells. As a result of this arrangement, the capillaries are close to squamous cells of adjacent alveoli, separated from the epithelium only by the sparse connective tissue. In routine preparation of lung tissue, it is difficult to distinguish between the nuclei of squamous cells, endothelial cells, and fibroblasts (6).

At the free ends of the interalveolar septa and around the open ends of the alveoli are narrow bands of smooth muscle (2), which is a continuation from the muscle layer of the respiratory bronchiole.

PLATE 86

LUNG

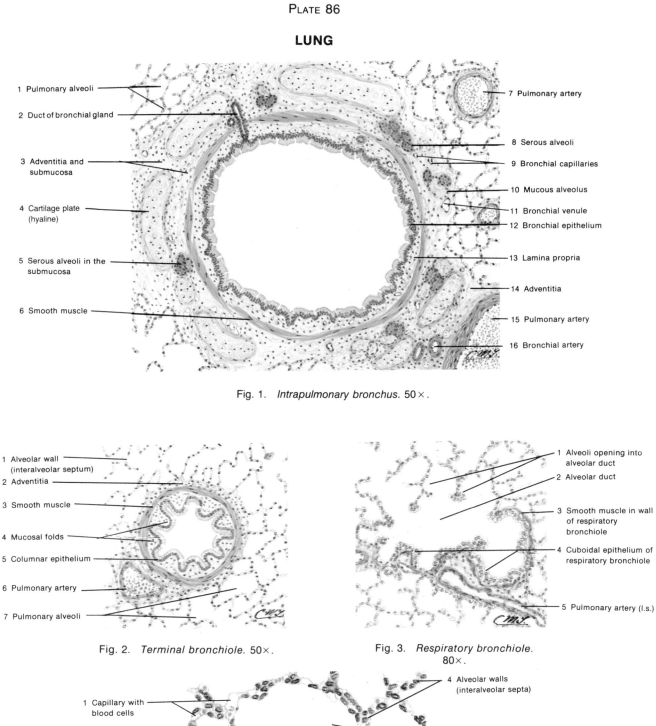

1 Pulmonary alveoli
2 Duct of bronchial gland
3 Adventitia and submucosa
4 Cartilage plate (hyaline)
5 Serous alveoli in the submucosa
6 Smooth muscle

7 Pulmonary artery
8 Serous alveoli
9 Bronchial capillaries
10 Mucous alveolus
11 Bronchial venule
12 Bronchial epithelium
13 Lamina propria
14 Adventitia
15 Pulmonary artery
16 Bronchial artery

Fig. 1. *Intrapulmonary bronchus.* 50×.

1 Alveolar wall (interalveolar septum)
2 Adventitia
3 Smooth muscle
4 Mucosal folds
5 Columnar epithelium
6 Pulmonary artery
7 Pulmonary alveoli

Fig. 2. *Terminal bronchiole.* 50×.

1 Alveoli opening into alveolar duct
2 Alveolar duct
3 Smooth muscle in wall of respiratory bronchiole
4 Cuboidal epithelium of respiratory bronchiole
5 Pulmonary artery (l.s.)

Fig. 3. *Respiratory bronchiole.* 80×.

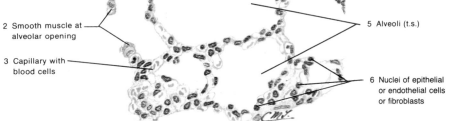

1 Capillary with blood cells
2 Smooth muscle at alveolar opening
3 Capillary with blood cells
4 Alveolar walls (interalveolar septa)
5 Alveoli (t.s.)
6 Nuclei of epithelial or endothelial cells or fibroblasts

Fig. 4. *Alveolar walls (interalveolar septa).* Stain: hematoxylin-eosin. 700×.

PLATE 87

KIDNEY: CORTEX AND ONE PYRAMID (PANORAMIC VIEW)

The kidney is divided into an outer region, the cortex (20) and an inner region, the medulla (21). The cortex is covered with a connective tissue capsule (19) and perirenal connective and adipose tissues (18).

The cortex contains convoluted tubules (3), glomeruli (2, 8), areas of straight tubules (4), and medullary rays (5). The substance of the cortex consists of renal corpuscles (glomerular or Bowman's capsules and glomeruli), adjacent proximal and distal convolutions (3) of the nephrons, and the interlobular arteries and veins (6, 7). The medullary rays (5) contain straight portions of nephrons and collecting tubules. Medullary rays do not reach the kidney capsule because of a narrow zone of convoluted tubules (1).

The medulla is composed of a number of renal pyramids. Each pyramid lies with its base adjacent to the cortex (11) and its apex directed inward. The apices of renal pyramids form the papilla (16), which projects into a minor calyx (14).

The medulla contains loops of Henle (straight or descending segments of proximal tubules, thin segments, and straight or ascending segments of distal tubules) and collecting tubules. The collecting tubules join each other in the medulla to form large papillary ducts (see Plate 89).

The papilla is usually covered with a simple columnar epithelium (12). As this epithelium reflects onto the outer wall of the calyx, it becomes transitional epithelium (13). A thin layer of connective tissue and smooth muscle (not illustrated) underlies this epithelium (14), which then merges with the connective tissue of the renal sinus (17).

In the renal sinus, between the pyramids, are branches of the renal artery and vein (15), the interlobar vessels. These vessels enter the kidney and then arch over the base of the pyramid at the corticomedullary junction as the arcuate vessels (9). The arcuate vessels give rise to smaller, interlobular arteries and veins (6, 7, 10). The arcuate arteries pass radially into the kidney cortex and give off numerous afferent glomerular arterioles to the glomeruli.

PLATE 87

KIDNEY: CORTEX AND ONE PYRAMID (PANORAMIC VIEW)

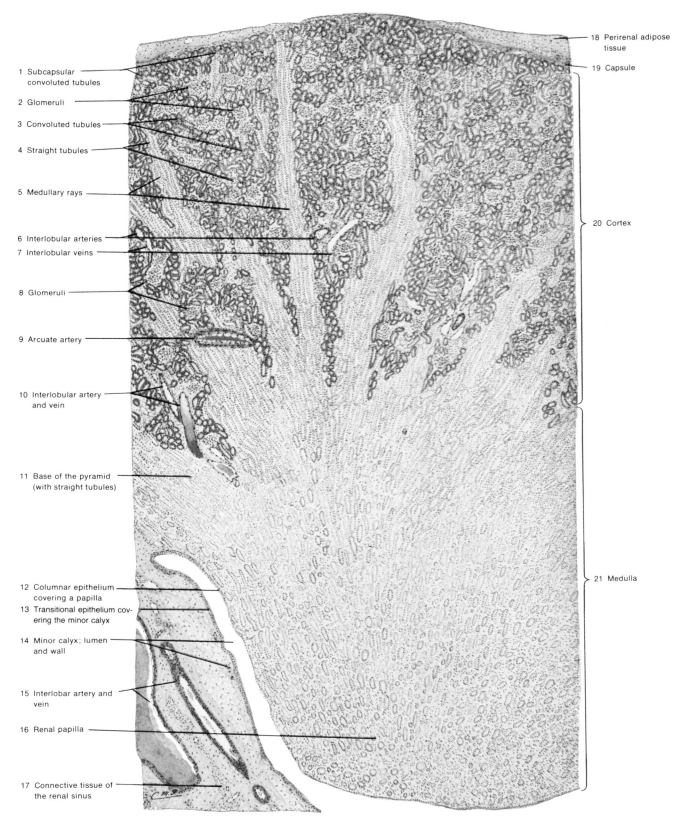

1 Subcapsular convoluted tubules

2 Glomeruli

3 Convoluted tubules

4 Straight tubules

5 Medullary rays

6 Interlobular arteries

7 Interlobular veins

8 Glomeruli

9 Arcuate artery

10 Interlobular artery and vein

11 Base of the pyramid (with straight tubules)

12 Columnar epithelium covering a papilla

13 Transitional epithelium covering the minor calyx

14 Minor calyx; lumen and wall

15 Interlobar artery and vein

16 Renal papilla

17 Connective tissue of the renal sinus

18 Perirenal adipose tissue

19 Capsule

20 Cortex

21 Medulla

Stain: hematoxylin-eosin. 25×.

PLATE 88 (Fig. 1)

KIDNEY: DEEP CORTICAL AREA AND OUTER MEDULLA

A higher magnification of the kidney cortex reveals greater details of the renal corpuscle. Each corpuscle consists of a glomerulus (3) and a glomerular or Bowman's capsule (2, 17). The glomerulus (3) is a tuft of capillaries formed from the afferent glomerular arterioles and supported by fine connective tissue.

The visceral layer (17) of the Bowman's capsule consists of modified epithelial cells called the podocytes. These cells closely follow the contours of the glomerulus and invest the capillary tufts. At the vascular pole, the visceral epithelium reflects to become the parietal or outer layer of the Bowman's capsule (17). The space between the visceral and parietal layers of Bowman's capsule is the Bowman's or capsular space. The capsular space becomes continuous with the lumen of the proximal convoluted tubule at the urinary pole (see Fig. 2). The squamous epithelium of the parietal layer changes to the cuboidal of the proximal convoluted tubule (9).

Numerous tubules, sectioned in various planes, lie adjacent to the renal corpuscles. The tubules are primarily of two types, the proximal convoluted (4, 10, 15, 21) and distal convoluted (1, 14, 21); these tubules are the initial and terminal segments of the nephron, respectively. The proximal convoluted tubules are numerous in the cortex, exhibit a small, uneven lumen, and contain a single layer of large cuboidal cells with intensely eosinophilic, granular cytoplasm. The well-developed brush borders (15) are present but are not always well preserved in sections.

Distal convoluted tubules (14) are fewer in number and exhibit a larger lumen with smaller, cuboidal cells. The cytoplasm stains less intensely and the brush borders are not present (14, compare with 15).

Renal corpuscles and their associated tubules constitute the kidney cortex. The cortex surrounds the medullary rays, which are composed of straight portions of the nephrons and collecting tubules.

The medullary rays include three types of tubules. The straight (descending) segments of the proximal tubules (6), the straight (ascending) segments of the distal tubules (11, 20), and the collecting tubules (5, 19). The straight segments of the proximal tubules are similar to the proximal convoluted tubules and the straight segments of the distal tubules are similar to distal convoluted tubules, respectively. Collecting tubules (5,19) are distinct because of lightly stained cuboidal cells and visible cell membranes.

The medulla contains only straight portions of tubules and thin segments of Henle's loops. In the outer medullary region are illustrated thin segments of Henle's loops (13, 23) lined with squamous epithelium, straight segments of distal tubules (20), and the collecting tubules (12, 22).

PLATE 88 (Fig. 2)

KIDNEY CORTEX: THE JUXTAGLOMERULAR APPARATUS

A small area of the kidney cortex at a higher magnification illustrates the renal corpuscle, adjacent tubules, and juxtaglomerular apparatus.

The renal corpuscle exhibits the glomerular capillaries (2), parietal (10a) and visceral (10b) epithelium of glomerular (Bowman's) capsule (10), and the capsular space (13). Conspicuous brush borders and acidophilic cells distinguish the proximal convoluted tubules (6, 14) from the distal convoluted tubules (1, 15) whose smaller, less intensely stained cells lack brush borders. The cells of the collecting tubules (8) are cuboidal, with distinct cell outlines and clear, pale cytoplasm. Distinct basement membranes (9) surround these tubules.

Each renal corpuscle exhibits a vascular pole on one side where the afferent glomerular arterioles (12) enter and efferent glomerular arterioles exit. On the opposite side of the corpuscle is the urinary pole (11), where the capsular space (13) becomes continuous with the lumen of the proximal convoluted tubule (6, 14). The plane of section through the renal corpuscle, as illustrated in this figure, is seen only occasionally in the kidney cortex; however, this type of section represents an important structural association of the renal corpuscle with blood filtration and initial stages of urine formation.

At the vascular pole, the smooth muscle cells in the tunica media of the afferent glomerular arteriole (12) are replaced by highly modified epithelioid cells with cytoplasmic granules. These are the juxtaglomerular cells (4). In the adjacent segment of the distal convoluted tubules, the cells that border the juxtaglomerular area are narrower and more columnar than elsewhere in the tubules. This area of darker, more compact cell arrangement is called the macula densa (5). The juxtaglomerular cells in the afferent glomerular arteriole and the macula densa cells in the distal convoluted tubule together constitute the juxtaglomerular apparatus.

PLATE 88

KIDNEY

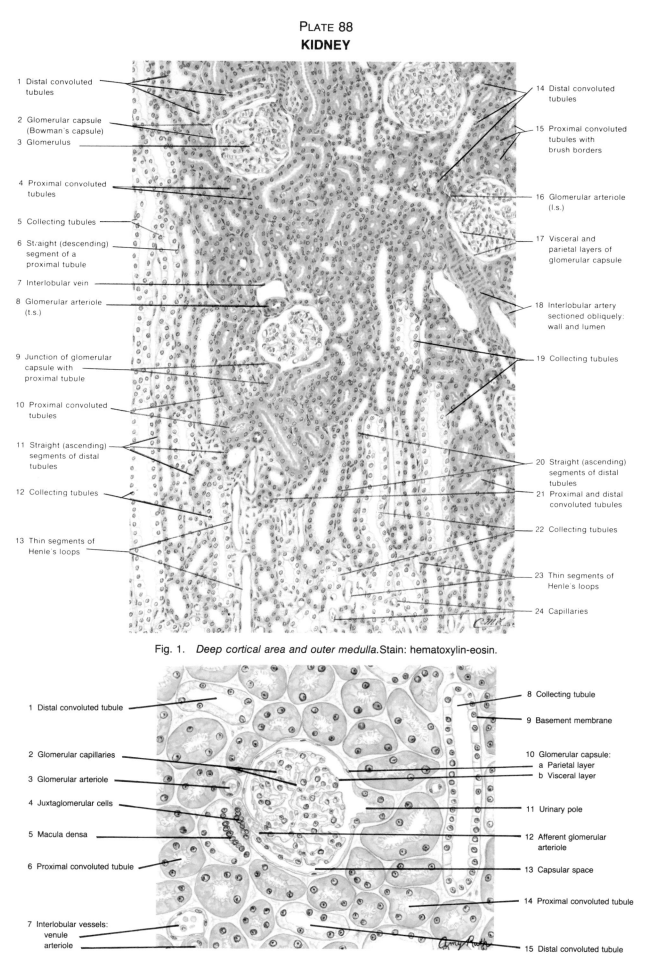

1 Distal convoluted
  tubules

2 Glomerular capsule
  (Bowman's capsule)
3 Glomerulus

4 Proximal convoluted
  tubules

5 Collecting tubules

6 Straight (descending)
  segment of a
  proximal tubule

7 Interlobular vein

8 Glomerular arteriole
  (t.s.)

9 Junction of glomerular
  capsule with
  proximal tubule

10 Proximal convoluted
   tubules

11 Straight (ascending)
   segments of distal
   tubules

12 Collecting tubules

13 Thin segments of
   Henle's loops

14 Distal convoluted
   tubules

15 Proximal convoluted
   tubules with
   brush borders

16 Glomerular arteriole
   (l.s.)

17 Visceral and
   parietal layers of
   glomerular capsule

18 Interlobular artery
   sectioned obliquely:
   wall and lumen

19 Collecting tubules

20 Straight (ascending)
   segments of distal
   tubules
21 Proximal and distal
   convoluted tubules

22 Collecting tubules

23 Thin segments of
   Henle's loops

24 Capillaries

Fig. 1.   *Deep cortical area and outer medulla.* Stain: hematoxylin-eosin.

1 Distal convoluted tubule

2 Glomerular capillaries

3 Glomerular arteriole

4 Juxtaglomerular cells

5 Macula densa

6 Proximal convoluted tubule

7 Interlobular vessels:
    venule
    arteriole

8 Collecting tubule

9 Basement membrane

10 Glomerular capsule:
   a Parietal layer
   b Visceral layer

11 Urinary pole

12 Afferent glomerular
   arteriole

13 Capsular space

14 Proximal convoluted tubule

15 Distal convoluted tubule

Fig. 2.   *Kidney cortex: The juxtaglomerular apparatus.* Stain: hematoxylin-eosin.

PLATE 89 (Fig. 1)

KIDNEY MEDULLA: PAPILLA (TRANSVERSE SECTION)

The papilla of the kidney contains the terminal portions of the collecting tubules, the papillary ducts (2, 5, 6). These ducts have large diameters and wide lumina and are lined by tall, pale-staining columnar cells. Also seen in this region are cross sections of the thin segments of the loops of Henle (3, 8) and the ascending straight portions of the distal tubules (1, 7). Connective tissue (10) is more abundant in this region than elsewhere in the kidney, and the collecting tubules are not as close together. Numerous small blood vessels (4, 9) are present. The thin segments of Henle's loop in cross section (3, 8) resemble the capillaries or venules (4, 9). In certain slide preparations, the numerous capillaries or venules (4, 9) can contain blood cells in their lumina, whereas the lumina of the thin segments of Henle's loop remain empty (3, 8).

PLATE 89 (Fig. 2)

PAPILLA ADJACENT TO A CALYX
(LONGITUDINAL SECTION)

Several collecting tubules merge in the medulla to form large, straight tubules called papillary ducts (5), which open at the tip of the papilla. Their numerous openings on the surface of the papilla produce a sieve-like appearance; this is the area cribrosa. In this illustration, the papilla is covered by a stratified cuboidal epithelium (8). At the area cribrosa, however, the covering epithelium is usually a simple columnar which is continuous with the lining of the papillary ducts. Also illustrated are thin segments of Henle's loops (3, 4, 6) and ascending straight portion of the distal tubule (1). Abundant connective tissue (7) and many capillaries (2) are also seen.

PLATE 89

KIDNEY MEDULLA: PAPILLA

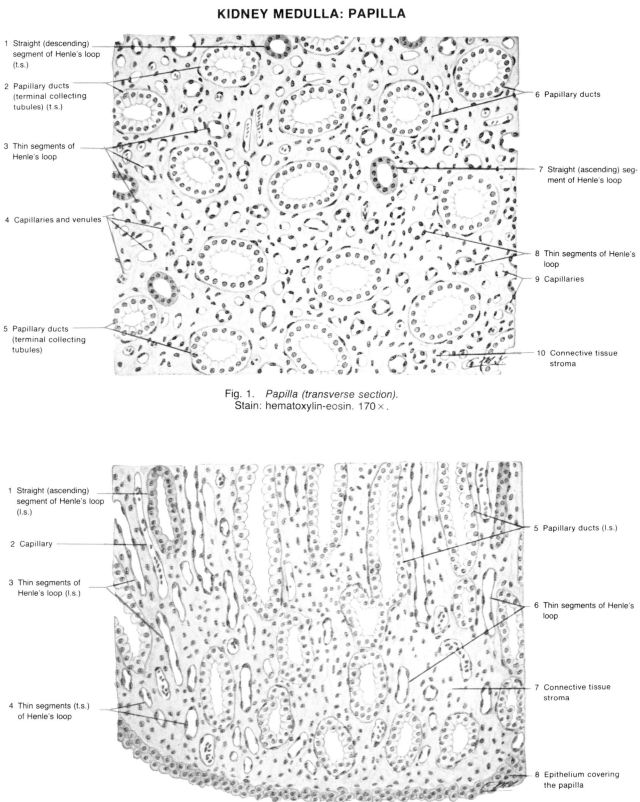

1 Straight (descending) segment of Henle's loop (t.s.)

2 Papillary ducts (terminal collecting tubules) (t.s.)

3 Thin segments of Henle's loop

4 Capillaries and venules

5 Papillary ducts (terminal collecting tubules)

6 Papillary ducts

7 Straight (ascending) segment of Henle's loop

8 Thin segments of Henle's loop

9 Capillaries

10 Connective tissue stroma

Fig. 1. *Papilla (transverse section).*
Stain: hematoxylin-eosin. 170 ×.

1 Straight (ascending) segment of Henle's loop (l.s.)

2 Capillary

3 Thin segments of Henle's loop (l.s.)

4 Thin segments (t.s.) of Henle's loop

5 Papillary ducts (l.s.)

6 Thin segments of Henle's loop

7 Connective tissue stroma

8 Epithelium covering the papilla

Fig. 2. *Papilla adjacent to a calyx, longitudinal section.*
Stain: hematoxylin-eosin. 120 ×.

PLATE 90 (Fig. 1)

URETER: TRANSVERSE SECTION

The undistended ureter exhibits a highly convoluted lumen; the convolutions are formed by the longitudinal mucosal folds. The wall of the ureter consists of mucosa, muscularis, and adventitia.

The mucosa consists of transitional epithelium (9, 10) and a wide lamina propria (5). The epithelium has several cell layers, with the outermost layer characterized by large cuboidal cells (9). The intermediate cells are polyhedral in shape, whereas the basal cells are low columnar or cuboidal (10). The basal surface of the epithelium is smooth; there are no connective tissue papillae indentations.

The wide lamina propria (5) contains fibroelastic connective tissue, which is denser, with more fibroblasts under the epithelium and looser near the muscularis. Diffuse lymphatic tissue and occasional small lymphatic nodules may be observed in the lamina propria.

In the upper part of the ureter, the muscularis consists of an inner longitudinal (3) and an outer circular smooth muscle layer (2); these layers are not always distinct. An additional outer, longitudinal layer of smooth muscle is present in the lower third of the ureter.

The adventitia (6) is continuous with the surrounding fibroelastic connective tissue and adipose tissue (1, 12), which contains numerous blood vessels (8, 11) and small nerves (7).

PLATE 90 (Fig. 2)

URETER WALL: TRANSVERSE SECTION

A higher magnification of the ureter wall illustrates in greater detail the structure of different layers. The transitional epithelium (8, 9, 10) exhibits the same cell layers as described in Figure 1. The outermost cells often stain deeper than the remaining cells. The surface membrane, illustrated as a narrow acidophilic band (9), serves as an osmotic barrier between urine and tissue fluids.

In the lamina propria (12), fibroblasts are more numerous in the connective tissue under the epithelium than in the deeper region.

The smooth muscle in the muscularis layer appears often in the form of loosely arranged bundles with abundant connective tissue, as illustrated in the inner longitudinal layer (11).

The adventitia (5) merges with the connective tissue (6) of the posterior abdominal wall in which the ureter is embedded.

PLATE 90

URETER

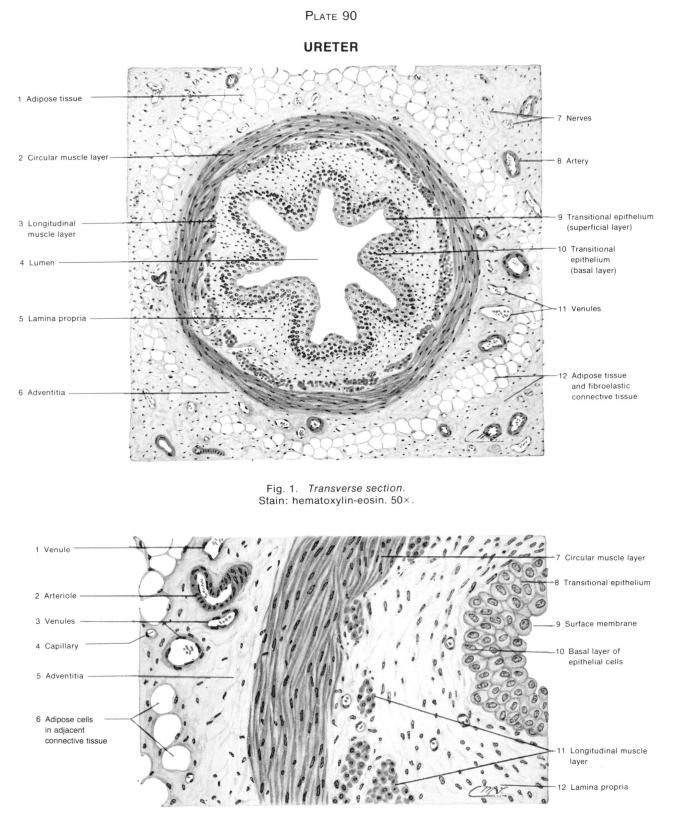

1 Adipose tissue

2 Circular muscle layer

3 Longitudinal muscle layer

4 Lumen

5 Lamina propria

6 Adventitia

7 Nerves

8 Artery

9 Transitional epithelium (superficial layer)

10 Transitional epithelium (basal layer)

11 Venules

12 Adipose tissue and fibroelastic connective tissue

Fig. 1. *Transverse section.*
Stain: hematoxylin-eosin. 50×.

1 Venule

2 Arteriole

3 Venules

4 Capillary

5 Adventitia

6 Adipose cells in adjacent connective tissue

7 Circular muscle layer

8 Transitional epithelium

9 Surface membrane

10 Basal layer of epithelial cells

11 Longitudinal muscle layer

12 Lamina propria

Fig. 2. *Ureter wall, transverse section.*
Stain: hematoxylin-eosin. 150×.

PLATE 91 (Fig. 1)

URINARY BLADDER, SUPERIOR SURFACE: WALL (TRANSVERSE SECTION)

The different layers in the bladder wall are similar to those observed in the ureter except for the thicker muscular wall (1).

The bladder wall consists of a mucosa (6–8), a muscularis (1, 9) and a serosa on the superior surface. The lower surface of the bladder is covered by adventitia, which merges with the connective tissue of adjacent structures.

The mucosa in an empty bladder exhibits numerous folds (6); however, these folds disappear during bladder distension. The transitional epithelium (7) has more cell layers and the lamina propria (8) is wider than that observed in the ureter. The loose connective tissue in the deeper zone contains more elastic fibers.

The muscularis (1, 9) is a thick layer, and in the neck of the bladder three layers are arranged in anastomosing bundles (1) between which is found loose connective tissue (2). In this section, the groups of muscle bundles are seen in various planes of section (1) and the three distinct muscle layers are difficult to distinguish. The interstitial connective tissue merges with the connective tissue of the serosa (4); mesothelium (5) is the outermost layer.

PLATE 91 (Fig. 2)

URINARY BLADDER: MUCOSA (TRANSVERSE SECTION)

The mucosa of the bladder is illustrated at a higher magnification.

In an empty bladder, the superficial cells of the transitional epithelium are low cuboidal or columnar (6). When the bladder is full or when the transitional epithelium is stretched over a fold, the cells exhibit a squamous appearance (9). The acidophilic surface membrane (7) of the superficial cells may be prominent. The deeper layers of cells are round (5) and basal cells more columnar (see also Plate 4).

In the lamina propria (2) are seen two zones, as in the ureter, but more pronounced. The subepithelial region is denser, with fine fibers and numerous fibroblasts (2, upper leader). The deeper zone (2, lower leader) contains typical loose or moderately dense irregular connective tissue which extends between the muscle fibers as interstitial connective tissue.

PLATE 91

URINARY BLADDER (SUPERIOR SURFACE)

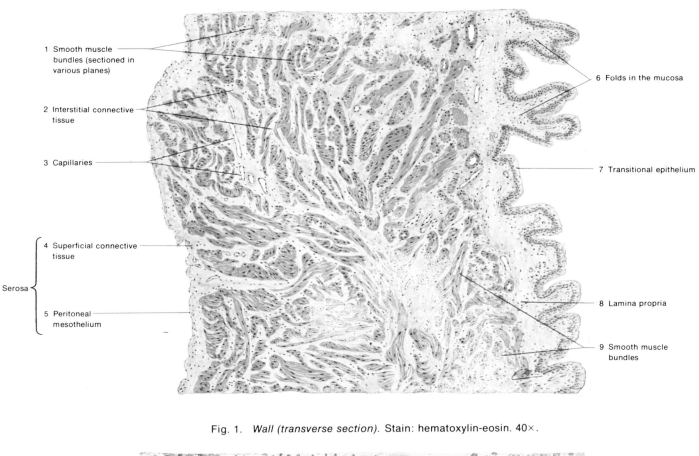

1 Smooth muscle bundles (sectioned in various planes)

2 Interstitial connective tissue

3 Capillaries

Serosa

4 Superficial connective tissue

5 Peritoneal mesothelium

6 Folds in the mucosa

7 Transitional epithelium

8 Lamina propria

9 Smooth muscle bundles

Fig. 1. *Wall (transverse section).* Stain: hematoxylin-eosin. 40×.

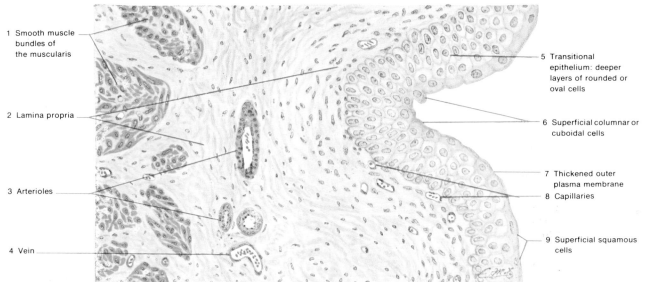

1 Smooth muscle bundles of the muscularis

2 Lamina propria

3 Arterioles

4 Vein

5 Transitional epithelium: deeper layers of rounded or oval cells

6 Superficial columnar or cuboidal cells

7 Thickened outer plasma membrane

8 Capillaries

9 Superficial squamous cells

Fig. 2. *Mucosa (transverse section).* Stain: hematoxylin-eosin. 160×.

PLATE 92 (Fig. 1)

HYPOPHYSIS (PITUITARY GLAND): PANORAMIC VIEW
(SAGITTAL SECTION)

The hypophysis consists of several different divisions: pars distalis (anterior lobe) (5), pars nervosa or infundibular process (11), pars intermedia (10), and pars tuberalis (9). The latter enfolds the infundibular stalk (8) and is therefore seen above and below the stalk in the sagittal plane of section.

The pars distalis (5) constitutes the largest of the four divisions of the hypophysis. Its glandular parenchyma is composed of two main types of cells, the chromophobe cells (1) and chromophil cells (3, 4). The chromophils are subdivided into acidophils (alpha) (3) and basophils (beta) cells (4). (See Fig. 2, below.) It is currently believed that the chromophobes represent acidophils or basophils in an inactive state following degranulation.

The pars nervosa (11) is the second largest of the four divisions. Pars nervosa and pars intermedia form the posterior lobe of the hypophysis, which consists primarily of unmyelinated nerve fibers and cells, the pituicytes. Numerous small connective tissue septa (12), arising from the capsule, penetrate into the gland.

The pars intermedia (10) is situated between the pars distalis and pars nervosa. This region contains colloid-filled cysts lined with different cells, with basophils predominant.

The pars tuberalis (9) surrounds the infundibular stalk (8), extending higher on the anterior than the posterior surface of the hypophysis. The infundibular stalk (8) connects the hypophysis with the central nervous system (base of the brain).

The pars nervosa is part of a larger region of the hypophysis, the neurohypophysis, which includes also the tuber cinerum of the median eminence and the infundibular stalk. The neurohypophysis develops as ventral evagination or extension from the floor of brain. On the other hand, the adenohypophysis develops from the oral ectoderm diverticulum, the pouch of Rathke, and includes the following divisions: pars distalis (5), pars intermedia (10), and par tuberalis (9).

PLATE 92 (Fig. 2)

HYPOPHYSIS (PITUITARY GLAND): SECTIONAL VIEW

Under higher magnification, different type of cells in the pars distalis are distinguished. The chromophobe cells (4) exhibit a light-staining, homogeneous cytoplasm. These cells are normally smaller than the chromophils and, in groups, their nuclei are closer together. The cytoplasm of chromophils stains red in acidophils (3) and blue in basophils (5).

Numerous sinusoidal capillaries (6) form a network in the pars distalis.

In pars intermedia are seen colloid-filled cysts or vesicles (7) lined by low columnar cells; some cells contain basophilic granules and others do not exhibit any granules in their cytoplasm. Follicles lined with basophils (8) are often present in pars intermedia. Some of the cells contain secretory granules in their cytoplasm (8, lower leader).

The pars nervosa is characterized by the presence of unmyelinated axons and cytoplasmic processes of the pituicytes, both of which stain lightly (9). Oval nuclei of the pituicytes are seen (10), but the scanty cytoplasm is usually not visible.

PLATE 92

HYPOPHYSIS (PITUITARY GLAND)

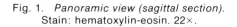

1 Group of chromophobe
  cells

2 Capsule

3 Cell group with
  predominance of
  acidophilic cells

4 Cell group with
  predominance of
  basophilic cells

5 Pars distalis

6 Sinusoidal capillaries

7 Veins

8 Infundibular stalk

9 Pars tuberalis

10 Pars intermedia with colloid
   vesicles

11 Pars nervosa
   (infundibular process)

12 Connective
   tissue septum

13 Blood vessels in
   the capsule

Fig. 1. *Panoramic view (sagittal section).*
Stain: hematoxylin-eosin. 22×.

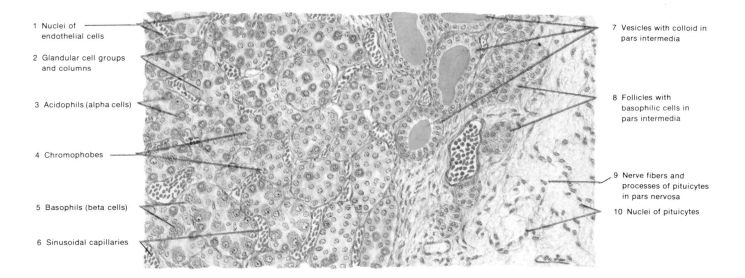

1 Nuclei of
  endothelial cells

2 Glandular cell groups
  and columns

3 Acidophils (alpha cells)

4 Chromophobes

5 Basophils (beta cells)

6 Sinusoidal capillaries

7 Vesicles with colloid in
  pars intermedia

8 Follicles with
  basophilic cells in
  pars intermedia

9 Nerve fibers and
  processes of pituicytes
  in pars nervosa

10 Nuclei of pituicytes

Fig. 2. *Sectional view.*
Stain: hematoxylin-eosin. 200×.

PLATE 93 (Fig. 1)

HYPOPHYSIS: PARS DISTALIS (AZAN STAIN)

Different cell types in the pars distalis are readily identified after the use of special fixatives and /or special stains. In the illustration, a corrosive sublimate mixture was used as a fixative. The section was then stained with azocarmine and differentiated with aniline oil. Phosphotungstic acid was then used to destain the connective tissue, followed by aniline blue and orange G as cytoplasmic stains. The cytoplasmic granules stain red, orange, or blue, depending on their respective affinities; the nuclei of all cells stain orange.

Chromophobes (3) usually stain light after any stain. Their nuclei stain pale and the cytoplasm pale orange, and the cell outlines remain poorly defined. The aggregation of chromophobes into groups or clumps is apparent in the illustration.

Two types of acidophils can be distinguished (although not as clearly as after other specific stains) by their staining reaction; cells with coarse granules stain red with azocarmine (1) and those with smaller granules stain with orange G (6).

Typical basophils are readily recognized by their blue-stained granules (2, 5), whereas the different types of basophils are not distinguishable. The degree of granularity and the stain density varies in different basophil cells.

PLATE 93 (Fig. 2)

HYPOPHYSIS: CELL GROUPS (AZAN STAIN)

Characteristic cells of the hypophysis after azan staining, as in Figure 1, are illustrated at higher magnification. Nuclei of all cells are stained orange-red.

In chromophobes (a), the light orange stain of the cytoplasm indicates its nongranular character and the indistinct cell boundaries. In the oval acidophils (b), the cytoplasmic granules stain intense red and the cell outlines are distinct. A sinusoid capillary is in close proximity to the acidophils.

The illustrated basophils (c) exhibit variable round, polyhedral, or angular shapes. The blue granules vary in size and are not as compact as in the acidophils.

The pituicytes (d) of pars nervosa exhibit variations in the shape and size of the cells and nuclei (1). The small, orange-stained cytoplasm sends out diffuse cytoplasmic processes (2) for varying distances.

PLATE 93

HYPOPHYSIS

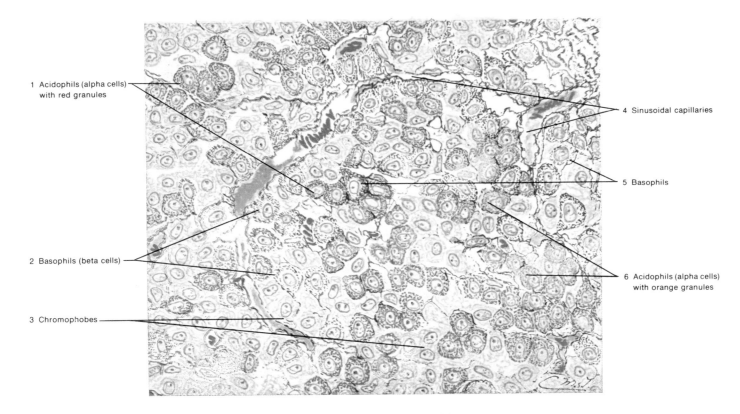

1 Acidophils (alpha cells) with red granules

4 Sinusoidal capillaries

5 Basophils

2 Basophils (beta cells)

6 Acidophils (alpha cells) with orange granules

3 Chromophobes

Fig. 1.   *Pars distalis (azan stain).*

Sectional view. Nuclei: orange; cytoplasmic granules of alpha cells: red or orange; cytoplasmic granules of beta cells: deep blue; collagenous and reticular fibers: blue; erythrocytes: bright red; hemolyzed blood: deep yellow. About 500×.

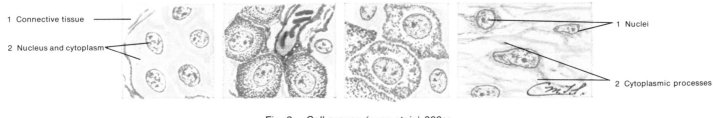

1 Connective tissue

2 Nucleus and cytoplasm

1 Nuclei

2 Cytoplasmic processes

Fig. 2.   *Cell groups (azan stain) 800×.*

a Chromophobes   b Acidophils (alpha cells)   c Basophils (beta cells)   d Pituicytes

PLATE 94 (Fig. 1)

THYROID GLAND (GENERAL VIEW)

The thyroid gland consists of various-sized, spherical follicles (1, 2, 5) that usually contain acidophilic colloid (2) material in their lumina. The follicular epithelium is simple columnar or cuboidal and consists primarily of the follicular or principal cells with large round nuclei. In routine histologic preparations, the colloid material often retracts from the follicular wall (1). Between the follicles are seen groups of cells without a lumen; these are the tangential sections through the follicular wall (4).

Connective tissue septa (6) arising from the thyroid gland capsule penetrate and divide the gland into groups of follicles or lobules. Relatively little connective tissue is found between individual follicles (6). In the connective tissue are found well developed capillary plexuses (3) closely associated with the follicular epithelium.

PLATE 94 (Fig. 2)

THYROID GLAND: FOLLICLES (SECTIONAL VIEW)

At a higher magnification, the epithelium of different follicles exhibits variable height; in some follicles, the cells are flattened (1), whereas in others, they are cuboidal or low columnar; the nuclei are vesicular. The appearance of the epithelium, the amount of colloid, and the size of the follicles vary with functional states of the gland.

As illustrated in Figure 1, most follicles are filled with acidophilic colloid material (5). In some follicles, the colloid is retracted (4); in others, the colloid contains vacuoles (7). Tangential sections through the walls of follicles (8) are seen as discrete clumps of cells within the interfollicular connective tissue. Capillaries (3) are prominent in the thyroid gland.

PLATE 94 (Fig. 3)

THYROID GLAND: PARAFOLLICULAR CELLS

Several follicles are illustrated at a higher magnification.

In addition to the follicular cells, the thyroid gland also contains parafollicular (3, 4) cells. These cells exhibit comparatively sparse distribution throughout the gland.

The parafollicular cells occur singly (3) or in groups (4) in the gland. They are situated within the follicles between the follicular cells and the basement membrane or in the interfollicular connective tissue. The parafollicular cells are larger than the follicular cells and oval or of variable shape, containing light, finely granular cytoplasm; they do not border directly on the follicular lumina.

PLATE 94

THYROID GLAND

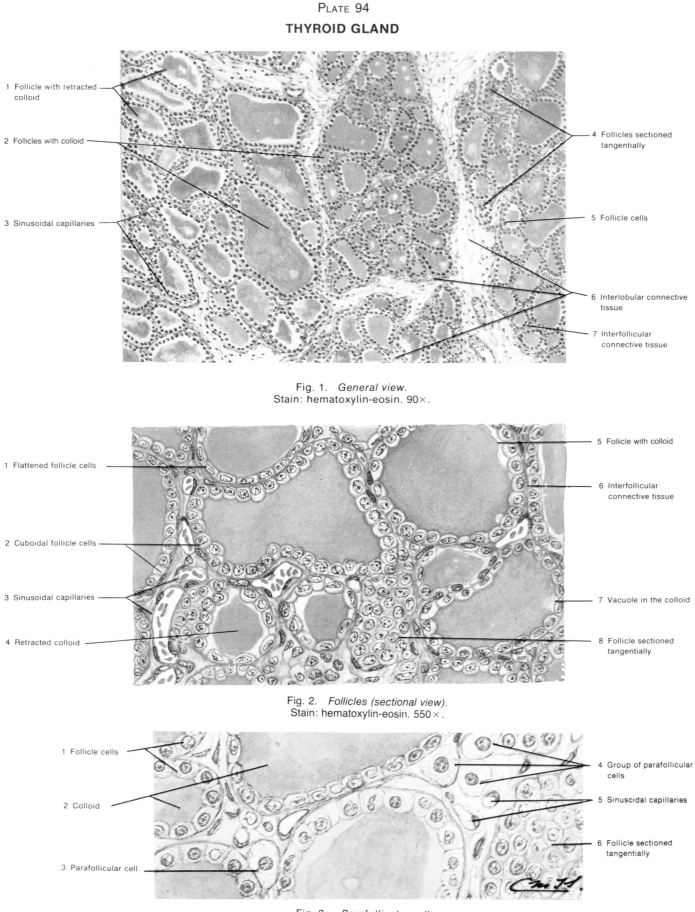

1 Follicle with retracted colloid

2 Follicles with colloid

3 Sinusoidal capillaries

4 Follicles sectioned tangentially

5 Follicle cells

6 Interlobular connective tissue

7 Interfollicular connective tissue

Fig. 1. *General view.*
Stain: hematoxylin-eosin. 90×.

1 Flattened follicle cells

2 Cuboidal follicle cells

3 Sinusoidal capillaries

4 Retracted colloid

5 Follicle with colloid

6 Interfollicular connective tissue

7 Vacuole in the colloid

8 Follicle sectioned tangentially

Fig. 2. *Follicles (sectional view).*
Stain: hematoxylin-eosin. 550×.

1 Follicle cells

2 Colloid

3 Parafollicular cell

4 Group of parafollicular cells

5 Sinusoidal capillaries

6 Follicle sectioned tangentially

Fig. 3. *Parafollicular cells.*
Stain: hematoxylin-eosin. 600×.

PLATE 95 (Fig. 1)

THYROID AND PARATHYROID GLANDS

The anatomical proximity of these two glands allows examination in the same section of their structural relationships and histologic differences.

A small section of the thyroid gland (7) is illustrated in the upper region. The various-sized follicles (1) contain colloid material and the surrounding connective tissue exhibits rich capillary network.

The thin connective tissue capsule (2, 8) of the thyroid gland separates the thyroid from the parathyroid (9) gland. This capsule also binds them together. From the capsule, trabeculae extend into the parathyroid gland (5, 6) and bring in the larger blood vessels (6), which then branch into an extensive capillary network among the parathyroid cells. Nerves accompany the blood vessels and the trabeculae may contain adipose cells (5).

The cells in the parathyroid gland are not arranged into follicles as seen in the thyroid gland; the cells are single and exhibit close arrangement. The majority of the cells, distributed in groups of various sizes, are the principal or chief cells (3). The larger oxyphil cells (4), seen in smaller groups, appear less frequent than the chief cells.

PLATE 95 (Fig. 2)

PARATHYROID GLAND

The characteristic features of the parathyroid gland are illustrated at a higher magnification.

The principal (chief) cells (1, 7) are the most numerous and are arranged in groups; capillaries course among the cell groups (5). The principal cells are round and exhibit a pale, slightly acidophilic cytoplasm; the nuclei are vesicular. Lighter, inactive principal (chief) cells and the darker, active principal cells (not illustrated) can be distinguished. Oxyphils (3, 6) occur singly or in small clusters. These cells are larger than the principal cells and exhibit granular, acidophilic cytoplasm and smaller, darker-staining nuclei. In adults, transitional forms are seen between oxyphils and principal cells. Oxyphil cells are not normally present in children under 4 years.

Colloid vesicles (2) are occasionally recorded in the gland.

Connective tissue trabeculae are present (4, 8), but do not form distinct lobules as in the thyroid gland.

PLATE 95

THYROID AND PARATHYROID GLANDS

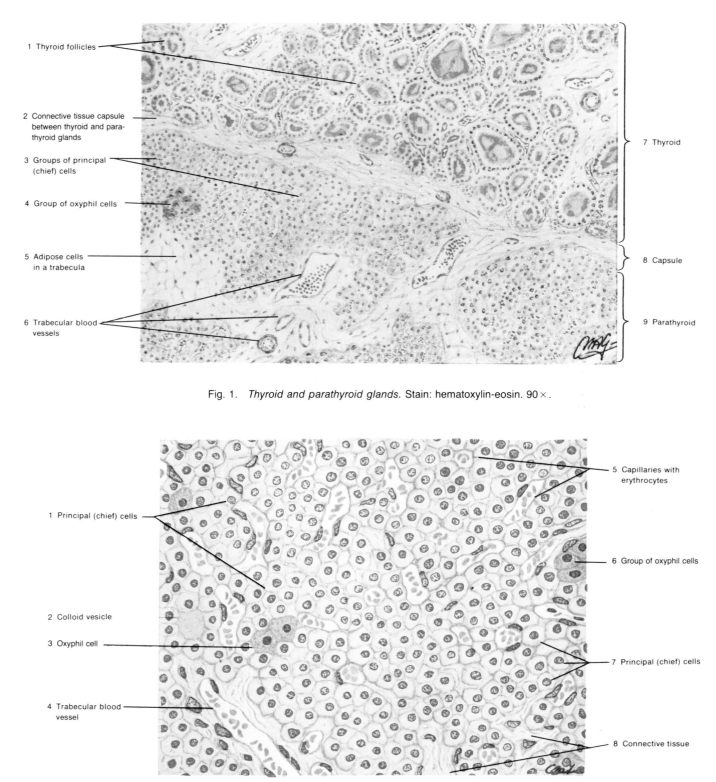

1 Thyroid follicles

2 Connective tissue capsule between thyroid and para- thyroid glands

3 Groups of principal (chief) cells

4 Group of oxyphil cells

5 Adipose cells in a trabecula

6 Trabecular blood vessels

7 Thyroid

8 Capsule

9 Parathyroid

Fig. 1. *Thyroid and parathyroid glands.* Stain: hematoxylin-eosin. 90 × .

1 Principal (chief) cells

2 Colloid vesicle

3 Oxyphil cell

4 Trabecular blood vessel

5 Capillaries with erythrocytes

6 Group of oxyphil cells

7 Principal (chief) cells

8 Connective tissue

Fig. 2. *Parathyroid gland.* Stain: hematoxylin-eosin. 550× .

PLATE 96

ADRENAL (SUPRARENAL) GLAND

The adrenal gland is encased in a thick connective tissue capsule (1) which contains branches of the main adrenal arteries, nerves (largely unmyelinated) (5), venules and lymphatics. Connective tissue trabeculae from the interior of the capsule pass into the cortex of the gland. The larger trabeculae carry arteries (4) to the medulla. Sinusoidal capillaries (7, 9) are found throughout the cortex and medulla.

The adrenal gland consists of an outer cortex (2) and an inner medulla (3).

The adrenal cortex is subdivided into three concentric zones which are not sharply demarcated from each other. The outer zone is the zona glomerulosa (2a), whose cells are arranged into ovoid groups. The cytoplasm of these cells (6) contains sparse lipid droplets which appear as vacuoles in the hematoxylin-eosin preparations; the nuclei stain dark. Sinusoidal capillaries (7) course between the cell groups. The middle layer is the zona fasciculata (2b). The cells of this layer (2b) are arranged into columns or plates with radial arrangement. Increased amount of lipid droplets in the cytoplasm give the cells a vacuolated appearance (8) after normal histologic preparation; the term spongiocytes is derived from this appearance of the cells (8). The nuclei are vesicular. Sinusoidal capillaries (9) between the cell columns follow a similar radial course. The layer bordering the adrenal medulla is the zona reticularis (2c). Cells of this layer form anastomosing cords and are frequently filled with lipofuscin pigment (11). The capillaries exhibit an irregular arrangement.

The medulla is not sharply demarcated from the cortex. The cells that constitute the majority of the medulla (3, 14) are arranged in groups. The cytoplasm is clear (14); however, following tissue fixation in potassium bichromate, fine brown granules become visible. This cellular alteration, termed the chromaffin reaction, indicates the presence of the catecholamines epinephrine and norepinephrine in the granules. The medulla also contains sympathetic ganglion cells (13), seen singly or in small groups. They exhibit the characteristic vesicular nucleus, prominent nucleolus, and a small amount of peripheral chromatin. Sinusoidal capillaries are also present in the medulla and drain its contents into the medullary veins (12).

PLATE 96

ADRENAL (SUPRARENAL) GLAND

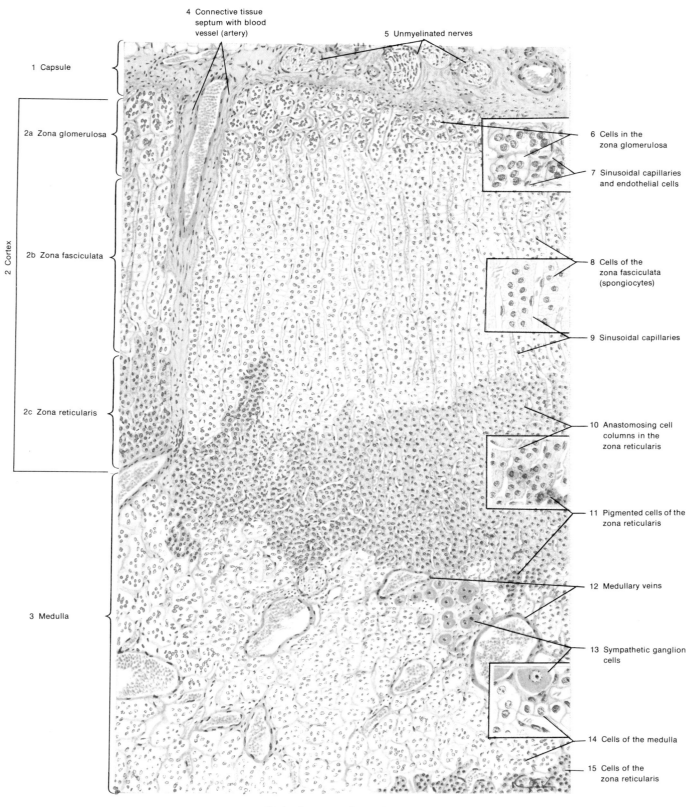

4 Connective tissue septum with blood vessel (artery)

5 Unmyelinated nerves

1 Capsule

2 Cortex

2a Zona glomerulosa

2b Zona fasciculata

2c Zona reticularis

3 Medulla

6 Cells in the zona glomerulosa

7 Sinusoidal capillaries and endothelial cells

8 Cells of the zona fasciculata (spongiocytes)

9 Sinusoidal capillaries

10 Anastomosing cell columns in the zona reticularis

11 Pigmented cells of the zona reticularis

12 Medullary veins

13 Sympathetic ganglion cells

14 Cells of the medulla

15 Cells of the zona reticularis

Stain: hematoxylin-eosin. 200×.

PLATE 97 (Fig. 1)

TESTIS

The testis is enclosed in a thick, connective tissue capsule, the tunica albuginea (1). Internal to this capsule is a layer of loose connective tissue with numerous blood vessels, the tunica vasculosa (2). This layer merges with the stroma of the testis, the interstitial connective tissue (7), which is rich in blood vessels (10). The connective tissue binds and supports the seminiferous tubules (3, 4, 9).

The seminiferous tubules are long, convoluted tubules that can be seen sectioned in various planes in a given section of the testis (3, 4, 9). They are lined with a specialized stratified epithelium called the germinal epithelium, which consists of two types of cells, the spermatogenic cells and the Sertoli cells. These cells rest on a thin basement membrane (5). (See Plate 98 for detailed structure.)

In the interstitial connective tissue between the seminiferous tubules are groups of endocrine cells, the interstitial cells or Leydig cells (8). These cells secrete the male sex hormone, testosterone.

PLATE 97 (Fig. 2)

SEMINIFEROUS TUBULES, STRAIGHT TUBULES, RETE TESTIS AND DUCTULI EFFERENTES (EFFERENT DUCTS)

The illustration includes a section through the mediastinum of the testis, a small section of the testis proper, and the ductuli efferentes.

Seminiferous tubules (1) are illustrated on the left, lined with spermatogenic cells and the supporting Sertoli cells. The interstitial connective tissue is continuous with the connective tissue of the mediastinum (3). In the mediastinum, the seminiferous tubules of each lobule converge to form straight tubules (2), which are short, narrow ducts lined with cuboidal or low columnar epithelium.

The straight tubules pass into the tubules of rete testis (4) located in the connective tissue of the mediastinum (3). The rete testis are irregular, anastomosing tubules with wide lumina lined by a single layer of low cuboidal or low columnar epithelium (6); the tubules become wider near the ductuli efferentes (efferent ducts) (5) into which they empty. The ductuli efferentes are straight; however, as they pass into the head of the epididymis, they become highly convoluted. (See Plate 99, Fig. 1.)

PLATE 97

TESTIS

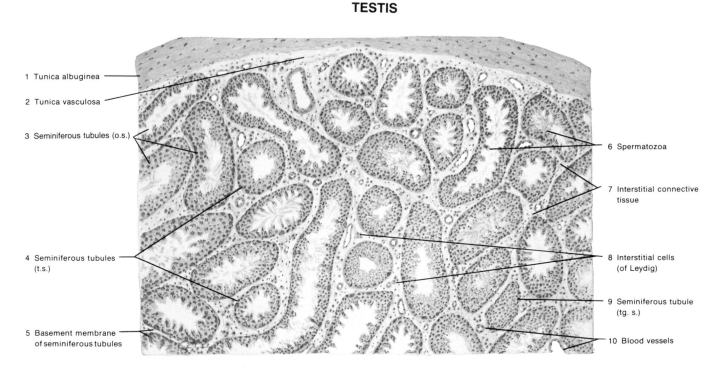

1 Tunica albuginea

2 Tunica vasculosa

3 Seminiferous tubules (o.s.)

4 Seminiferous tubules (t.s.)

5 Basement membrane of seminiferous tubules

6 Spermatozoa

7 Interstitial connective tissue

8 Interstitial cells (of Leydig)

9 Seminiferous tubule (tg. s.)

10 Blood vessels

Fig. 1. *Testis. Sectional view.* Stain: hematoxylin-eosin. 70×.

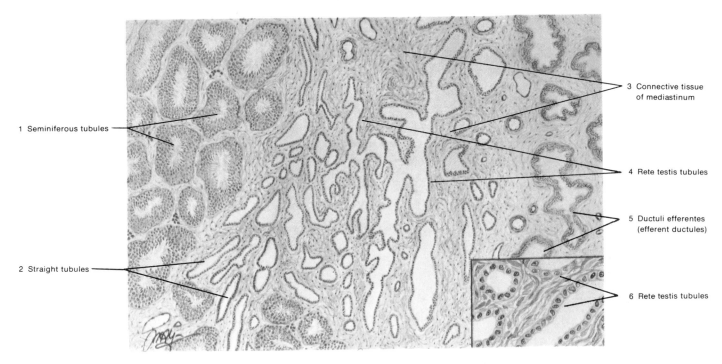

1 Seminiferous tubules

2 Straight tubules

3 Connective tissue of mediastinum

4 Rete testis tubules

5 Ductuli efferentes (efferent ductules)

6 Rete testis tubules

Fig. 2. *Seminiferous tubules, straight tubules, rete testis, and ductuli efferentes (efferent ducts).* Stain: hematoxylin-eosin. 60× and 400×.

PLATE 98

TESTIS: SEMINIFEROUS TUBULES (TRANSVERSE SECTION)

Transverse sections of several seminiferous tubules are illustrated. Between the tubules in the interstitial connective tissue are fibroblasts (2), blood vessels (4, 12, 25), nerves, and lymphatics. Also present between the seminiferous tubules are the interstitial cells (Leydig cells), which occur singly or in groups (3). These cells are large, round, or polygonal with granular cytoplasms and distinct, round nuclei (3). The interstitial cells constitute the endocrine component of the testis because they synthesize and secrete the male sex hormone testosterone.

Each seminiferous tubule is surrounded by an outer layer of compact connective tissue with flattened fibroblasts and an inner basement membrane (6). Enclosed by the basement membrane is the specialized germinal epithelium of the seminiferous tubules consisting of two cell types, namely, the supporting or Sertoli cells and the spermatogenic cells. These cells are clearly seen in a transverse section of the seminiferous tubule (5).

The Sertoli cells are slender, elongated cells with very irregular outlines extending from the basement membrane to the free luminal surface (19, 32). The distinctive nucleus is ovoid or angular in shape, clearly outlined with fine, sparse chromatin and contains one or more prominent nucleoli; the nucleoli may vary in position in different cells. In tangential sections of the tubules (15), the Sertoli cells are seen as round cross sections (16).

Spermatogenic cells are arranged in rows between and around the Sertoli cells; in different sections, the spermatogenic cells often appear superimposed on Sertoli cells, obscuring their cytoplasm (8, 13). The most primitive or immature spermatogenic cells, the spermatogonia (17, 18), are situated adjacent to the basement membrane of the seminiferous tubules. Spermatogonia divide mitotically (1, 21) to produce several generations of cells. Viewed under high magnification, three types of spermatogonia are usually recognized in the human testis. The pale type A (27) spermatogonia exhibit a light-staining cytoplasm and a round or ovoid nucleus with pale-staining, finely granular chromatin dispersed throughout the nucleus. One or two nucleoli may be attached to the nuclear membrane. A second, dark type A spermatogonia (not illustrated) is similar, but the chromatin stains darker. In type B spermatogonia (28), the chromatin granules in the spherical nucleus vary in size and are distributed along the nuclear membrane. A central nucleolus (not illustrated) is centrally located.

Type A spermatogonia serve as stem cells and give rise to other type A and type B spermatogonia. The final mitosis of type B spermatogonia gives rise to primary spermatocytes (11, 22), which become situated adjacent to the spermatogonia and nearer to the tubular lumen. Their nuclei have variable appearances (11, 22) due to different states of activity of the chromatin. These cells promptly enter the first meiotic division, and representative meiotic figures (7) are prevalent in the tubules. The reorganization of their chromatin into thin chromosomes indicates the leptotene stage (29). An increase in size and thickening of the chromosomes (and darker staining) due to pairing indicates the zygotene stage (30). The pachytene stage (31) is characterized by further increase in cell size and shorter, thicker, and more obvious chromosome strands. Primary spermatocytes, the largest germ cells in the seminiferous tubules, occupy the middle of the germinal epithelium. The primary spermatocytes, by meiotic division, give rise to secondary spermatocytes.

The secondary spermatocytes are distinctly smaller than the primary spermatocytes and the nuclear chromatin is less dense (23, 33). These cells divide soon after their formation and are not frequently seen in stained sections. This second meiotic (maturation) division gives rise to spermatids.

The spermatids are smaller cells (24) with small nuclei containing fine as well as larger chromatin granules. These cells lie in groups in the luminal portion of the seminiferous tubule epithelium (24). The cells become closely associated with the surface of Sertoli cells, and in this environment differentiate into spermatozoa (26; 34a, b, c) by a process called spermiogenesis.

The small, deep-staining heads of spermatozoa are embedded in the cytoplasm of the Sertoli cells (20), while their tails extend into the lumen of the seminiferous tubule. A mature spermatozoan in profile and frontal view is illustrated (35a and b).

PLATE 98

TESTIS: SEMINIFEROUS TUBULES (TRANSVERSE SECTION)

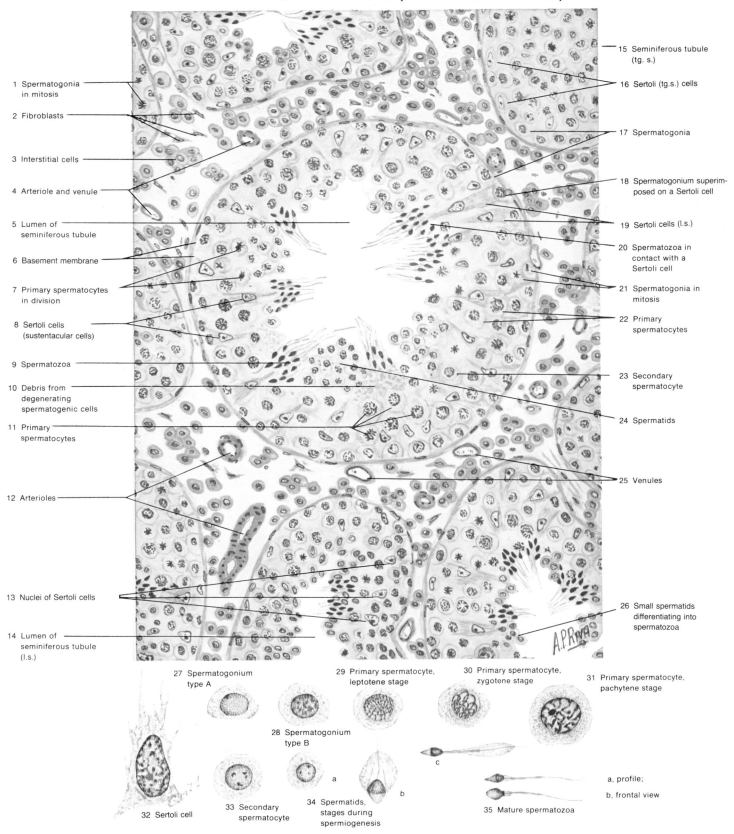

1 Spermatogonia in mitosis

2 Fibroblasts

3 Interstitial cells

4 Arteriole and venule

5 Lumen of seminiferous tubule

6 Basement membrane

7 Primary spermatocytes in division

8 Sertoli cells (sustentacular cells)

9 Spermatozoa

10 Debris from degenerating spermatogenic cells

11 Primary spermatocytes

12 Arterioles

13 Nuclei of Sertoli cells

14 Lumen of seminiferous tubule (l.s.)

15 Seminiferous tubule (tg. s.)

16 Sertoli (tg.s.) cells

17 Spermatogonia

18 Spermatogonium superimposed on a Sertoli cell

19 Sertoli cells (l.s.)

20 Spermatozoa in contact with a Sertoli cell

21 Spermatogonia in mitosis

22 Primary spermatocytes

23 Secondary spermatocyte

24 Spermatids

25 Venules

26 Small spermatids differentiating into spermatozoa

27 Spermatogonium type A

28 Spermatogonium type B

29 Primary spermatocyte, leptotene stage

30 Primary spermatocyte, zygotene stage

31 Primary spermatocyte, pachytene stage

32 Sertoli cell

33 Secondary spermatocyte

34 Spermatids, stages during spermiogenesis

35 Mature spermatozoa

a, profile;

b, frontal view

Stain: hematoxylin-eosin. 300× and 1000×.

PLATE 99 (Fig. 1)

DUCTULI EFFERENTES AND TRANSITION TO DUCTUS EPIDIDYMIS

The ductuli efferentes or efferent ducts (1, 5) emerge from the mediastinum on the posterior-superior surface of the testis and connect the rete testis with the ductus epididymis. The ductuli efferentes are located in the connective tissue and form a portion of the head of the epididymis (2). Due to the tortuous, spiral course of the tubules, they are seen as isolated tubules cut in various planes of section (1, 5).

The lumina of the ducts exhibit a characteristic irregular contour (4). The lining epithelium is simple, consisting of alternating groups of tall ciliated and shorter nonciliated cells (4), which are believed to be absorptive. Occasional basal cells may be present, giving the epithelium a pseudo-stratified appearance. The basal surface of the tubules has a smooth contour. Located under the basement membrane is a thin layer of connective tissue containing a thin layer of circularly arranged smooth muscle fibers (3).

The distal ends of the tubules near the epididymis are lined with columnar cells only (6), and the lumina exhibit an even contour. As the ductuli efferentes terminate in the ductus epididymis, there is an abrupt transition of the epithelium to tall pseudostratified columnar type.

PLATE 99 (Fig. 2)

DUCTUS EPIDIDYMIS

The ductus epididymis is a long, highly convoluted tubule surrounded by the connective tissue. A transverse section of the epididymis illustrates the convoluted tubules as varied individual sections (2, 5, 6) surrounded by smooth muscle fibers (7) and connective tissue (1). Both the internal and external surfaces of epithelium have smooth contours.

The tubular epithelium is pseudostratified (4), consisting of very tall columnar principal cells (9) with long, nonmotile stereocilia (8) and small basal cells (10). The function of the columnar principal cells (9) with stereocilia (8) is primarily absorption of the tubular fluid; the function of the basal cells is not known. The stereocilia (8) are long, branched microvilli.

The basement membrane (3) surrounding the tubules is distinct. The lamina propria with the circularly arranged smooth muscle fibers (7) is thin and more pronounced than in the ductuli efferentes.

Spermatozoa clumps are seen in the lumina of some of the tubules.

PLATE 99

TESTIS

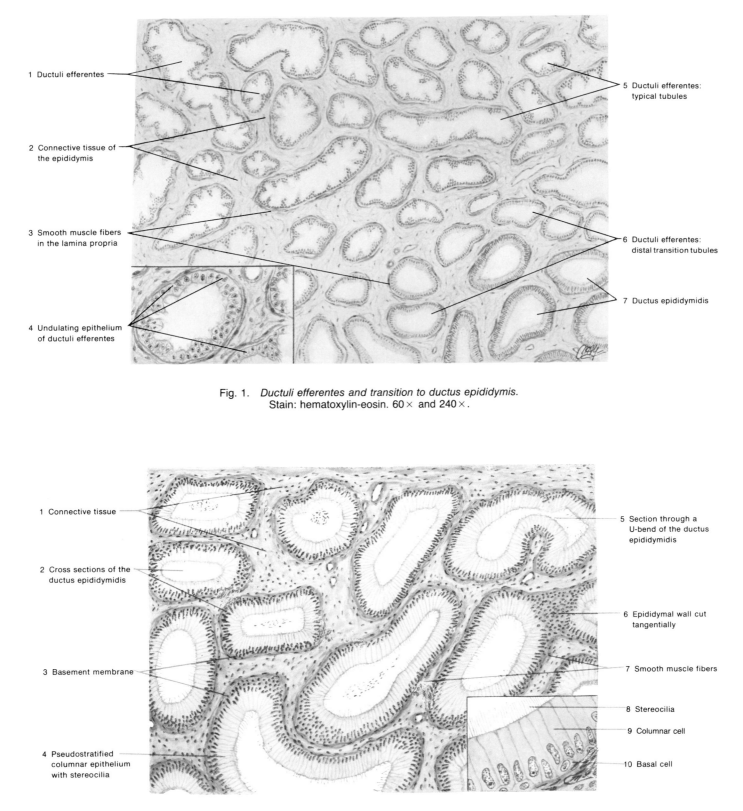

1 Ductuli efferentes

2 Connective tissue of
the epididymis

3 Smooth muscle fibers
in the lamina propria

4 Undulating epithelium
of ductuli efferentes

5 Ductuli efferentes:
typical tubules

6 Ductuli efferentes:
distal transition tubules

7 Ductus epididymidis

Fig. 1. *Ductuli efferentes and transition to ductus epididymis.*
Stain: hematoxylin-eosin. 60× and 240×.

1 Connective tissue

2 Cross sections of the
ductus epididymidis

3 Basement membrane

4 Pseudostratified
columnar epithelium
with stereocilia

5 Section through a
U-bend of the ductus
epididymidis

6 Epididymal wall cut
tangentially

7 Smooth muscle fibers

8 Stereocilia

9 Columnar cell

10 Basal cell

Fig. 2. *Ductus epididymis.* Stain: hematoxylin-eosin. 90×.

PLATE 100 (Fig. 1)

TESTIS: DUCTUS DEFERENS (TRANSVERSE SECTION)

The ductus deferens exhibits a narrow, irregular lumen, a thin mucosa, and a thick muscularis surrounded by adventitia. The irregular outline of the lumen is due to longitudinal folds of the lamina propria (5, 6) which, in transverse section, appear as crests or papillae (6).

The epithelium is pseudostratified columnar (7) but is lower than in the ductus epididymis. The epithelium rests on a thin basement membrane and stereocilia is usually present on the cells. The thin lamina propria (5, 6) contains compact collagenous fibers and fine elastic network.

The muscularis consists of a thin inner longitudinal layer (3), a thick middle circular layer (2), and a thin outer longitudinal smooth muscle layer (1). The muscularis is surrounded by adventitia (4), which contains abundant blood vessels and nerves. The adventitia merges with the connective tissue surrounding the spermatic cord.

PLATE 100 (Fig. 2)

AMPULLA OF THE DUCTUS DEFERENS

The terminal portion of ductus deferens forms an enlargement, the ampulla. The ampulla differs from the ductus deferens mainly in the structure of its mucosa.

The lumen of the ampulla is larger and the mucosa exhibits numerous thin, irregular, branching folds (6) with diverticula or crypts (5, 9) located between them. The epithelium lining the lumen and the crypts is simple columnar or cuboidal (7) and is secretory in nature.

The muscularis is similar to the ductus deferens: a thin outer longitudinal layer (3), thick middle layer (2), and thin inner longitudinal layer (1) adjacent to the lamina propria.

PLATE 100

TESTIS

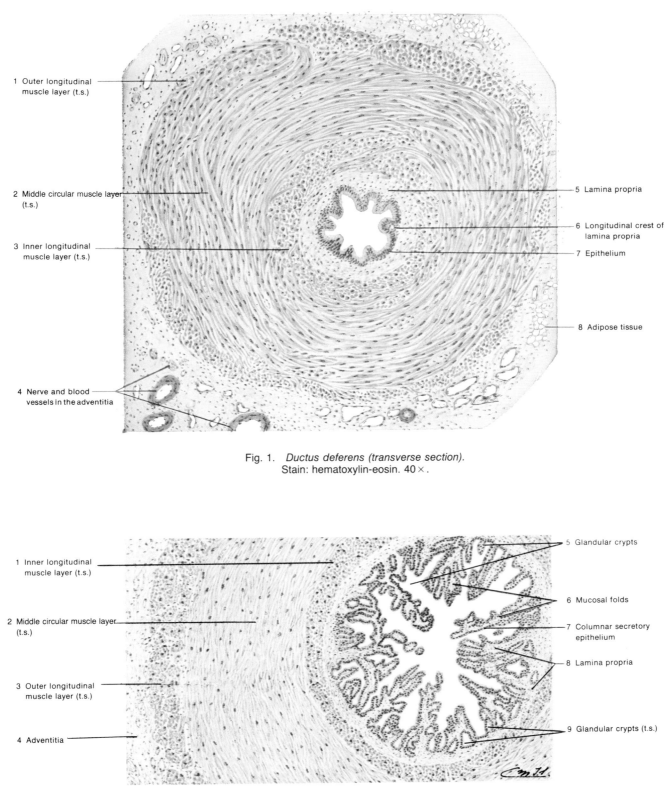

Fig. 1. *Ductus deferens (transverse section).*
Stain: hematoxylin-eosin. 40 ×.

1 Outer longitudinal muscle layer (t.s.)

2 Middle circular muscle layer (t.s.)

3 Inner longitudinal muscle layer (t.s.)

4 Nerve and blood vessels in the adventitia

5 Lamina propria

6 Longitudinal crest of lamina propria

7 Epithelium

8 Adipose tissue

Fig. 2. *Ampulla of the ductus deferens (transverse section).*
Stain: hematoxylin-eosin. 60 ×.

1 Inner longitudinal muscle layer (t.s.)

2 Middle circular muscle layer (t.s.)

3 Outer longitudinal muscle layer (t.s.)

4 Adventitia

5 Glandular crypts

6 Mucosal folds

7 Columnar secretory epithelium

8 Lamina propria

9 Glandular crypts (t.s.)

PLATE 101 (Fig. 1)

PROSTATE GLAND WITH PROSTATIC URETHRA

Illustrated in Figure 1 are the prostate gland, prostatic urethra, colliculus seminalis, and prostatic utricle.

In the prostate gland, the alveoli (4, 5) are part of the many small, irregular branched tubuloalveolar glands; the alveoli vary in size (4, 5). The larger-sized alveoli exhibit wide, irregular lumina (4) and variable epithelium (see Fig. 2).

The glands are embedded in a characteristic, fibromuscular stroma (3, 6) in which strands of smooth muscle (6), collagen, and elastic fibers are oriented in various directions.

The prostatic urethra (1) is illustrated as a crescent-shaped structure with small diverticula along its lumen (8); the diverticula are especially prominent in the urethral recesses (9).

The epithelium in the prostatic urethra is usually transitional. The fibromuscular stroma of the prostate gland surrounds the urethra; however, a thin lamina propria may be present.

A ridge of dense fibromuscular stroma without glands, the colliculus seminalis (2), protrudes into the urethral lumen, giving it a crescent shape. The prostatic utricle (10) is situated in the mass of the colliculus and is often dilated at its distal end (7) before entering the urethra. Its thin mucous membrane is typically folded and the epithelium is usually simple secretory or pseudostratified columnar.

The ejaculatory ducts (11) enter the prostate gland, course beside the utriculus (10) and open into the prostatic urethra.

PLATE 101 (Fig. 2)

PROSTATE GLAND: SECTIONAL VIEW
(SECTION FROM MAIN PROSTATIC GLANDS IN FIG. 1)

A small section of the prostate gland from Figure 1 is illustrated at a higher magnification to show more detail in the glands and stroma.

The alveolar (1) size is variable and the lumina are wide and typically irregular due to the epithelium-covered connective tissue folds (5) which protrude into their lumina. A characteristic feature in the alveoli are the spherical prostatic concretions (8) formed by concentric layers of condensed prostatic secretions. The number of prostatic concretions increases with the age of the individual, and they may become calcified.

Although the epithelium (4) in the glands is usually simple columnar or pseudostratified and the cells are light-staining in the distal regions, there is considerable variation. In some regions, the epithelium may be squamous or cuboidal.

Ducts of the glands may resemble the alveoli, and it is often difficult to distinguish the difference between the two structures. In the terminal portions of the ducts, the epithelium is usually columnar and stains darker (7) before entering the urethra.

The fibromuscular stroma (6) is a characteristic feature of the prostate gland. Smooth muscle fibers (3) and the connective tissue (9) can, at times, be distinguished; however, they blend together in the stroma (6) and are distributed throughout the gland.

PLATE 101

PROSTATE GLAND

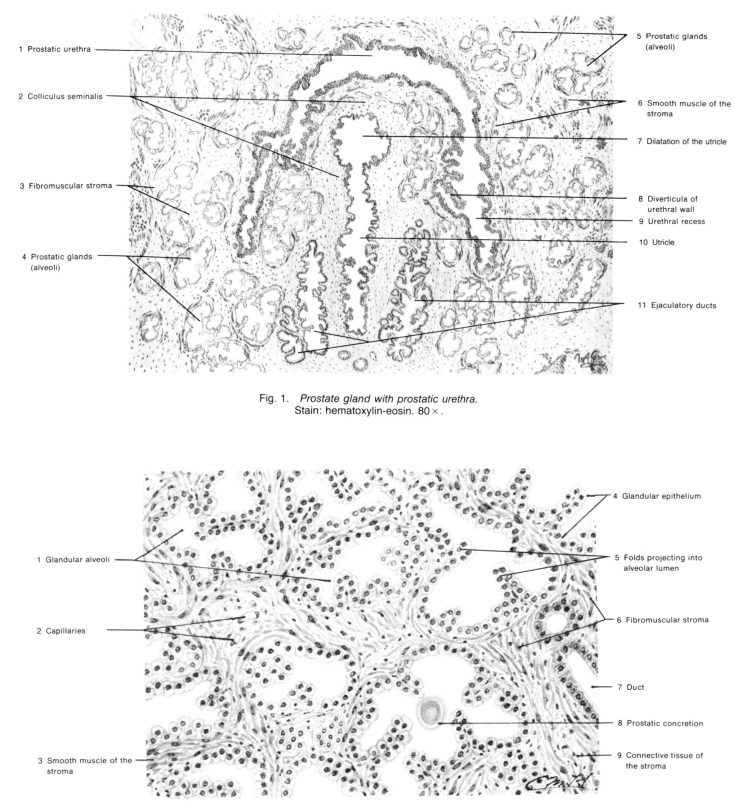

1 Prostatic urethra

2 Colliculus seminalis

3 Fibromuscular stroma

4 Prostatic glands (alveoli)

5 Prostatic glands (alveoli)

6 Smooth muscle of the stroma

7 Dilatation of the utricle

8 Diverticula of urethral wall

9 Urethral recess

10 Utricle

11 Ejaculatory ducts

Fig. 1. *Prostate gland with prostatic urethra.*
Stain: hematoxylin-eosin. 80 ×.

1 Glandular alveoli

2 Capillaries

3 Smooth muscle of the stroma

4 Glandular epithelium

5 Folds projecting into alveolar lumen

6 Fibromuscular stroma

7 Duct

8 Prostatic concretion

9 Connective tissue of the stroma

Fig. 2. *Prostate gland: sectional view (section from main prostatic glands in Fig. 1).* Stain: hematoxylin-eosin. 180 ×.

PLATE 102 (Fig. 1)

SEMINAL VESICLE

The seminal vesicles are elongated bodies or sacs with highly convoluted and irregular lumina. A section through the wall illustrates the complexity of the primary folds (5). These branch into numerous secondary folds (6) which frequently anastomose, forming crypts and cavities (1). Lamina propria forms the core of the larger folds (5) and thin stroma of smaller folds (6). The folds extend far into the lumen of the seminal vesicle.

The epithelium (4) varies in appearance but is usually low pseudostratified with basal cells and low columnar or cuboidal secretory cells. The thin lamina propria (7) projects into the folds.

The muscularis (2) consists of inner circular and outer longitudinal muscle layers. This arrangement is often difficult to observe due to the complex folding of the mucosa. The adventitia (3) surrounds the muscularis and blends with the surrounding connective tissue.

PLATE 102 (Fig. 2)

BULBOURETHRAL GLAND

This is a compound tubuloalveolar gland. One lobule and portions of other lobules of the gland are illustrated in this figure. The gland is surrounded by skeletal muscle (2) and connective tissue. Skeletal and some smooth muscle fibers are also present in the interlobular septa (3).

The secretory units vary in structure and size. Most of the units have an alveolar shape (4) and others exhibit tubular (5) or various other shapes. The secretory product is primarily mucus (4). The secretory cells are cuboidal, low columnar or squamous, and light-staining. Interspersed among the secretory cells are darker-staining acidophilic cells.

Smaller excretory ducts may be lined with secretory cells, and the larger ducts (6) exhibit pseudostratified or stratified columnar epithelium.

PLATE 102

SEMINAL VESICLE AND BULBOURETHRAL GLAND

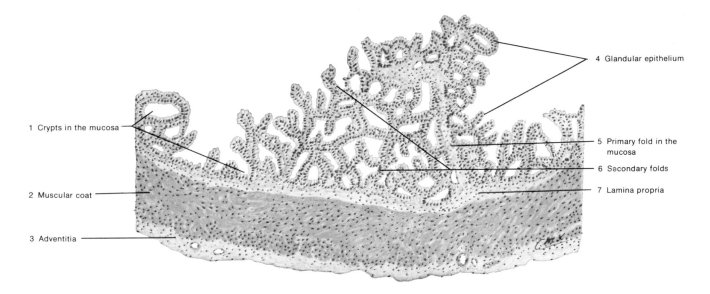

1 Crypts in the mucosa

4 Glandular epithelium

5 Primary fold in the mucosa

6 Secondary folds

2 Muscular coat

7 Lamina propria

3 Adventitia

Fig. 1. *Seminal vesicle.* Stain: hematoxylin-eosin. 60×.

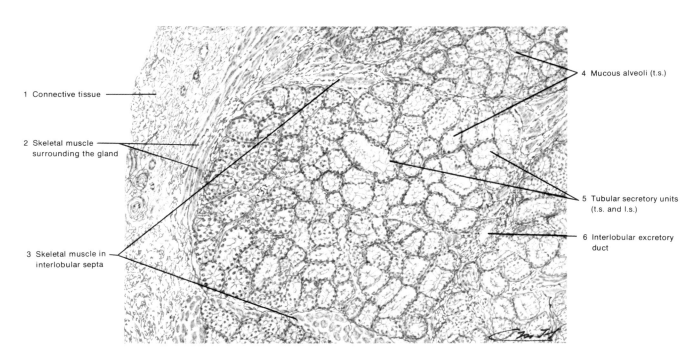

1 Connective tissue

4 Mucous alveoli (t.s.)

2 Skeletal muscle surrounding the gland

5 Tubular secretory units (t.s. and l.s.)

6 Interlobular excretory duct

3 Skeletal muscle in interlobular septa

Fig. 2. *Bulbourethral gland. Sectional view.*
Stain: Masson's stain. 350×.

PLATE 103 (Fig. 1)

HUMAN PENIS (TRANSVERSE SECTION)

A cross section of the penis illustrates the three cavernous bodies: the two adjacent corpora cavernosa (9) and a single corpus spongiosum (16) around the urethra (15). Surrounding the two larger corpora cavernosa is a thick, fibrous connective tissue capsule, the tunica albuginea (5), which also extends between the two corpora cavernosa as the median septum (10) of the penis. This septum is better developed at the posterior end of the penis than at the anterior end. The tunica albuginea surrounding the corpus spongiosum (6) is thinner than that around the corpora cavernosa and contains smooth muscle and elastic fibers.

All three cavernous bodies are surrounded by loose connective tissue, the deep penile fascia (Buck's fascia) (4) which, in turn, is surrounded by the connective tissue of the dermis (2) which lies under the epidermis (1). Strands of smooth muscle, the dartos tunic (3), and an abundance of peripheral blood vessels are located in the dermis. Sebaceous glands (7) are present in the dermis on the ventral side of the penis.

The core of each corpus cavernosum is occupied by numerous trabeculae (14) which consist of collagenous, elastic and smooth muscle fibers. These surround the cavernous cavities or sinuses (veins) (12) of corpora cavernosa. Nerves and blood vessels are found in the trabeculae. The cavities or sinuses of the corpora cavernosa (12) are lined with endothelium and receive blood from the dorsal (8) and deep arteries (11). Arterial branches of the latter open into the cavernous cavities. The corpus spongiosum (corpora cavernosa urethrae) receives its blood supply largely from the bulbourethral artery, a branch of the internal pudendal artery. Blood that leaves the cavernous cavities exits mainly through the superficial veins (13) in the vascularized dermis (2) and the deep dorsal vein.

The urethra is designated as the spongiosa (15) or cavernous urethra. Toward the base of the penis, the urethra is lined with pseudostratified or stratified columnar epithelium; however, at the external orifice, the epithelium becomes stratified squamous.

Not apparent at this magnification are the numerous small but deep invaginations of the mucous membrane, the urethral lacunae of Morgagni, which contain mucous cells. Branched tubular urethral glands of Littré open into these recesses (see Fig. 2).

PLATE 103 (Fig. 2)

CAVERNOUS URETHRA (TRANSVERSE SECTION)

A major portion of the cavernous urethra is illustrated; it has a pseudostratified or stratified columnar epithelium (5) lining. A thin lamina propria (3) merges with the surrounding connective tissue of the corpus spongiosum.

Numerous various-sized mucosal outpockets (3) give the urethral lumen (4) an irregular form. Some of these outpockets or lacunae of Morgagni contain mucous cells (9). The deeper lacunae (6) in the urethra give rise to branched tubular glands of Littré (7), which extend into lamina propria or corpus spongiosum (7, lowest leader).

The urethral glands are lined with the same type of epithelium as that which lines the lumen (stratified columnar in this illustration); the superficial cells are mucus-secreting.

The corpus spongiosum surrounds the urethra and its internal structure is similar to that of the corpora cavernosa described above in Figure 1. In the illustration are seen the characteristic trabeculae (1, 11) of connective tissue and smooth muscle between cavernous veins (2, 8, 10).

PLATE 103

PENIS AND CAVERNOUS URETHRA

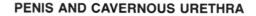

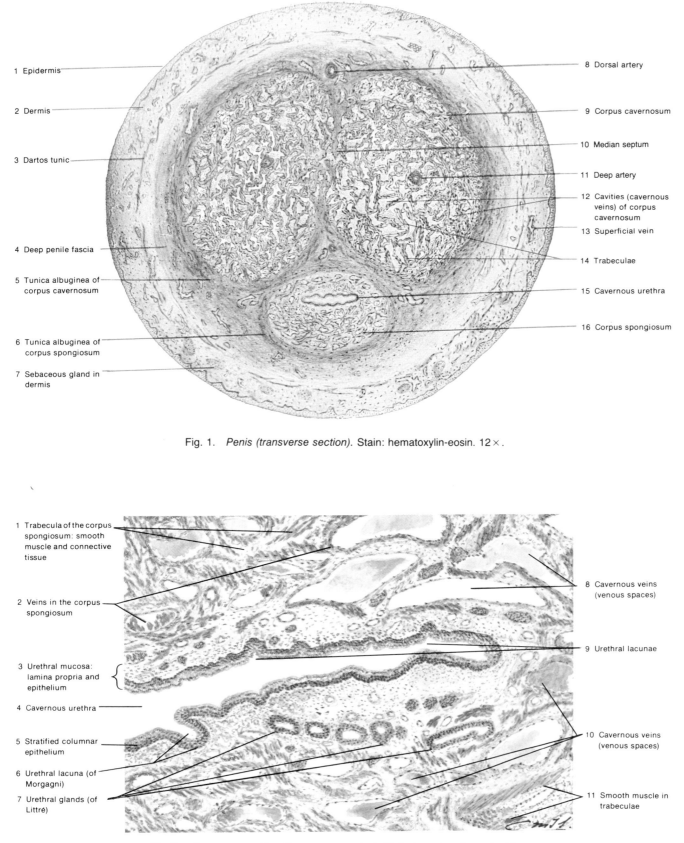

1 Epidermis

2 Dermis

3 Dartos tunic

4 Deep penile fascia

5 Tunica albuginea of corpus cavernosum

6 Tunica albuginea of corpus spongiosum

7 Sebaceous gland in dermis

8 Dorsal artery

9 Corpus cavernosum

10 Median septum

11 Deep artery

12 Cavities (cavernous veins) of corpus cavernosum

13 Superficial vein

14 Trabeculae

15 Cavernous urethra

16 Corpus spongiosum

Fig. 1.   *Penis (transverse section).* Stain: hematoxylin-eosin. 12×.

1 Trabecula of the corpus spongiosum: smooth muscle and connective tissue

2 Veins in the corpus spongiosum

3 Urethral mucosa: lamina propria and epithelium

4 Cavernous urethra

5 Stratified columnar epithelium

6 Urethral lacuna (of Morgagni)

7 Urethral glands (of Littré)

8 Cavernous veins (venous spaces)

9 Urethral lacunae

10 Cavernous veins (venous spaces)

11 Smooth muscle in trabeculae

Fig. 2.   *Cavernous urethra (transverse section).* Stain: hematoxylin-eosin. 80×.

PLATE 104

OVARY (PANORAMIC VIEW)

The ovarian surface is covered by a single layer of low cuboidal or squamous cells called the germinal epithelium (1). This layer is continuous with the mesothelium of the visceral peritoneum (14). Beneath the epithelium is a dense, connective tissue layer, the tunica albuginea (2).

The ovary has a peripheral cortex and a central medulla. The cortex occupies the greater part of the ovary and its connective tissue stroma (8) contains large, spindle-shaped fibroblasts. Coursing in all directions in the cortex are compact, fine collagenous and reticular fibers.

The medullary stroma (24) is a typical dense, irregular connective tissue which is continuous with that of the mesovarium (13). Numerous blood vessels in the medulla (10) distribute smaller vessels to all parts of the cortex. The mesovarium is covered by ovarian germinal epithelium (12) and peritoneal mesothelium (14).

Numerous ovarian follicles in various stages of development are located in the stroma of the cortex (3, 4, 7, 9, 16–20, 22, 28, 29). The detailed structure of some of these follicles is illustrated in Plate 105. The most numerous follicles are the primordial (3; 29, lower leader), located in the periphery of the cortex and under the tunica albuginea (2); these follicles are the smallest and simplest in structure. The largest of the follicles (16–20) is the mature follicle. Its various parts are: the theca interna and externa (16), the granulosa cells (17), a large antrum (18) filled with liquor folliculi (follicular fluid), and the cumulus oophorus (19), which contains the primary oocyte (20). The smaller follicles with stratified granulosa cells around the oocyte are the growing follicles (4, lower leader). Larger follicles with antral cavities of various sizes are called secondary or vesicular follicles (7, 9, 28). These follicles are situated deeper in the cortex and are surrounded by modified stromal cells, the theca folliculi (6), which differentiate into an inner secretory theca interna and an outer connective tissue, the theca externa (16). Most of the illustrated follicles contain a primary oocyte (6, 20, 28) and its nucleus. In the primordial follicles, the oocyte is small but gradually increases in size in the primary, growing, and vesicular follicles.

Most follicles never attain maturity and undergo degeneration (atresia) during various stages of growth, thus becoming atretic follicles (11, 21, 26, 30; see also Plate 106). The atretic follicles are gradually replaced by the stroma.

Following ovulation, the follicular wall collapses into folds and the corpus luteum is formed. Successive stages in corpus luteum regression are indicated (15, 27, 23, 5). Plates 106 and 107 illustrate these changes at a higher magnification.

PLATE 104

OVARY (PANORAMIC VIEW)

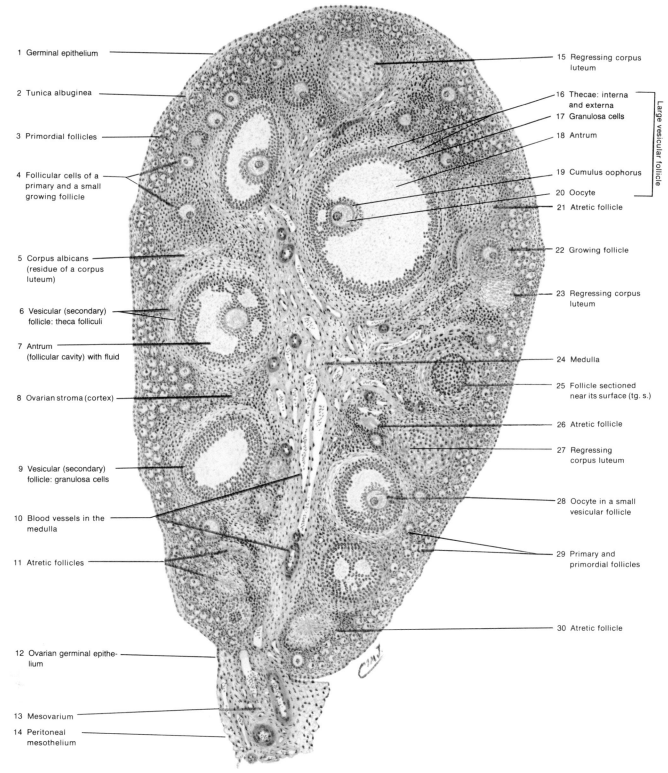

1 Germinal epithelium

2 Tunica albuginea

3 Primordial follicles

4 Follicular cells of a primary and a small growing follicle

5 Corpus albicans (residue of a corpus luteum)

6 Vesicular (secondary) follicle: theca folliculi

7 Antrum (follicular cavity) with fluid

8 Ovarian stroma (cortex)

9 Vesicular (secondary) follicle: granulosa cells

10 Blood vessels in the medulla

11 Atretic follicles

12 Ovarian germinal epithelium

13 Mesovarium

14 Peritoneal mesothelium

15 Regressing corpus luteum

16 Thecae: interna and externa

17 Granulosa cells

18 Antrum

19 Cumulus oophorus

20 Oocyte

21 Atretic follicle

Large vesicular follicle

22 Growing follicle

23 Regressing corpus luteum

24 Medulla

25 Follicle sectioned near its surface (tg. s.)

26 Atretic follicle

27 Regressing corpus luteum

28 Oocyte in a small vesicular follicle

29 Primary and primordial follicles

30 Atretic follicle

Ovary (dog). Stain: hematoxylin-eosin. 60×.

PLATE 105 (Fig. 1)

OVARY: OVARIAN CORTEX, PRIMARY AND GROWING FOLLICLES

The cuboidal germinal epithelium (1) lines the ovarian surface. Beneath the epithelium is the tunica albuginea (2), a layer of dense connective tissue.

Numerous primordial follicles (5, 6) are located in the outer zone of the ovarian stroma, immediately below the tunica albuginea (2). Each primordial follicle consists of a primary oocyte (5) surrounded by a single layer of a squamous follicular cells (6). In larger primary follicles, the follicular cells change to cuboidal or low columnar (7).

In growing follicles, the follicular cells, by mitotic (3) proliferation, form layers of cuboidal cells called the granulosa cells (10) and surround the primary oocyte (4, 11). The innermost layer of the granulosa cells surrounding the oocyte differentiates into the corona radiata (13); these cells are more columnar than the other granulosa cells. Between the corona radiata and the oocyte is the noncellular glycoprotein layer, the zona pellucida (12). Stromal cells arranged around the follicular cells form the theca interna (9); at this stage of development, theca externa has not differentiated. The oocyte (4) has a large eccentric nucleus (11) with a conspicuous nucleolus.

An atretic follicle (15) is illustrated with the remnants of hypertrophied zona pellucida.

PLATE 105 (Fig. 2)

OVARY: WALL OF A MATURE FOLLICLE

Figure 2 illustrates a portion of the mature follicle with an oocyte. The area represented in this figure is comparable to the area in Plate 104 that illustrates the mature follicle, the cumulus oophorus with its oocyte (19, 20), and the different thecae layers.

The granulosa cells (6), formed by the hypertrophied follicular cells, enclose the central cavity or antrum (8) of the follicle. The antrum (8) is filled with follicular fluid secreted by the granulosa cells. Smaller isolated accumulations of the follicular fluid may also occur among the granulosa cells (14); these round vacuoles, which appear clear or faintly acidophilic, are the Call-Exner bodies (3, 7); their origin and function are not known.

A local thickening of the granulosa cells on one side encloses the oocyte (11) and projects into the antrum, forming a hillock called the cumulus oophorus (12). The oocyte is surrounded by a prominent noncellular zona pellucida (10) and a single layer of radially arranged corona radiata (9) cells that are attached to the zona pellucida.

The basal row of granulosa cells rests on a thin basement membrane (5). Adjacent to this membrane is the theca interna (4), an inner layer of vascularized, secretory cells, and the theca externa (2), an outer layer of connective tissue cells.

PLATE 105

OVARY

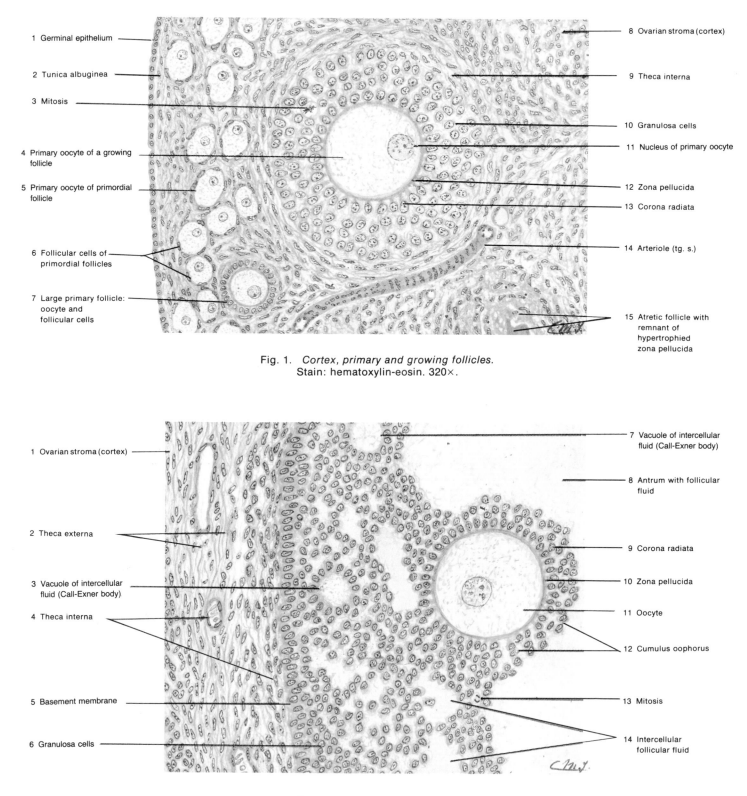

1 Germinal epithelium
2 Tunica albuginea
3 Mitosis
4 Primary oocyte of a growing follicle
5 Primary oocyte of primordial follicle
6 Follicular cells of primordial follicles
7 Large primary follicle: oocyte and follicular cells

8 Ovarian stroma (cortex)
9 Theca interna
10 Granulosa cells
11 Nucleus of primary oocyte
12 Zona pellucida
13 Corona radiata
14 Arteriole (tg. s.)
15 Atretic follicle with remnant of hypertrophied zona pellucida

Fig. 1. *Cortex, primary and growing follicles.*
Stain: hematoxylin-eosin. 320×.

1 Ovarian stroma (cortex)
2 Theca externa
3 Vacuole of intercellular fluid (Call-Exner body)
4 Theca interna
5 Basement membrane
6 Granulosa cells

7 Vacuole of intercellular fluid (Call-Exner body)
8 Antrum with follicular fluid
9 Corona radiata
10 Zona pellucida
11 Oocyte
12 Cumulus oophorus
13 Mitosis
14 Intercellular follicular fluid

Fig. 2. *Wall of a mature follicle.*
Stain: hematoxylin-eosin. 320×.

PLATE 106

OVARY: CORPORA LUTEA AND FOLLICULAR ATRESIA
(HUMAN OVARY)

Illustrated in this figure are a newly formed corpus luteum, corpora lutea in various stages of regression, and several stages of follicular atresia.

The ovarian surface is covered by a single layer of germinal epithelium (1). Lying directly underneath this layer is a thin connective tissue, the tunica albuginea. The cortex (2, 18) constitutes the greater portion of the ovary and contains the follicles and corpora lutea. The medulla (7) occupies the central region of the ovary and contains larger blood vessels, which supply the cortical region.

The newly formed corpus luteum (3) is a large structure. It is formed after the rupture of the mature follicle and the collapse of its walls. The thin zone of theca lutein cells (4), formed from the theca interna cells, is located on the periphery of the corpus luteum and the contours of its folds. (See Plate 107 for details.) The mass of the corpus luteum wall is formed from the granulosa lutein cells (5), which are the hypertrophied granulosa cells of the follicle. The connective tissue has proliferated from the theca externa cells, forming the stroma for capillaries in the wall of corpus luteum and filling the former follicular cavity (6).

Also illustrated in the ovary is a portion of corpus luteum in moderate regression (10), with the plane of section passing through its outer wall. The granulosa lutein cells are smaller and the nuclei are pyknotic (10a), and larger blood vessels are growing in from the stroma (10b). Theca lutein cells are not visible.

A later stage of corpus luteum regression (16) indicates further shrinkage of lutein cells and pyknosis of nuclei (16b) and a fibrous central core (16a). Connective tissue invades the regressing luteal cells and replaces them as they degenerate. The stroma forms a capsule (16c) around the regressing corpus luteum; however, this is not a constant feature. Replacement by the connective tissue of all lutein cells leaves a fibrous, hyalinized scar, the corpus albicans (15).

A large, normal follicle (17) exhibits the theca interna (17a) and the thick granulosa cell layer (17b); a thin basement membrane separates the two layers. The cumulus oophorus (17d) contains a normal oocyte (17e), and the antrum is filled with follicular fluid (17c).

Numerous follicles undergo degenerative changes called atresia at any time before reaching maturity. Atresia in large follicles is gradual; however, serial changes can be recognized by noting follicles in different stages of atresia. A follicle in an early stage of atresia is illustrated (14). The theca interna (14a) and the granulosa cells (14b) are intact, however, some of the cells are beginning to slough off into the antrum (14e), which still contains follicular fluid (14d). Also, a disruption of cumulus oophorus has taken place and degeneration of the oocyte is advanced. A remnant of the oocyte, surrounded by thickened zona pellucida (14c), is seen in the antrum.

A follicle in a more advanced stage of atresia is also illustrated (13). The theca interna (13a) is still visible; however, the cells appear somewhat hypertrophied. The granulosa cells are no longer present; all of the cells have sloughed off and have been resorbed. The basement membrane between these two layers has thickened and folded and is now called the hypertrophied glassy membrane (13b). Loose connective tissue is growing in from the stroma (13e) and has partially filled the reduced follicular cavity (13d), in which follicular fluid (13c) is still present.

With further atresia, connective tissue stroma replaces the theca interna cells (9a). The hypertrophied glassy membrane (9b) becomes thicker and more folded and the loose connective tissue with small blood vessels completely fills the former antrum (9c). In the last stages of atresia, the entire follicle is replaced by stroma; the hypertrophied and folded glassy membrane (11) remains for some time as the only indication of a follicle.

PLATE 106

OVARY: CORPORA LUTEA AND FOLLICULAR ATRESIA

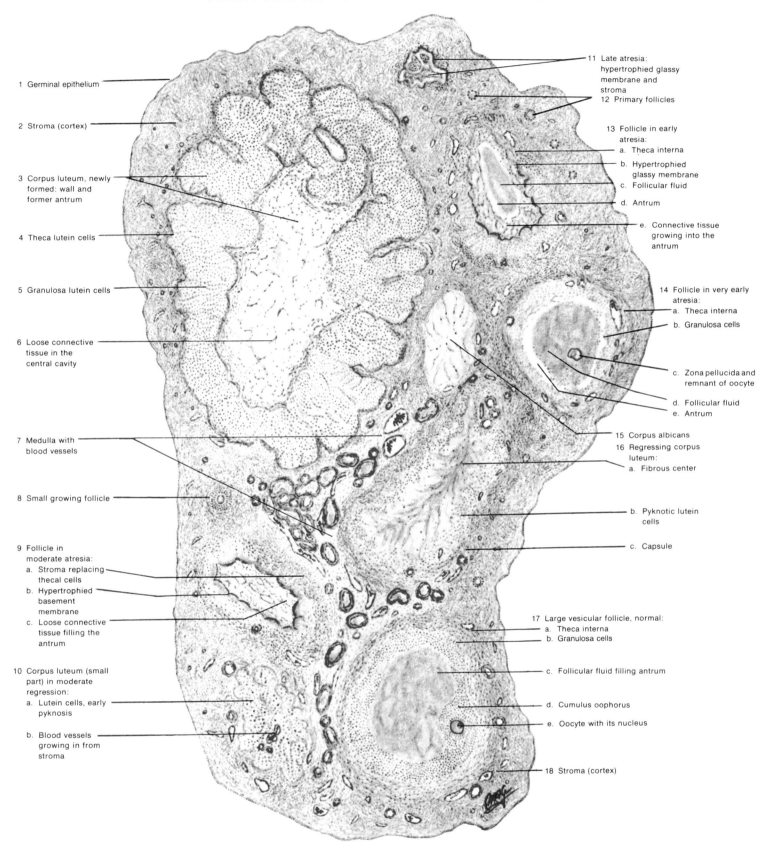

1 Germinal epithelium

2 Stroma (cortex)

3 Corpus luteum, newly formed: wall and former antrum

4 Theca lutein cells

5 Granulosa lutein cells

6 Loose connective tissue in the central cavity

7 Medulla with blood vessels

8 Small growing follicle

9 Follicle in moderate atresia:
   a. Stroma replacing thecal cells
   b. Hypertrophied basement membrane
   c. Loose connective tissue filling the antrum

10 Corpus luteum (small part) in moderate regression:
   a. Lutein cells, early pyknosis
   b. Blood vessels growing in from stroma

11 Late atresia: hypertrophied glassy membrane and stroma
12 Primary follicles

13 Follicle in early atresia:
   a. Theca interna
   b. Hypertrophied glassy membrane
   c. Follicular fluid
   d. Antrum
   e. Connective tissue growing into the antrum

14 Follicle in very early atresia:
   a. Theca interna
   b. Granulosa cells
   c. Zona pellucida and remnant of oocyte
   d. Follicular fluid
   e. Antrum

15 Corpus albicans
16 Regressing corpus luteum:
   a. Fibrous center
   b. Pyknotic lutein cells
   c. Capsule

17 Large vesicular follicle, normal:
   a. Theca interna
   b. Granulosa cells
   c. Follicular fluid filling antrum
   d. Cumulus oophorus
   e. Oocyte with its nucleus

18 Stroma (cortex)

Human Ovary. Stain: hematoxylin-eosin. 80×.

PLATE 107 (Fig. 1)

CORPUS LUTEUM (PANORAMIC VIEW)

The corpus luteum, in cross section, appears as a highly folded, thick mass of glandular tissue (3). The central core contains remnants of follicular fluid, serum, occasionally blood, and loose connective tissue (8, 9).

The glandular tissue is composed of anastomosing epithelioid cells (3) consisting primarily of granulosa lutein cells (3, upper leader) and peripheral theca lutein cells (3, lower leader) which extend along the connective tissue septa (7) between the folds of the wall (6).

The cells of theca externa form a poorly defined capsule (1) around the developing corpus luteum. Thin septa of connective tissue from theca externa extend into the depressions between the folds (2, 7).

The core of the corpus luteum (the former follicular cavity) fills with loose connective tissue from the theca externa which has proliferated and penetrated the layers of the glandular tissue. The connective tissue covers the inner surface of the luteal cells (8) and then spreads throughout the core of the corpus luteum (9).

The ovarian stroma (4) around the corpus luteum is highly vascular (5).

PLATE 107 (Fig. 2)

PERIPHERAL WALL

Granulosa lutein (7) cells constitute the mass of the corpus luteum. These cells are the hypertrophied former granulosa cells of the mature follicle. The cells are large and lightly stained due to lipid inclusions, and have large vesicular nuclei. The theca lutein cells (2), the former theca interna cells, remain external to the granulosa lutein cells on the periphery of the corpus luteum and in the depressions between the folds. Theca lutein cells (2) are smaller than the granulosa lutein cells. Their cytoplasm stains deeper and the nuclei are smaller and darker.

Numerous capillaries (8) within fine connective tissue septa (6) have proliferated inward from the theca externa (5) and are observed between the anastomosing columns of lutein cells (6, 8).

The connective tissue capsule (5) around the corpus luteum is poorly defined and the surrounding stroma remains highly vascular (1, 3, 4).

PLATE 107

CORPUS LUTEUM

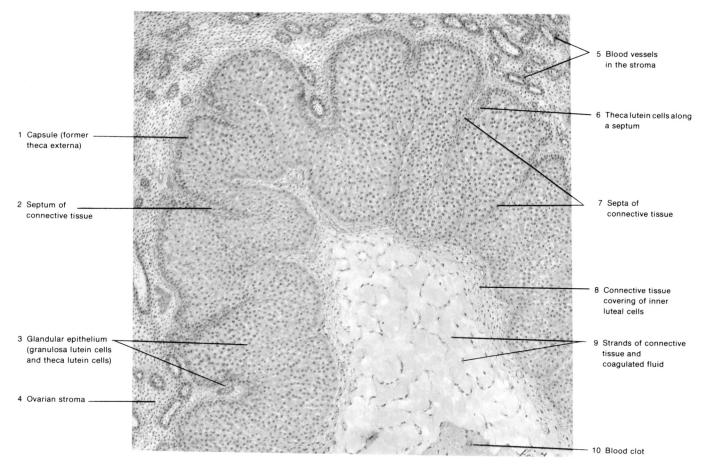

1 Capsule (former theca externa)

2 Septum of connective tissue

3 Glandular epithelium (granulosa lutein cells and theca lutein cells)

4 Ovarian stroma

5 Blood vessels in the stroma

6 Theca lutein cells along a septum

7 Septa of connective tissue

8 Connective tissue covering of inner luteal cells

9 Strands of connective tissue and coagulated fluid

10 Blood clot

Fig. 1. *Panoramic view.*
Stain: hematoxylin-eosin. 80×.

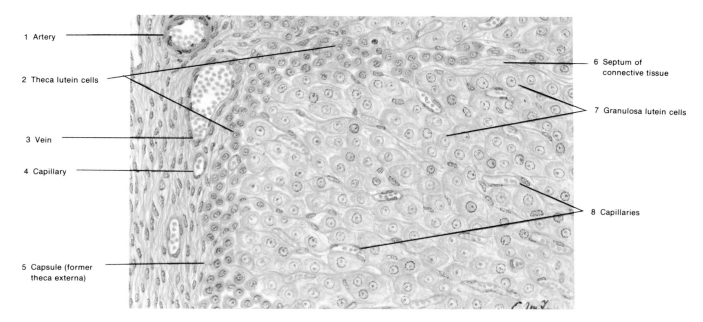

1 Artery

2 Theca lutein cells

3 Vein

4 Capillary

5 Capsule (former theca externa)

6 Septum of connective tissue

7 Granulosa lutein cells

8 Capillaries

Fig. 2. *Peripheral wall.*
Stain: hematoxylin-eosin. 250×.

PLATE 108 (Fig. 1)

UTERINE TUBE: AMPULLA (PANORAMIC VIEW, TRANSVERSE SECTION)

Extensive ramification of tall mucosal folds (9) forms an irregular luminal contour in the uterine tube (Fallopian tube). The lumen extends between the prominent mucosal folds and forms deep grooves in the tube. The lining epithelium (10) is simple columnar and the lamina propria (8) is a well vascularized, loose connective tissue. The muscularis consists of two smooth muscle layers, an inner circular (1) and an outer longitudinal layer (6). The interstitial connective tissue (2) is abundant and, as a result, the muscle layers are not distinct, especially the outer layer. Serosa (7) forms the outermost layer on the uterine tube.

PLATE 108 (Fig. 2)

UTERINE TUBE: MUCOSAL FOLDS (EARLY PROLIFERATIVE PHASE)

The lining epithelium is simple but may appear pseudostratified. It is composed of ciliated (1) and nonciliated, secretory cells. During the early proliferative phase of the menstrual cycle, the ciliated cells hypertrophy, exhibit cilia growth, and become the predominant cells. There is evidence of increased secretory activity in the nonciliated cells during the follicular phase. The epithelium shows cyclic changes and the proportion of ciliated and nonciliated cells varies with different stages of menstrual cycle.

The lamina propria (2) is a highly cellular, loose connective tissue with fine collagenous and reticular fibers. The abundant large fibroblasts are apparently less differentiated than the typical fibroblasts. In tubal pregnancy, this connective tissue reacts like the uterine endometrium and numerous fibroblasts become decidual cells.

PLATE 108 (Fig. 3)

UTERINE TUBE: MUCOSAL FOLDS (EARLY PREGNANCY)

During the luteal phase of the menstrual cycle and early pregnancy, the secretory cells (2) are predominant. These cells appear slender with elongated nuclei and apices that protrude into tubular lumina. The secretory cells (2) intermix with ciliated cells (3) in the uterine tube.

PLATE 108

UTERINE TUBE: AMPULLA

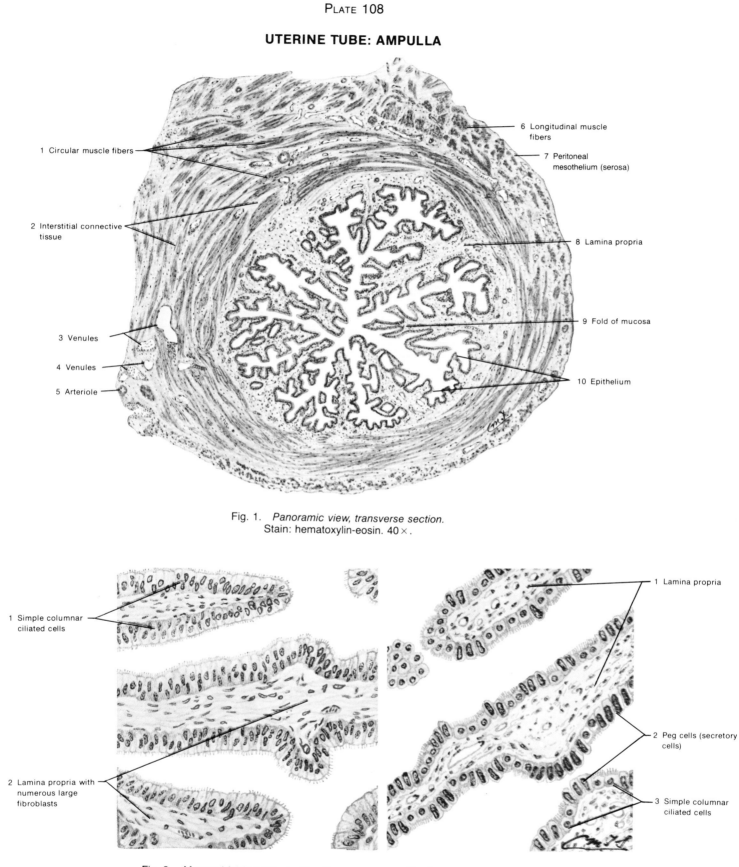

1 Circular muscle fibers

2 Interstitial connective tissue

3 Venules

4 Venules

5 Arteriole

6 Longitudinal muscle fibers

7 Peritoneal mesothelium (serosa)

8 Lamina propria

9 Fold of mucosa

10 Epithelium

Fig. 1.   *Panoramic view, transverse section.*
Stain: hematoxylin-eosin. 40×.

1 Simple columnar ciliated cells

2 Lamina propria with numerous large fibroblasts

1 Lamina propria

2 Peg cells (secretory cells)

3 Simple columnar ciliated cells

Fig. 2.   *Mucosal folds (early proliferative phase).* Stain: hematoxylin-eosin. 320×.

Fig. 3.   *Mucosal folds (early pregnancy).* Stain: hematoxylin-eosin. 320×.

PLATE 109

UTERUS: PROLIFERATIVE (FOLLICULAR) PHASE

During a normal menstrual cycle, the uterine endometrium undergoes a sequence of changes that are closely correlated with the ovarian function. Cyclic activities in a nonpregnant uterus are divided into three distinct phases: a proliferative or follicular phase, a secretory or luteal phase, and a menstrual phase. The structure of the uterine wall during each phase is illustrated in Plates 109, 110, and 111, respectively.

The uterine wall consists of three layers: the inner endometrium or mucosa (1–4), the middle muscular or myometrium (5, 6, 12, 13), and the outer serous membrane or perimetrium.

The endometrium is normally subdivided into two zones or layers: a narrow, deep layer, the stratum basale or basalis (4, 15); and a wider, superficial layer above the stratum basalis that extends to the lumen of the uterus, the stratum functionale or functionalis (1, 2, 3, 14). The endometrium consists of a simple columnar secretory epithelium (1) overlying the thick lamina propria, the endometrial stroma (2, 3, 4). The surface epithelium extends down into the stroma to form numerous long, tubular uterine glands (8). The uterine glands are usually straight in the superficial portion of the endometrium (8) but may exhibit bifurcation in the deep region near the myometrium. As a result, numerous glands are seen in cross sections (10) in the abundant endometrial stroma (3).

In the proliferative phase, cross sections of coiled arteries (9) are seen in the deeper regions of the endometrium, excluding the superficial third portion of the endometrium, which at this time contains veins and capillaries.

The endometrial stroma is cellular and resembles mesenchymal tissue. The branching fibroblasts are embedded in a network of reticular and fine collagenous fibers of the ground substance. The stroma is more compact in the basalis, which is not indicated in this illustration.

The endometrium is firmly attached to the underlying myometrium, which consists of compact bundles of smooth muscle fibers (5, 6, 13) separated by thin strands of connective tissue (12). Three poorly defined muscle layers can be distinguished. The myometrium is highly vascular (7).

PLATE 109

UTERUS: PROLIFERATIVE (FOLLICULAR) PHASE

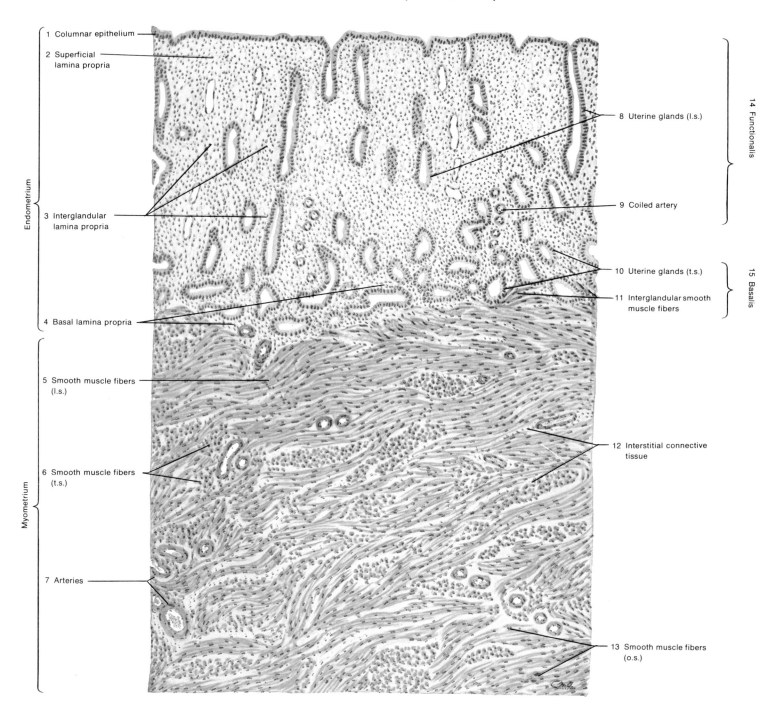

1 Columnar epithelium

2 Superficial lamina propria

3 Interglandular lamina propria

4 Basal lamina propria

5 Smooth muscle fibers (l.s.)

6 Smooth muscle fibers (t.s.)

7 Arteries

8 Uterine glands (l.s.)

9 Coiled artery

10 Uterine glands (t.s.)

11 Interglandular smooth muscle fibers

12 Interstitial connective tissue

13 Smooth muscle fibers (o.s.)

14 Functionalis

15 Basalis

Endometrium

Myometrium

Stain: hematoxylin-eosin. 45×.

PLATE 110

UTERUS: SECRETORY (LUTEAL) PHASE

During the secretory phase of the menstrual cycle, the endometrium thickens as a result of increased glandular secretion and stromal edema. The glandular cells hypertrophy (4) due to increased accumulation of large quantities of secretory product. The uterine glands become tortuous (3, 4, 9) and their dilated lumina contain secretory material (5, 10). In the endometrial stroma (8), increased accumulation of tissue fluid produces edema. The coiled arteries (7) now extend into the superficial portion of the endometrium, the functionalis layer.

The observed alterations in the uterine glands and endometrial stroma are characteristic features of the functionalis layer of the endometrium during secretory or lateral phase of the menstrual cycle. In the basal stratum or basalis layer (11) only minimal change is noted during the different phases of the menstrual cycle.

PLATE 110

UTERUS: SECRETORY (LUTEAL) PHASE

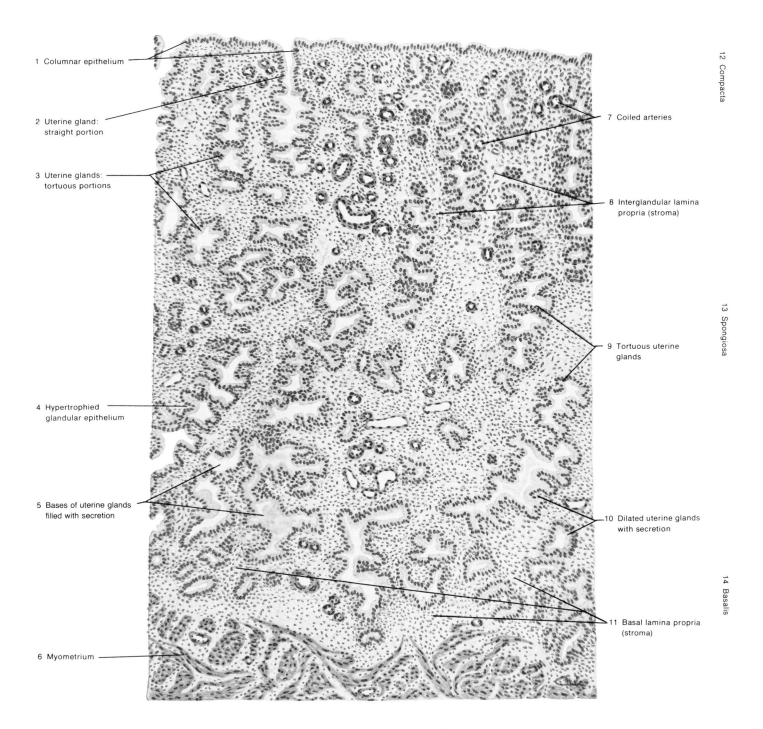

1 Columnar epithelium

2 Uterine gland:
straight portion

3 Uterine glands:
tortuous portions

4 Hypertrophied
glandular epithelium

5 Bases of uterine glands
filled with secretion

6 Myometrium

7 Coiled arteries

8 Interglandular lamina
propria (stroma)

9 Tortuous uterine
glands

10 Dilated uterine glands
with secretion

11 Basal lamina propria
(stroma)

12 Compacta

13 Spongiosa

14 Basalis

Stain: hematoxylin-eosin. 45×.

PLATE 111

UTERUS: MENSTRUAL PHASE

During the menstrual phase of the cycle, the endometrial surface (1) loses its epithelium and much of its underlying tissue. The stratum functionale or functionalis layer of the endometrium is sloughed off or shed during every menstrual cycle. The endometrial surface that is being shed contains blood clots (7), fragments of disintegrated stroma (6), and uterine glands. Some of the intact uterine glands are filled with blood (2). In the deeper layers of the endometrium, the stratum basale or the basalis layer, the bases of the uterine glands, remain intact (9) during the menstrual flow.

The endometrial stroma of most of the functionalis layer contains aggregations of free erythrocytes (8), which have been extruded from the disintegrating blood vessels. In addition, there is moderate infiltration of lymphocytes and neutrophils into the endometrial stroma. On the other hand, the basilar portion of the endometrial stroma remains generally unaffected (4) during this phase.

The distal or superficial portions of the coiled arteries become necrotic while the deeper parts of these vessels (3) remain intact.

PLATE 111

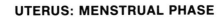

UTERUS: MENSTRUAL PHASE

1 Superficial
endometrium
without epithelium

2 Glandular lumen filled
with blood

3 Coiled arteries

4 Interglandular lamina
propria of basal region

5 Smooth muscle fibers
(myometrium)

6 Fragments of disintegrated
stroma

7 Blood clots

8 Erythrocytes in
lamina propria

9 Intact bases of
uterine glands

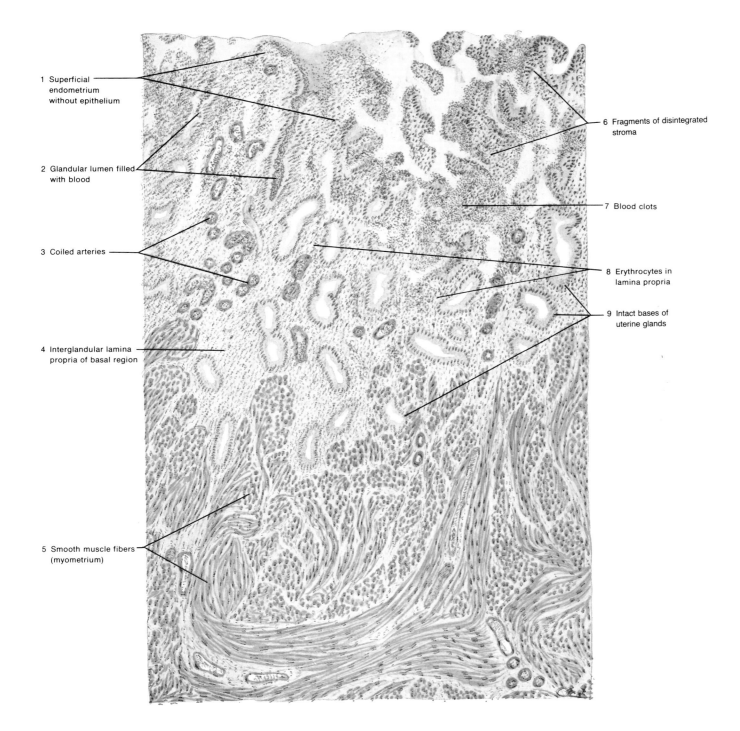

Stain: hematoxylin-eosin. 45×.

PLATE 112 (Fig. 1)

PLACENTA: FIVE MONTHS' PREGNANCY
(PANORAMIC VIEW)

The upper part of the plate represents the fetal portion of the placenta (10, 11), which also includes the chorionic plate and the villi arising from it. The maternal placenta is the decidua basalis (8) and includes the functionalis of the endometrium (12–14) which lies directly beneath the fetal placenta. Below this region is seen the basal portion of the endometrium containing the basal parts of the uterine glands (15); this region is not shed during parturition. A small section of the myometrium (17) is illustrated in the lower right field.

The surface of the amnion (1) is lined by the squamous epithelium. The underlying layer of the connective tissue (2) represents the merged connective tissue of the amnion and chorion. Below the connective tissue is the trophoblast of the chorion (3, 10), details of which are not distinguishable at this magnification. Trophoblast and the underlying connective tissue form the chorionic plate (10).

Anchoring villi arise from the chorionic plate (4, upper leader), extend to the uterine wall, and embed in the decidua basalis (7). This continuity is not seen in this illustration; however, larger units in the fetal placenta probably represent sections of the anchoring villi (4, lower leader). These increase in size and complexity during pregnancy.

Numerous floating villi are seen (chorion frondosum), sectioned in various planes (5, 11) due to their outgrowth in all directions from the anchoring villi. These villi "float" in the intervillous spaces (6), which are bathed in maternal blood. The detailed structure of these villi is further illustrated in Figure 2.

The maternal portion of the placenta or decidua basalis exhibits embedded anchoring villi (7), groups of large decidual cells (8), and typical stroma. Also seen here are the distal portions of the uterine glands in various stages of regression (14), which disappear later, and maternal blood vessels, recognized by their size or by red blood cells in their lumina (9). A maternal blood vessel is seen opening into an intervillous space (13).

Coiled arteries (16) and basal portions of the uterine glands (15) are present in the deep zone of the endometrium. Fibrin deposits appear on the surface of the decidua basalis (12) and increase in volume and extent as the pregnancy continues.

PLATE 112 (Fig. 2)

CHORIONIC VILLI (PLACENTA AT FIVE MONTHS)

The figure illustrates, at a higher magnification, several chorionic villi from placenta at 5 months of pregnancy. The trophoblast epithelium is composed of an outer layer of syncytial cells, the syncytiotrophoblast (1), and an inner layer of cells, the cytotrophoblast (2). The interior of the villus contains embryonic connective tissue (3) and fetal blood vessels (5) which are branches of umbilical arteries and veins; both nucleated and non-nucleated erythrocytes may be present. Intervillous spaces (4) are bathed by maternal blood and the erythrocytes are non-nucleated. One of the illustrated villi is attached to the endometrium (6), and several decidual cells (7) are seen in the stroma.

PLATE 112 (Fig. 3)

CHORIONIC VILLI (PLACENTA AT TERM)

This figure illustrates several chorionic villi from a placenta at term. In contrast to the villi illustrated in Figure 2, the chorionic epithelium in these villi is observed only as syncytiotrophoblast (1), whose syncytial character is more pronounced than in Figure 2. The connective tissue is more differentiated, illustrating more fibers, fewer typical fibroblasts, and numerous large, round cells (Hofbauer cells) (4) which are believed to be phagocytic. Fetal blood vessels are numerous (3), having increased in complexity of branching as pregnancy progressed.

PLATE 112

PLACENTA

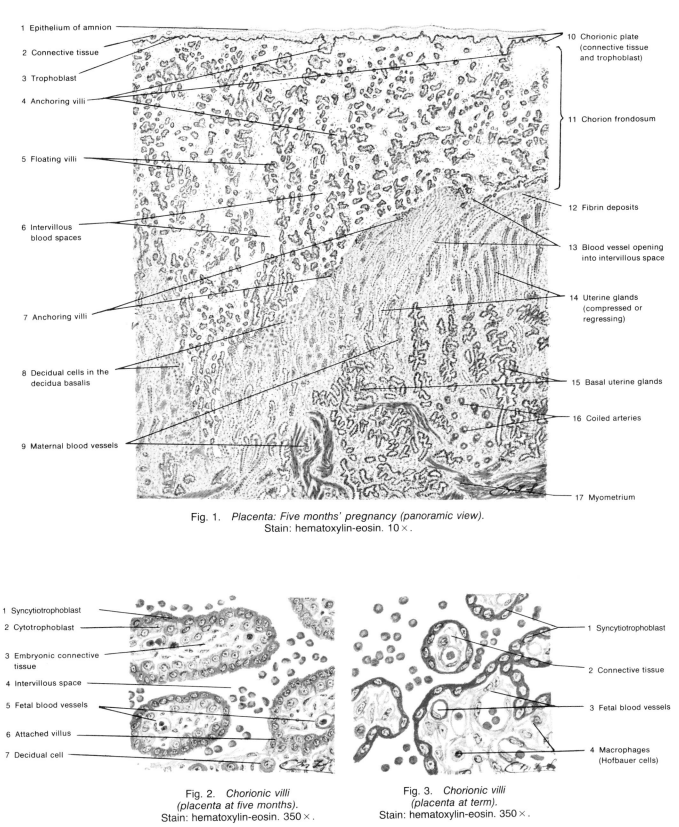

1 Epithelium of amnion

2 Connective tissue

3 Trophoblast

4 Anchoring villi

5 Floating villi

6 Intervillous blood spaces

7 Anchoring villi

8 Decidual cells in the decidua basalis

9 Maternal blood vessels

10 Chorionic plate (connective tissue and trophoblast)

11 Chorion frondosum

12 Fibrin deposits

13 Blood vessel opening into intervillous space

14 Uterine glands (compressed or regressing)

15 Basal uterine glands

16 Coiled arteries

17 Myometrium

Fig. 1. *Placenta: Five months' pregnancy (panoramic view).*
Stain: hematoxylin-eosin. 10 ×.

1 Syncytiotrophoblast

2 Cytotrophoblast

3 Embryonic connective tissue

4 Intervillous space

5 Fetal blood vessels

6 Attached villus

7 Decidual cell

Fig. 2. *Chorionic villi
(placenta at five months).*
Stain: hematoxylin-eosin. 350 ×.

1 Syncytiotrophoblast

2 Connective tissue

3 Fetal blood vessels

4 Macrophages (Hofbauer cells)

Fig. 3. *Chorionic villi
(placenta at term).*
Stain: hematoxylin-eosin. 350 ×.

PLATE 113

CERVIX: LONGITUDINAL SECTION

The mucosa of the endocervix (cervix uteri) is lined with tall, mucus-secreting columnar epithelium (1), differing from the uterine epithelium, with which it is continuous. Similar epithelium also lines the numerous, highly branched tubular cervical glands (2) which extend deep into the wide lamina propria (4). The lamina propria exhibits a highly "cellular" type of connective tissue in the body of the uterus, but a more fibrous type in the cervix.

In the lower part of the cervix, at the os cervix (5) or opening of the cervical canal into the vaginal canal, the columnar epithelium abruptly changes to stratified squamous (6). This epithelium then continues over the vaginal portion of the cervix, the portio vaginalis (6), and its external wall (8) in the vaginal fornix. At the base of the fornix (7), the epithelium reflects back to line the vaginal canal.

The muscularis (3, 10) is not as compact as in the body of the uterus; however, both the muscularis and the lamina propria are well vascularized.

PLATE 113

CERVIX: LONGITUDINAL SECTION

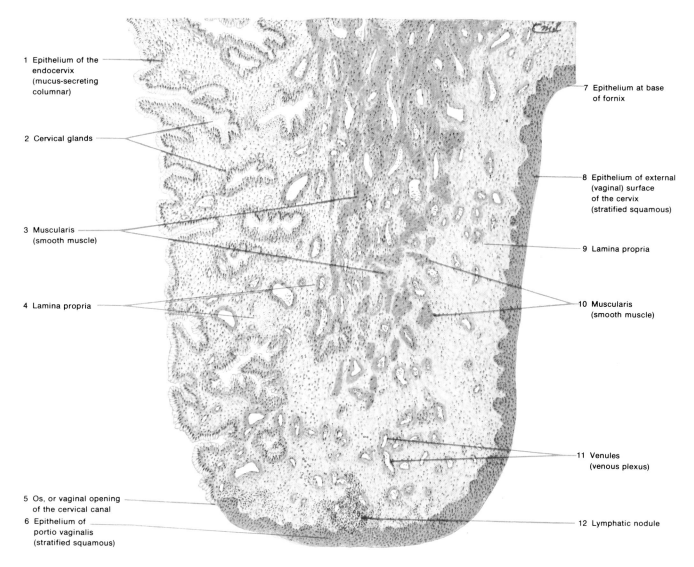

1 Epithelium of the
endocervix
(mucus-secreting
columnar)

2 Cervical glands

3 Muscularis
(smooth muscle)

4 Lamina propria

5 Os, or vaginal opening
of the cervical canal

6 Epithelium of
portio vaginalis
(stratified squamous)

7 Epithelium at base
of fornix

8 Epithelium of external
(vaginal) surface
of the cervix
(stratified squamous)

9 Lamina propria

10 Muscularis
(smooth muscle)

11 Venules
(venous plexus)

12 Lymphatic nodule

Stain: hematoxylin-eosin. 20×.

PLATE 114 (Fig. 1)

VAGINA: LONGITUDINAL SECTION

The vaginal mucosa exhibits numerous transverse folds (5). The surface epithelium is noncornified stratified squamous (1) whose cells have a rich glycogen content (see Fig. 2). Connective tissue papillae (2) are present and have variable height in the posterior region of the vaginal wall.

The wide lamina propria (4) contains moderately dense, irregular connective tissue that is rich in elastic fibers; however, it is looser in the deeper area, and fibrous extensions from this region pass into the muscularis. Diffuse lymphatic tissue and lymphatic nodules (3) are usually observed under the epithelium. Small blood vessels are numerous throughout the lamina propria.

The muscularis consists predominantly of longitudinal (6) and oblique (9) bundles of smooth muscle fibers. Circular muscle fibers (11) are less numerous and more frequently found in the inner layers. Interstitial connective tissue (8) is rich in elastic fibers.

The adventitia (7) contains numerous blood vessels (10) and nerve bundles.

PLATE 114 (Fig. 2)

GLYCOGEN IN HUMAN VAGINAL EPITHELIUM

Glycogen is a prominent component of the vaginal epithelium except in the deepest layers, where its content is minimal or completely lacking. Glycogen accumulates during the follicular phase of the menstrual cycle and reaches its maximum before ovulation. It can be demonstrated by iodine vapor or iodine solution in mineral oil (Mancini's method). Glycogen stains a reddish-purple.

The tissues in illustrations "a" and "b" were fixed in absolute alcohol and formaldehyde. The amount of glycogen present in the cells during the interfollicular phase of the cycle is then illustrated (a). During the follicular phase, the amount of glycogen increases, especially in the cells of the intermediate and the more superficial layers (b).

The tissue in illustration "c" is from the same specimen as "b," but it was fixed by the Altmann-Gersch method (freezing and drying in a vacuum). This method produces less tissue shrinkage and illustrates abundant glycogen during the follicular phase and its diffuse distribution throughout the vaginal cells' cytoplasm.

PLATE 114

VAGINA

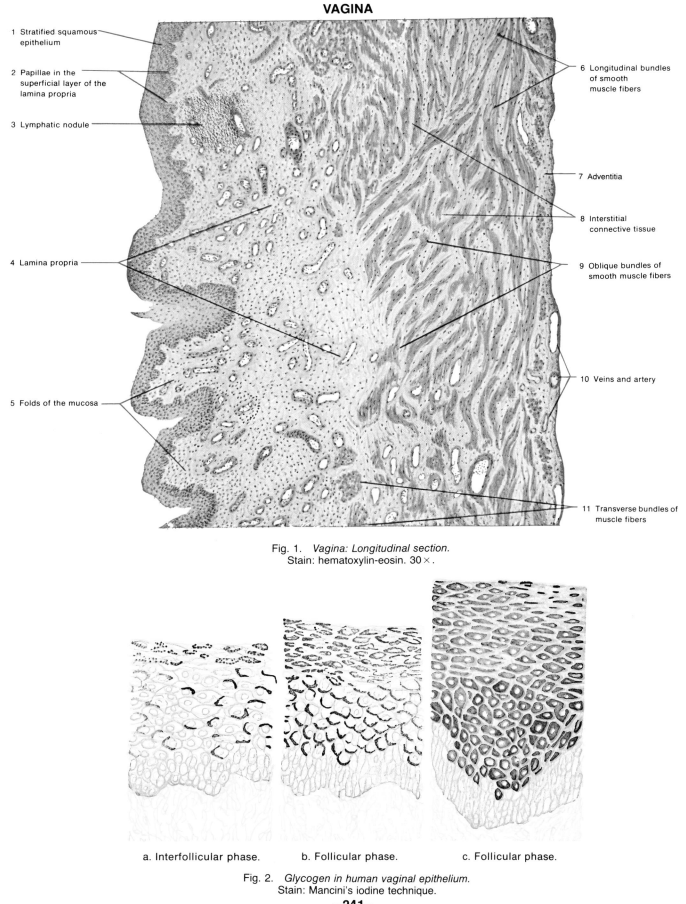

1 Stratified squamous epithelium

2 Papillae in the superficial layer of the lamina propria

3 Lymphatic nodule

4 Lamina propria

5 Folds of the mucosa

6 Longitudinal bundles of smooth muscle fibers

7 Adventitia

8 Interstitial connective tissue

9 Oblique bundles of smooth muscle fibers

10 Veins and artery

11 Transverse bundles of muscle fibers

Fig. 1. *Vagina: Longitudinal section.*
Stain: hematoxylin-eosin. 30 ×.

a. Interfollicular phase.   b. Follicular phase.   c. Follicular phase.

Fig. 2. *Glycogen in human vaginal epithelium.*
Stain: Mancini's iodine technique.

PLATE 115

VAGINA: EXFOLIATE CYTOLOGY (VAGINAL SMEARS)

This plate illustrates numerous examples of different cell types in vaginal smears obtained from normal women during different days of the menstrual cycle, early pregnancy, and menopause. The Shorr trichrome stain (Bierbrich Scarlet, Orange G, and Fast Green) plus Harris hematoxylin facilitates recognition of the different cell types.

In Figure 7 are illustrated individual cell types in a normal vaginal smear. The superficial acidophilic cell (a) of the vaginal mucosa is flat, somewhat irregular in outline, measures from 35 to 65 μm in diameter, exhibits a small nucleus, and contains ample cytoplasm stained light orange. At (b) is a similar superficial basophilic cell with blue-green cytoplasm. Illustrated at (c) is a cell from the intermediate stratum of the vaginal epithelium. It is flattened like the superficial cells but is smaller, measuring 20 to 40 μm, and has a basophilic blue-green cytoplasm. The nucleus is somewhat larger and often vesicular. The cells illustrated at (d) are intermediate cells in profile, characterized by their elongated form with folded borders and elongated, eccentric nucleus. At (e) are illustrated cells of the internal basal layers of the vaginal epithelium, the basal cells. The larger cells are from the external portion of the basal layers and the more superficial are the parabasal cells. All cells are oval, measure from 12 to 15 μm in diameter, and exhibit large nuclei with a more prominent chromatin. Most of these cells exhibit basophilic staining.

In Figure 1 is illustrated a vaginal smear from the fifth day of the menstrual cycle (postmenstrual phase). Predominant are intermediate cells (1) from the outer layers of the intermediate layer (transitions to the deeper superficial cells). A few superficial acidophilic and basophilic (2) cells and leukocytes are present.

Figure 2 represents a vaginal smear from the 14th day of the menstrual cycle (ovulatory phase), characterized by the predominance of large superficial acidophilic cells (8), the scarcity of superficial basophilic cells (10) and intermediate cells (9), and the absence of leukocytes. This smear is characteristic of the high estrogenic stimulation normally observed before ovulation and is called the "follicular smear." The superficial cells "mature" with increased estrogen levels and become acidophilic. A similar type of smear can be obtained from a menopausal individual treated with high doses of estrogen.

In Figure 3 is a representative of a smear taken from the 21st day of the cycle and represents the luteal (progestational) phase. This phase is indicative of increased levels of progesterone. Predominant are large cells from the intermediate layers (precornified superficial cells) with folded borders (3) that aggregate into clumps. Superficial acidophilic (4) cells, superficial basophilic (5) cells, and leukocytes are scarce.

The cells in Figure 4 represent the premenstrual stage of the 28th day of the cycle. This stage is characterized by a great predominance of grouped (14) intermediate cells with folded borders (13, 14), an increase of neutrophilic cells (12), a scarcity of superficial cells (11), and an abundance of mucus which blurs the preparations.

In Figure 5 is illustrated a smear from a 3-month pregnancy illustrating predominantly cells from the intermediate layers, many with folded borders (6). These cells typically form dense groups or conglomerations (7). Cells from superficial layers and neutrophilic cells are very scarce.

The vaginal smear during menopause (Fig. 6) is different from all smears in other phases. In a typical "atrophic" smear, the predominant cells are oval basal cells of various dimensions (17). Cells from the intermediate layers are scarce (15), and the neutrophilic cells are abundant (16). The menopausal smears, however, vary, depending on the stage of menopause and the estrogen levels.

The vaginal exfoliate cytology is correlated with the ovarian cycle. Understanding its characteristic features permits recognition of follicular activity during normal menstrual phases or after estrogenic and other therapy. Also, exfoliate cytology provides important information (together with cells from the endocervix) for detecting regional pathologic or malignant conditions.

PLATE 115

VAGINA: EXFOLIATE CYTOLOGY (VAGINAL SMEARS)

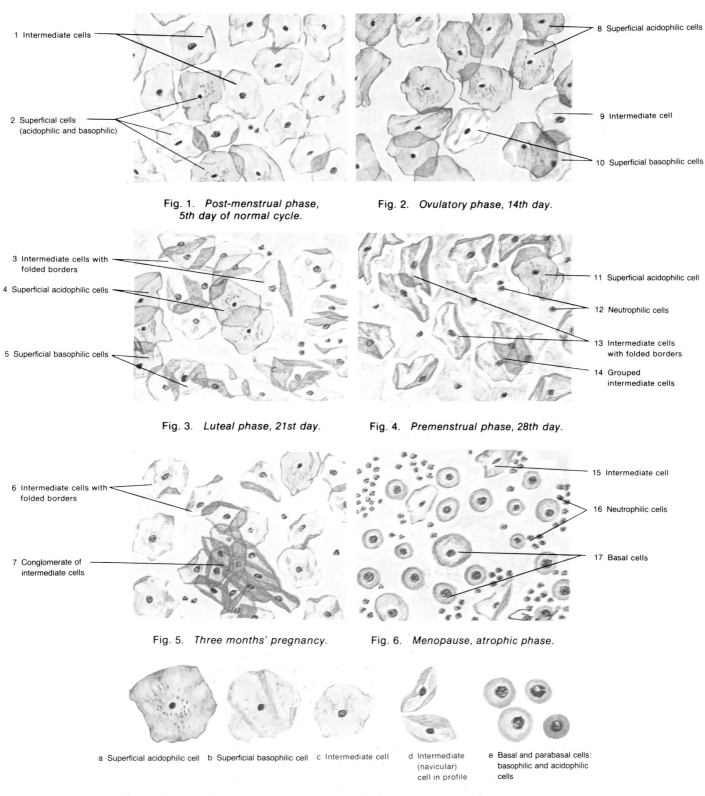

1 Intermediate cells

2 Superficial cells
(acidophilic and basophilic)

8 Superficial acidophilic cells

9 Intermediate cell

10 Superficial basophilic cells

Fig. 1. *Post-menstrual phase,
5th day of normal cycle.*

Fig. 2. *Ovulatory phase, 14th day.*

3 Intermediate cells with
folded borders

4 Superficial acidophilic cells

5 Superficial basophilic cells

11 Superficial acidophilic cell

12 Neutrophilic cells

13 Intermediate cells
with folded borders

14 Grouped
intermediate cells

Fig. 3. *Luteal phase, 21st day.*

Fig. 4. *Premenstrual phase, 28th day.*

6 Intermediate cells with
folded borders

7 Conglomerate of
intermediate cells

15 Intermediate cell

16 Neutrophilic cells

17 Basal cells

Fig. 5. *Three months' pregnancy.*

Fig. 6. *Menopause, atrophic phase.*

a Superficial acidophilic cell b Superficial basophilic cell c Intermediate cell   d Intermediate   e Basal and parabasal cells:
                                                                  (navicular)   basophilic and acidophilic
                                                                  cell in profile   cells

Fig. 7. Types of cells found in vaginal smears during different and normal reproductive phases.
Stain: Shorr's trichrome. 250× and 450×

PLATE 116 (Fig. 1)

MAMMARY GLAND, INACTIVE

The mammary gland (breast) consists of 15 to 25 lobes, each of which is an individual compound tubulo-alveolar type of gland (see pages 26 and 27). Each glandular lobe is separated by interlobar stroma and has its own lactiferous duct, which emerges independently onto the surface of the nipple. The interlobar stroma consists of dense connective tissue and varying amounts of fat. Each lobe contains similar interlobular connective tissue (2, 11) between individual lobules. Figure 1 illustrates one complete mammary gland lobule with its surrounding interlobular connective tissue and a portion of another (1).

The inactive mammary gland contains an abundance of connective tissue and a minimum of glandular elements. The lobules contain groups of small tubules lined with cuboidal or low columnar epithelium (3, 10). These tubules resemble ducts and remain in this state as long as the mammary gland remains inactive. Some cyclic changes may be seen in the mammary gland; however, these regress at the end of the menstrual cycle. Occasionally a better defined tubule is seen which is a small intralobular duct (6) or a large intralobular excretory (8) duct that emerges from the lobule to join the interlobular duct. Potential tubules may be present as undifferentiated solid cords of cells (5).

The excretory tubules are surrounded by a loose, fine connective tissue, the intralobular connective tissue (4), which contains fibroblasts, lymphocytes, plasma cells, and eosinophils. Surrounding this region is the dense interlobular connective (2) and adipose (11) tissue.

PLATE 116 (Fig. 2)

MAMMARY GLAND DURING THE FIRST HALF OF PREGNANCY

The mammary gland exhibits extensive changes in preparation for lactation. During the first half of pregnancy, the intralobular ducts undergo rapid proliferation and form terminal buds which differentiate into alveoli (2, 6). Most of the alveoli are empty; however, some may contain a secretory product (5). At this stage of development, it is difficult to distinguish between small intralobular ducts (9) and alveoli (6). The ducts appear more regular in outline and have a more distinct epithelial lining (9).

The glandular lobules are filled with numerous alveoli and the loose intralobular connective tissue (7) appears relatively reduced. On the other hand, there is an increased infiltration of lymphocytes and other cells. The interlobular dense connective tissue (3) appears as septa between the developing lobules. The interlobular ducts (4) that are lined with taller columnar cells course in the interlobular septa and empty into the large lactiferous ducts (8), which are usually lined with low pseudostratified columnar epithelium. Each lactiferous duct collects the secretory product of a lobe and transports it to the nipple.

PLATE 116

MAMMARY GLAND

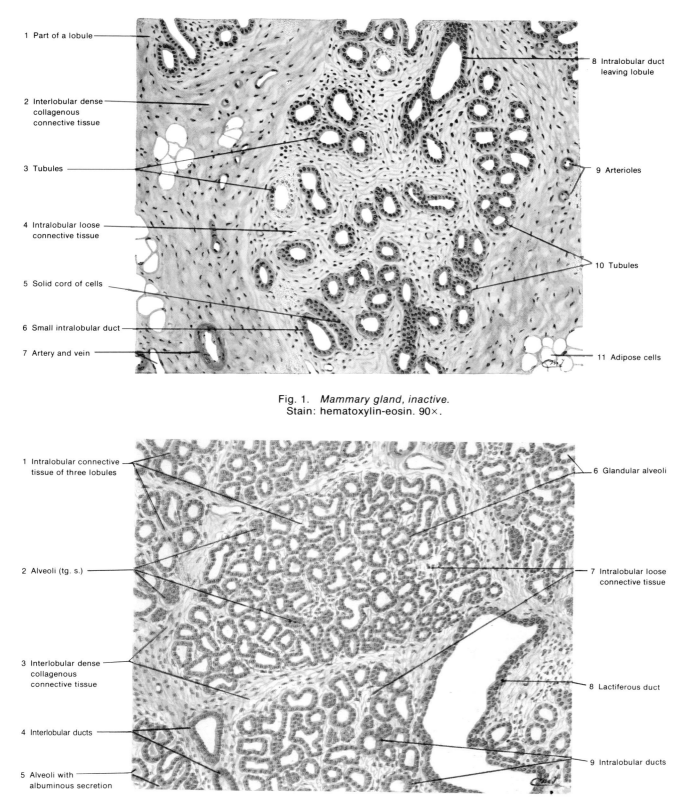

1 Part of a lobule

2 Interlobular dense collagenous connective tissue

3 Tubules

4 Intralobular loose connective tissue

5 Solid cord of cells

6 Small intralobular duct

7 Artery and vein

8 Intralobular duct leaving lobule

9 Arterioles

10 Tubules

11 Adipose cells

Fig. 1. *Mammary gland, inactive.*
Stain: hematoxylin-eosin. 90×.

1 Intralobular connective tissue of three lobules

2 Alveoli (tg. s.)

3 Interlobular dense collagenous connective tissue

4 Interlobular ducts

5 Alveoli with albuminous secretion

6 Glandular alveoli

7 Intralobular loose connective tissue

8 Lactiferous duct

9 Intralobular ducts

Fig. 2. *Mammary gland during the first half of pregnancy.*
Stain: hematoxylin-eosin. 90×.

PLATE 117 (Fig. 1)

MAMMARY GLAND, SEVENTH MONTH OF PREGNANCY

At 7 months of pregnancy, the glandular alveoli enlarge and the cells become secretory (1) with the secretory product often present in some alveolar lumina. Because the intralobular ducts also contain secretory material (6), the distinction between the alveoli and ducts remains difficult. In some sections, round alveoli (7) can be seen opening directly into an elongated excretory duct (6).

In later stages of pregnancy, there is a further relative reduction in the amount of intralobular (3) and interlobular connective tissue (5). The latter contains interlobular ducts (2) and a lactiferous duct (4) with secretory product in its lumen.

PLATE 117 (Fig. 2)

MAMMARY GLAND DURING LACTATION

This illustration depicts a few lobules in an active mammary gland during lactation at low (left) and higher (right) magnifications. The illustrated structures are generally similar to those represented in Figure 1.

The major difference in the lactating mammary gland is the presence of large number of distended alveoli filled with milk secretion (2) and showing irregular branching patterns (3). Also, there is a reduction of interlobular connective tissue septa (4).

During lactation, however, the histology of individual alveoli varies; all of the alveoli do not exhibit the same state of activity. The active alveoli are lined by low epithelium and their lumina are filled with milk, which appears as eosinophilic material containing large vacuoles of dissolved fat droplets (2, 9). Some active alveoli accumulate secretory product in their cytoplasm (8) and their cell apices appear vacuolated due to fat removal. Other alveoli exhibit a resting, inactive condition (6, 11); their lumina are empty, and their epithelium appears taller.

In the mammary gland, myoepithelial cells (not illustrated) are present between the alveolar cells and the basal lamina (see Plates 56, 57, 58); their contractions assist in expelling the milk into excretory ducts. The interlobular ducts (5, 7) are embedded in the connective tissue septa, which contain numerous adipose cells (1, 12).

PLATE 117

MAMMARY GLAND

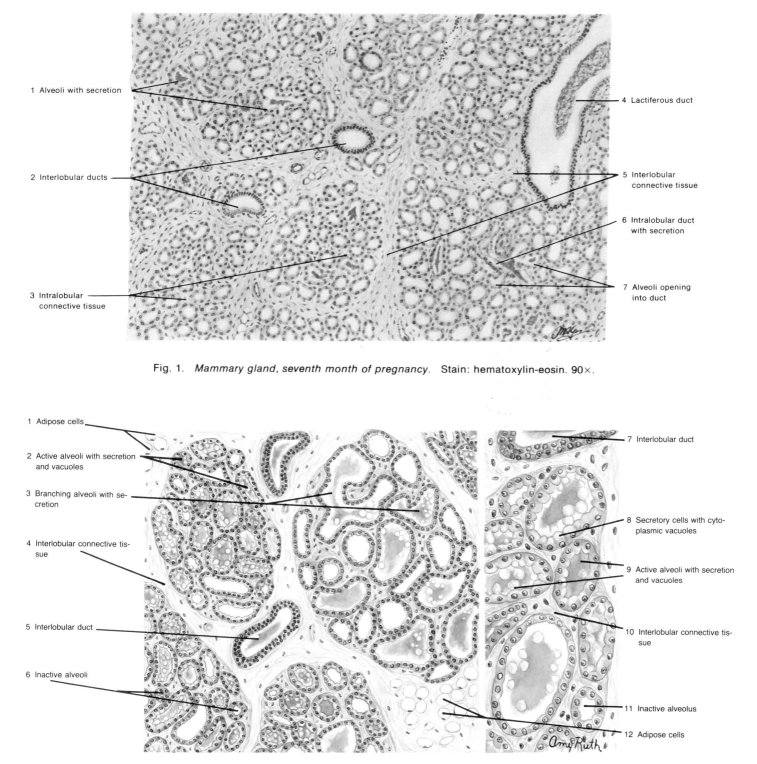

1 Alveoli with secretion

2 Interlobular ducts

3 Intralobular connective tissue

4 Lactiferous duct

5 Interlobular connective tissue

6 Intralobular duct with secretion

7 Alveoli opening into duct

Fig. 1.   *Mammary gland, seventh month of pregnancy.*   Stain: hematoxylin-eosin. 90×.

1 Adipose cells

2 Active alveoli with secretion and vacuoles

3 Branching alveoli with secretion

4 Interlobular connective tissue

5 Interlobular duct

6 Inactive alveoli

7 Interlobular duct

8 Secretory cells with cytoplasmic vacuoles

9 Active alveoli with secretion and vacuoles

10 Interlobular connective tissue

11 Inactive alveolus

12 Adipose cells

Fig. 2.   *Mammary gland during lactation.*   Stain: hematoxylin-eosin. 90× and 200×.

PLATE 118

EYELID (SAGITTAL SECTION)

The outer layer of the eyelid is illustrated on the left and the inner layer, which is adjacent to the eyeball, on the right.

The outer layer is thin skin and the epidermis consists of a stratified squamous epithelium with some papillae. The dermis contains hair follicles (1, 4) and sebaceous and sweat glands (2).

The inner layer is a mucous membrane, the palpebral conjunctiva (17). The lining epithelium is a low stratified columnar type (14) with goblet cells scattered among the epithelial cells. The stratified squamous epithelium of the skin continues over the margin of the eyelid and is transformed into the stratified columnar type. The thin lamina propria of the palpebral conjunctiva (17) contains connective tissue with elastic and collagenous fibers. Beneath the lamina propria is a plate of dense, collagenous connective tissue, the tarsus (16), which contains large, specialized sebaceous glands, the tarsal (Meibomian) glands (15). The alveoli of these glands open into a long central duct (18) which runs parallel to the conjunctiva surface and opens at the lid margin.

The free end of the eyelid contains eyelashes which arise from large, long hair follicles (20). Associated with the eyelashes are small sebaceous glands (9). Between the hair follicles are large sweat glands, the glands of Moll (8).

Three sets of muscles are present in the eyelid: the extensive palpebral portion of the skeletal muscle, the orbicularis oculi (5), the skeletal ciliary muscle (of Riolan) (19) in the region of the hair follicles of the eyelashes and tarsal glands, and the smooth, superior tarsal muscle (of Müller) (10).

The accessory lacrimal gland (12) lies in the connective tissue behind the conjunctiva of the fornix. Diffuse lymphatic tissue (13) is prevalent in this region. In addition to the main lacrimal gland, numerous small, accessory tarsal lacrimal glands are found in the connective tissue above the tarsal plate. These glands are scattered, vary in number, and are not seen in every section of the eyelid.

PLATE 118

EYELID (SAGITTAL SECTION)

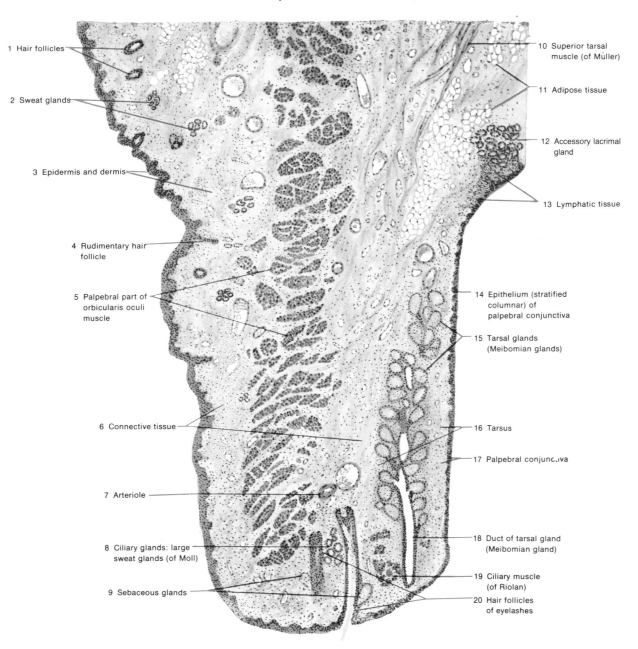

1 Hair follicles

2 Sweat glands

3 Epidermis and dermis

4 Rudimentary hair follicle

5 Palpebral part of orbicularis oculi muscle

6 Connective tissue

7 Arteriole

8 Ciliary glands: large sweat glands (of Moll)

9 Sebaceous glands

10 Superior tarsal muscle (of Müller)

11 Adipose tissue

12 Accessory lacrimal gland

13 Lymphatic tissue

14 Epithelium (stratified columnar) of palpebral conjunctiva

15 Tarsal glands (Meibomian glands)

16 Tarsus

17 Palpebral conjunctiva

18 Duct of tarsal gland (Meibomian gland)

19 Ciliary muscle (of Riolan)

20 Hair follicles of eyelashes

Stain: hematoxylin-eosin. 20×.

PLATE 119 (Fig. 1)

LACRIMAL GLAND

The lacrimal gland is a tear-secreting gland composed of several tubuloalveolar glands. The alveoli (1, 8) vary in size and shape and resemble the serous type; however, their lumina are larger and may contain irregular outpocketings of cells (5) into the lumina. The alveolar cells are more columnar than pyramidal, contain large secretory granules and lipid droplets, and stain lightly. Myoepithelial cells (basket cells) (3) are present around individual alveoli.

The smaller intralobular excretory ducts (2, lower leader) are lined with simple cuboidal or columnar epithelium. The larger ducts (2, upper leader) and the interlobular ducts (7, 11) are lined with two layers of low columnar or pseudostratified epitheliium.

Interalveolar (intralobular) connective tissue is sparse; however, interlobular connective tissue (4) is abundant and may contain adipose tissue.

PLATE 119 (Fig. 2)

CORNEA (TRANSVERSE SECTION)

The anterior surface of the cornea is covered with nonpapillated, stratified squamous nonkeratinized epithelium (1, 6, 7). The lowest or basal cell layer is columnar and rests on thin basement membrane. Beneath the corneal epithelium is a thick, homogeneous anterior limiting membrane (Bowman's) (2), which is derived from the underlying corneal stroma or substantia propria (3). The stroma forms the body of the cornea and consists of parallel bundles of collagenous fibers which form thin lamellae (9) and layers of flat, branching fibroblasts, the keratocytes (8), between the collagenous fibers. The corneal keratocytes are modified fibroblasts.

The posterior surface of the cornea is covered with a very low cuboidal epithelium, the posterior epithelium (5, 10), which is also the corneal endothelium. The posterior limiting membrane (Descemet's membrane) (4) is wide and constitutes the basement membrane of the posterior corneal epithelium. It rests on the posterior portion of the corneal stroma.

PLATE 119

EYE

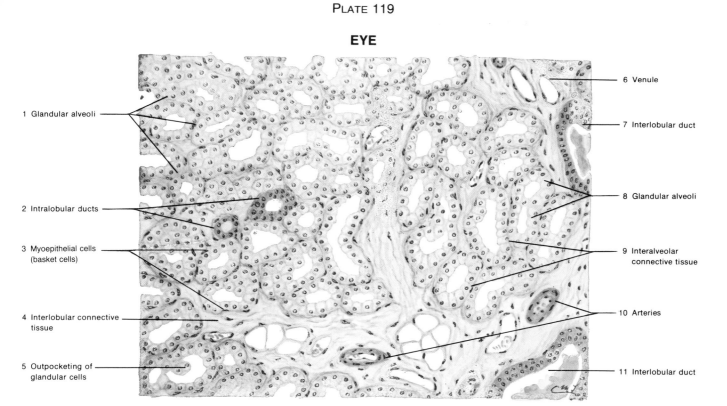

1 Glandular alveoli

2 Intralobular ducts

3 Myoepithelial cells
(basket cells)

4 Interlobular connective
tissue

5 Outpocketing of
glandular cells

6 Venule

7 Interlobular duct

8 Glandular alveoli

9 Interalveolar
connective tissue

10 Arteries

11 Interlobular duct

Fig. 1.   *Lacrimal gland.* Stain: hematoxylin-eosin. 180 ×.

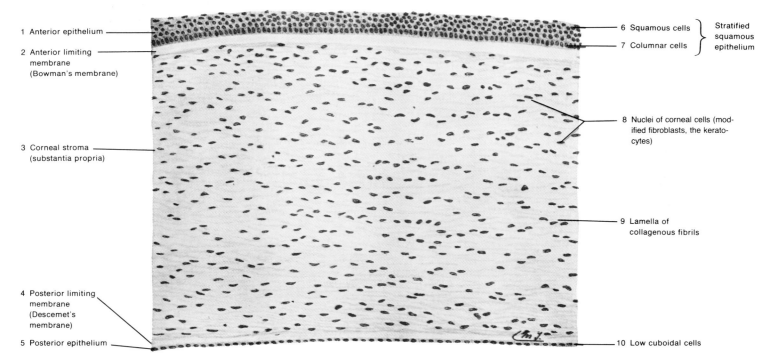

1 Anterior epithelium

2 Anterior limiting
membrane
(Bowman's membrane)

3 Corneal stroma
(substantia propria)

4 Posterior limiting
membrane
(Descemet's
membrane)

5 Posterior epithelium

6 Squamous cells

7 Columnar cells

Stratified
squamous
epithelium

8 Nuclei of corneal cells (modified fibroblasts, the keratocytes)

9 Lamella of
collagenous fibrils

10 Low cuboidal cells

Fig. 2.   *Cornea (transverse section).* Stain: hematoxylin-eosin. 180 ×.

PLATE 120

EYE (SAGITTAL SECTION)

The capsule of the eyeball consists of three concentric layers: an outer, tough, fibrous tunic composed of the cornea (1) and the sclera (3, 9, 23); a middle vascular layer or the uvea, composed of the choroid (8, 21), the ciliary body (4, 17) and the iris (15); and an innermost layer of photosensitive nerve tissue, the retina (7, 18, 20).

The cornea (1) is a transparent layer and its histologic details are illustrated in Plate 119, Figure 2.

The sclera (3, 9, 23) is white, opaque, and tough connective tissue layer composed of densely woven collagenous fibers. The sclera aids in maintaining the rigidity of the eyeball and appears as the "white" of the eye. The junction or transition between the cornea and sclera is the limbus (13). The region where the optic nerve (27) emerges from the ocular capsule marks the site of the continuation of sclera (9) with the dura mater (11) of the central nervous system.

The choroid (8, 21) and the ciliary body of the uvea lie adjacent to the sclera (9, 23). In sagittal section, the ciliary body appears triangular in shape. It is composed of the ciliary muscle (4) and the ciliary processes (17). Smooth muscle fibers constitute the ciliary muscle and are disposed in longitudinal, circular and radial directions. The folded and highly vascular extensions of the ciliary body constitute the ciliary processes (17). These processes are attached to the equator of the lens (6) by suspensory ligament of the lens (5) or the zonular fibers. Contraction of the ciliary muscle reduces the tension on the suspensory ligament and allows the lens (6) to assume a more convex shape.

The iris (15) is the colored portion of the eye as seen in situ. The circular and radial arrangement of smooth muscle fibers forms the pupil. The anterior chamber (12) of the eye is situated between the iris and cornea while the posterior chamber (16) lies between the iris and the lens. Both the anterior and posteriors chambers are filled with a fluid, the aqueous humor. Located behind the lens is the vitreous chamber (22), which is filled with a gelatinous substance, the vitreous humor.

The inner tunic or retina (7, 18, 20) of the eyeball is the photoreceptive region of the eye; however, it is not light-receptive throughout. In an anterior hemisection of the eyeball, the posterior rim of the ciliary body appears scalloped. The ora serrata (19) is the sharp, serrated, anterior delimitation of the sensory part of the retina. Posterior to the ora serrata is the optic retina (7, 20), which consists of numerous cell layers, one of which contains the light-receptive cells, the rods and cones (see page 121, Fig. 2). Anterior to the ora serrata is the blind or nonsensitive retina, which, as a simplified pigment layer, extends to the tip of the iris. The section of the blind retina adjacent to the ciliary body is the ciliary retina (18), and that adjacent to the iris is the iridial retina (not labeled). These portions of the retina are not photosensitive.

On the posterior wall of the eye are situated two landmarks, the macula lutea (25) and the optic papilla (26) or disk. The macula lutea is a small greenish-yellow spot that varies in diameter from 1.05 to 5.00 mm. In its center is a depression called the fovea centralis, which represents the area of most acute vision. The center of the fovea is devoid of rods and blood vessels but contains an abundance of cone cells.

The optic papilla (26) is the site of exit of the optic nerve. This region lacks both the rods and cones and constitutes the "blind spot" of the eye.

The extensive histologic details of the retina are illustrated in Plate 121.

The outer limit of the sclera is contiguous with orbital fatty tissue (24), which is composed of loose connective tissue, fat cells, nerves, blood and lymphatic vessels, and glands.

PLATE 120

EYE (SAGITTAL SECTION)

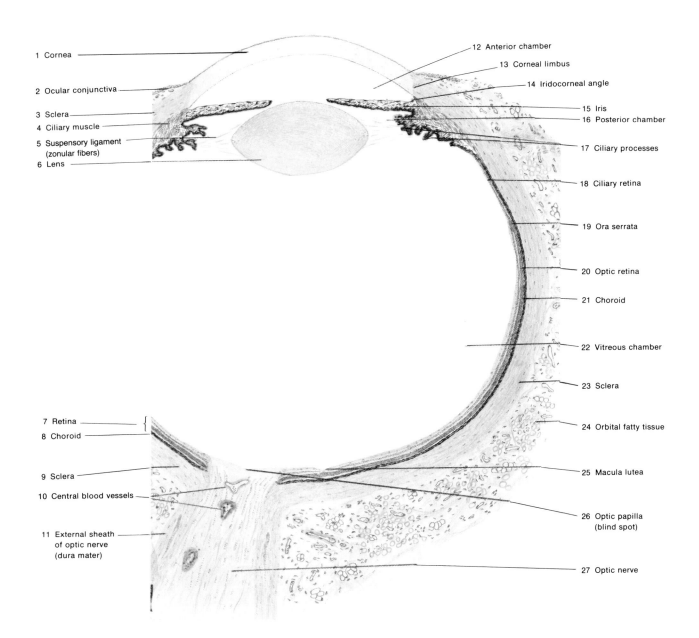

1 Cornea

2 Ocular conjunctiva

3 Sclera

4 Ciliary muscle

5 Suspensory ligament
(zonular fibers)

6 Lens

7 Retina

8 Choroid

9 Sclera

10 Central blood vessels

11 External sheath
of optic nerve
(dura mater)

12 Anterior chamber

13 Corneal limbus

14 Iridocorneal angle

15 Iris

16 Posterior chamber

17 Ciliary processes

18 Ciliary retina

19 Ora serrata

20 Optic retina

21 Choroid

22 Vitreous chamber

23 Sclera

24 Orbital fatty tissue

25 Macula lutea

26 Optic papilla
(blind spot)

27 Optic nerve

Stain: hematoxylin-eosin. 15×.

PLATE 121 (Fig. 1)

RETINA, CHOROID, AND SCLERA: PANORAMIC VIEW

For most of its extent, the wall of each eyeball is composed of three coats: the sclera (1), the choroid (2), and the retina (3).

In this illustration, only the deeper portion of the sclera (1) is illustrated. The stroma of the sclera is composed of dense collagenous fibers (4) that course parallel to the surface of the eyeball. Between the collagen bundles is a delicate network of elastic fibers. Flattened or elongated fibroblasts are present throughout the sclera and the melanocytes (5) are found in the deepest layer.

The layers comprising the choroid are described in detail in the following paragraphs.

The human retina has been divided into 10 layers except in the specialized regions. These are listed in order in Figure 1 (7–16).

PLATE 121 (Fig. 2)

LAYERS OF THE CHOROID AND RETINA IN DETAIL

The choroid is subdivided into the following layers: the suprachoroid lamina (17), the vessel layer (18), the choriocapillary layer (19), and the transparent limiting membrane, the glassy membrane (Bruch's membrane).

The suprachoroid lamina (17) consists of lamellae of fine collagenous fibers, a rich network of elastic fibers, fibroblasts, and numerous large melanocytes. The vessel layer (18) contains large and medium-sized vessels (1). In the the loose connective tissue between the blood vessels are numerous, large flat melanocytes (2) that give this layer its chracteristic black color. The choriocapillary layer (19) contains a network of capillaries with large lumina in a stroma of fine collagenous and elastic fibers. The innermost layer of the choroid, the glassy membrane, lies adjacent to the pigment epithelium of the retina (3).

The outermost layer of the retina is the pigment epithelium (3) and its basement membrane forms the innermost layer of the glassy membrane of the choroid. The cuboidal cells of the pigment epithelium contain melanin (pigment) granules in apical regions of the cytoplasm; processes with pigment granules extend into the layer of rods and cones (20).

Adjacent to the pigment epithelium is a layer of slender rods (4, 22) and thicker cones (5, 21) situated next to the outer limiting membrane (6, 23), which is formed by the processes of the neuroglial cells, the Müller's cells (30).

The outermost nuclear layer contains nuclei of the rods (8, 25) and cones (7, 24) and the outermost processes of Müller's cells (26). In the outer plexiform layer (9), the axons of rods and cones synapse with the dendrites of bipolar (28) and horizontal cells (27).

The inner nuclear layer (10) contains the nuclei of bipolar (29), horizontal, amacrine (31) and neuroglial Müller's cells (30). The horizontal and amacrine cells are association cells. In the inner plexiform layer (11), the axons of bipolar cells (29) synapse (32) with the dendrites of the ganglion and amacrine cells.

The ganglion cell layer (12) contains the cell bodies of ganglion cells (33) and scattered neuroglial cells. Dendrites from the ganglion cells synapse in the inner plexiform layer (32).

The nerve fiber layer (13, 14) contains the vertically and horizontally directed axons of the ganglion cells (14) and the inner fiber network of Müller's cells (13, 37). Axons of the ganglion cells (14, 33) converge toward the optic disk to form the optic nerve. The terminations of the inner fibers of Müller's cells expand to form the inner limiting membrane (15, 36) of the retina.

Blood vessels of the retina course in the nerve fiber layer and penetrate as far as the inner nuclear layer (10). Sections of some of the vessels' various planes can be seen (unlabeled) in this layer.

PLATE 121

RETINA, CHOROID, AND SCLERA

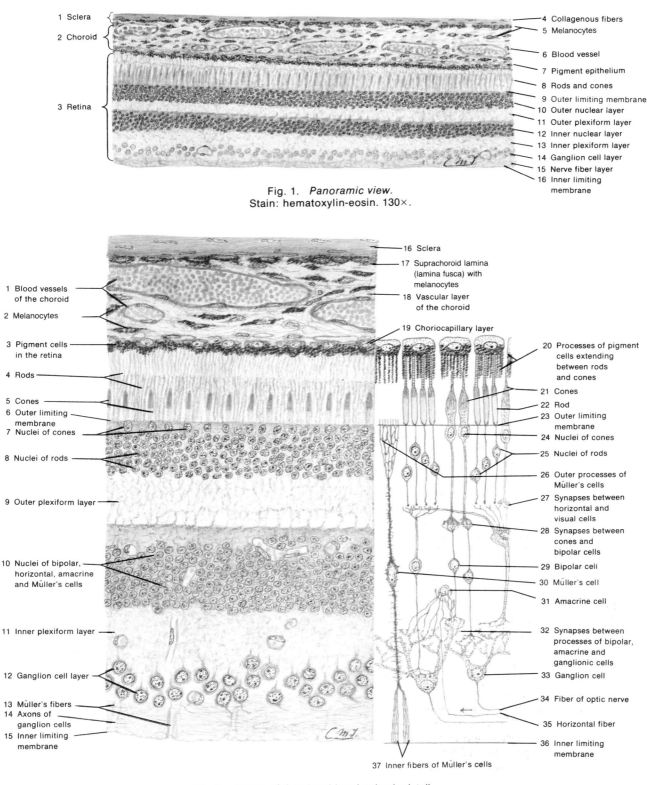

1 Sclera

2 Choroid

3 Retina

4 Collagenous fibers
5 Melanocytes
6 Blood vessel
7 Pigment epithelium
8 Rods and cones
9 Outer limiting membrane
10 Outer nuclear layer
11 Outer plexiform layer
12 Inner nuclear layer
13 Inner plexiform layer
14 Ganglion cell layer
15 Nerve fiber layer
16 Inner limiting membrane

Fig. 1. *Panoramic view.*
Stain: hematoxylin-eosin. 130×.

16 Sclera
17 Suprachoroid lamina (lamina fusca) with melanocytes
18 Vascular layer of the choroid
19 Choriocapillary layer

1 Blood vessels of the choroid
2 Melanocytes
3 Pigment cells in the retina
4 Rods
5 Cones
6 Outer limiting membrane
7 Nuclei of cones
8 Nuclei of rods
9 Outer plexiform layer
10 Nuclei of bipolar, horizontal, amacrine and Müller's cells
11 Inner plexiform layer
12 Ganglion cell layer
13 Müller's fibers
14 Axons of ganglion cells
15 Inner limiting membrane

20 Processes of pigment cells extending between rods and cones
21 Cones
22 Rod
23 Outer limiting membrane
24 Nuclei of cones
25 Nuclei of rods
26 Outer processes of Müller's cells
27 Synapses between horizontal and visual cells
28 Synapses between cones and bipolar cells
29 Bipolar cell
30 Müller's cell
31 Amacrine cell
32 Synapses between processes of bipolar, amacrine and ganglionic cells
33 Ganglion cell
34 Fiber of optic nerve
35 Horizontal fiber
36 Inner limiting membrane

37 Inner fibers of Müller's cells

Fig. 2. *Layers of the choroid and retina in detail.*
Stain: hematoxylin-eosin. 400×.

PLATE 122 (Fig. 1)

INNER EAR: COCHLEA (VERTICAL SECTION)

The bony or osseous labyrinth of the cochlea (16, 18) is twisted in a spiral around a central axis of a spongy bone, the modiolus (17). Embedded in the bony modiolus is the spiral ganglion (14), which is composed of bipolar afferent neurons. Long central processes (axons) from these bipolar cells form part of the cochlear nerve (9); the short peripheral processes (dendrites) innervate the hair cells in the organ of Corti (13).

The bony labyrinth is divided into two major cavities by the osseous spiral lamina (8) and the basilar membrane (membranous spiral lamina) (7). The osseous spiral lamina (8) projects from the modiolus about halfway into the lumen of the cochlear canal. The basilar membrane (7) continues from the spiral lamina to the spiral ligament (6), which is a thickening of the periosteum on the outer bony wall of the cochlear canal (5). The cochlear canal is subdivided into a lower compartment, the scala tympani (4), and an upper compartment, the scala vestibuli (2). Both compartments pursue a spiral course to the apex of the cochlea, where they communicate through a small orifice called the helicotrema (1).

The vestibular membrane (Reissner's membrane) (10) separates the scala vestibuli (2) from the cochlear duct (scala media) (3) and forms the roof over the cochlear duct. The cells specialized for receiving sound vibrations and transmitting them as nerve impulses to the brain are located in the organ of Corti (13); this organ rests on the basilar membrane (7) on the floor of the cochlear duct. The tectorial membrane (12) overlies the cells in the organ of Corti.

PLATE 122 (Fig. 2)

COCHLEAR DUCT (SCALA MEDIA)

The cochlear duct is illustrated at higher magnification and in greater detail.

The outer wall of the cochlear duct is formed by the vascular area called the stria vascularis (16), which consists of columnar epithelium. The stratified epithelium covering the stria vascularis is unique in that it contains intraepithelial capillary network formed from the vessels located in the connective tissue of the spiral ligament (17). The lamina propria in this region is the spiral ligament (17, 19), which consists of collagenous fibers, pigmented fibroblasts, and numerous blood vessels.

The roof of the cochlear duct (9) is formed by the vestibular membrane (6), which separates it from the scala vestibuli (7). The vestibular membrane extends from the spiral ligament (17) of the outer wall of the cochlea, located at the upper extent of the vascular stria (15, 16), to the thickened periosteum of the osseous spiral lamina (4) near the limbus (5).

The spiral limbus (5) forms a part of the cochlear duct floor (9). The limbus is a thickened mass of periosteal connective tissue (4) of the osseous spiral lamina (1), which bulges into the cochlear duct. It is supported by a lateral extension of the osseous spiral lamina (1). The limbus is covered by an epithelium that appears columnar. The lateral extracellular extension of this epithelium beyond the vestibular lip of the limbus is the tectorial membrane (10), which overlies the inner spiral sulcus (8) and part of the organ of Corti (12), including its hair cells (11).

The basilar membrane (13) consists of a plate of vascularized connective tissue underlying a thinner plate of basilar fibers. The organ of Corti (12) rests on these basilar fibers. The organ extends from the spiral limbus (5) to the spiral ligament (17, 19).

The organ of Corti (12) consists of highly specialized sensory or hair cells (11), several types of supporting cells, and spaces and tunnels. The deeply staining cells to the left of the hair cells are the pillar cells surrounding the inner tunnel (not illustrated), which is within the organ of Corti. Various names are assigned to the other supporting cells.

From the bipolar cells of the spiral ganglion (3), peripheral (afferent) processes (2) course through the channels in the osseous spiral lamina to terminate (synapse) with the hair cells (11) of the organ of Corti (12).

PLATE 122

INNER EAR

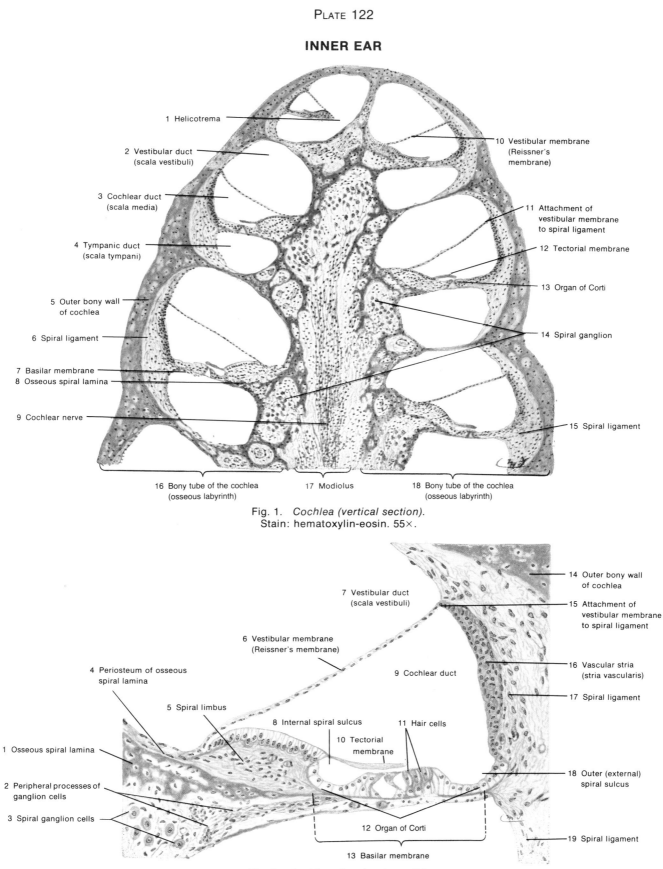

1 Helicotrema

2 Vestibular duct
(scala vestibuli)

3 Cochlear duct
(scala media)

4 Tympanic duct
(scala tympani)

5 Outer bony wall
of cochlea

6 Spiral ligament

7 Basilar membrane

8 Osseous spiral lamina

9 Cochlear nerve

10 Vestibular membrane
(Reissner's
membrane)

11 Attachment of
vestibular membrane
to spiral ligament

12 Tectorial membrane

13 Organ of Corti

14 Spiral ganglion

15 Spiral ligament

16 Bony tube of the cochlea
(osseous labyrinth)

17 Modiolus

18 Bony tube of the cochlea
(osseous labyrinth)

Fig. 1. *Cochlea (vertical section).*
Stain: hematoxylin-eosin. 55×.

7 Vestibular duct
(scala vestibuli)

6 Vestibular membrane
(Reissner's membrane)

9 Cochlear duct

4 Periosteum of osseous
spiral lamina

5 Spiral limbus

8 Internal spiral sulcus

11 Hair cells

10 Tectorial
membrane

1 Osseous spiral lamina

2 Peripheral processes of
ganglion cells

3 Spiral ganglion cells

14 Outer bony wall
of cochlea

15 Attachment of
vestibular membrane
to spiral ligament

16 Vascular stria
(stria vascularis)

17 Spiral ligament

18 Outer (external)
spiral sulcus

19 Spiral ligament

12 Organ of Corti

13 Basilar membrane

Fig. 2. *Cochlear duct (scala media).*
Stain: hematoxylin-eosin. 200×.

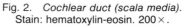

INDEX

Acidophilic cell (alpha cell) of
    hypophysis, 196–199
  (oxyphilic cell) of parathyroids, 202,
    203
Acinus, pancreatic, 172, 173
  serous, 124, 125, 172, 173
Adipose cells, 28–31, 34–35
Adipose tissue, 34, 35
Adrenal glands, 204, 205
Adventitia (tunica adventitia), of blood
    vessels, 86, 87
  of ductus deferens, 212, 213
  of esophagus, 130, 131
  of rectum, 160, 161
  of seminal vesicle, 216, 217
  of ureter, 192, 193
  of vagina, 240, 241
Alpha cell (acidophilic cell) of
    hypophysis, 196–199
Alveolar ducts, of lung, 182–185
  sac, 182, 183
Alveolar gland, compound, 26, 27
Alveolus, of lung, 182–185
  mucous, 126–129
  of mammary gland, 244–247
  of sebaceous glands, 108, 109
  of tooth, 122, 123
  serous, 125–129
Amacrine cell, 254, 255
Ameloblast, 122, 123
Ampulla of ductus deferens, 198, 199
  of uterine tube, 228, 229
Anal canal, 162, 163
Anal valve, 162, 163
Anorectal junction, 162, 163
Anterior chamber of eye, 252, 253
Anterior horn, 62–67, 78, 81
  (ventral) median fissure, 78–81
Anterior lateral column of the spinal
    cord, 78, 79
Aorta, orcein stain, 88, 89
Appendix, 158, 159
APUD cells, 140, 150
Aqueous humor, 252, 253
Arachnoid of spinal cord, 80, 81
Argentaffin cell, 150 (see APUD cells)
Arrector pili muscles, 104–111
Arteries, 72, 73, 86–89
  arcuate, 186, 187
  coiled, of uterus, 230–235
  elastic, 88, 89
  elastic membrane of, 72, 73, 86–89

endothelium of, 72, 73, 86–89
  hepatic, 164–167
  interlobular, of kidney, 186–189
  pulmonary, of heart, 92, 93
    of lung, 182–185
  renal, 186, 187
  transverse section of, 72, 73, 86–89
  tunica adventitia of, 72, 73, 86–89
  tunica media of, 72, 73, 86–89
Astrocytes (macroglia), 68–71
  perivascular, 70, 71
Atrium, left, 90, 91
Auerbach's plexus (myenteric plexus),
    138, 139, 146–151, 156–161
Axon, 66, 67, 72–75
  hillock, 66, 67

Basement membrane, of ductus
    epididymis, 210, 211
  of epithelium, 16–21
  of seminiferous tubules, 208, 209
Basilar membrane, 256, 257
Basket cell, 124, 126
Basophil, 52, 53, 58, 59
Basophilic cell (beta cell) of hypophysis,
    196–199
Beta cell (basophilic cell) of hypophysis,
    196–199
Bile canaliculi, 166, 167
Bile ducts, 164–167, 169
Billroth, cords of (splenic cords), 102
Bipolar cell of retina, 254, 255
Bladder, gall, 170, 171
  urinary, 194, 195
Blind spot, 252, 253
Blood cells, Celani's stain of, 54, 55
  development of, 56–59
  of bone marrow, 56–59
  of peripheral blood, 52–55
  Pappenheim's stain of, 54, 55
  supravital stain of, 54, 55
  vessels, 86, 87
Blood platelets, 52–59
Bone, 40–52
  cancellous, 42, 43
  compact, 40, 41, 48, 49
  development of, 42–51
  endochondral, 44–49
  epiphyses of, 50, 51
  intracartilaginous, 44–49
  intramembranous, 42, 43
  marrow, 56–59

Bowman's capsule, 188, 189
  membrane, 250, 251
Brain
  fibrous astrocytes of, 70, 71
  microglia of, 70, 71
  oligodendrocytes of, 70, 71
Bronchiole, 182–185
  respiratory, 182–185
  terminal, 182–185
Bronchi, 182–185
  epithelium of, 70, 71
Bruch's membrane, 254
Brunner's glands, 146–149
Brush border of kidney, 188–189
Buck's fascia, 219
Bulbourethral gland, 216, 217

Cajal's stain, 66, 67, 78, 79, 82, 83
Call-Exner bodies, 222, 223
Calyx, of kidney, 186, 187
Canal, central, 78, 79
Canaliculi, bile, of liver, 166, 167
  of bone, 40, 41
  of teeth, 120, 121
Cardia, 136, 137
Cardiac glands, 136, 137
Cartilage, 36–39
  articular, 50, 51
  elastic, 38, 39
  epiglottic, 176–179
  fibrous, 38, 39
  hyaline, 36, 37
  tracheal, 180, 181
Cells, amacrine, 254, 255
  argentaffin, 150
  bipolar, of the retina, 254, 255
  centroacinar, 172, 173
  enteroendocrine, 150, 151
  Kupffer, 166, 167
  Paneth, 150, 151
  parietal, 138–143
  Sertoli, 208, 209
Cementum of teeth, 120, 121
Centroacinar cell, 172, 173
Cerebellum, 82, 83
Cerebral cortex, layers of, 84, 85
Cervical glands, 238, 239
Cervix, 238, 239
Chief cells (principal cells), of
    parathyroids, 202, 203
  of stomach, 138–143
Chondroblasts, 35, 36
Chondrocytes, 36–39, 44, 45
Chorion, of placenta, 236, 237
Chorionic villi, 236, 237
Choroid layer of eye, 252–255
Chromaffin reaction, 204
Chromatophore, 254, 255
Chromophil cell, of hypophysis,
    196–199

Chromophobe cell, of hypophysis,
    196–199
Ciliary body, muscle, 252, 253
  of eye, 252, 253
  processes, 252, 253
Circumvallate (vallate) papilla, 116, 117
Cochlea, 256, 257
Coiled arteries, of uterus, 230–235
Colony Forming Unit (CFU), 58, 59
Collagenous fibers, 28–35
Collecting tubules of kidney, 186–191
Colon, 154–157
Column, anterior (ventral) of spinal
    cord, 78–81
  of Clarke, 80, 81
  posterior (dorsal), of spinal cord,
      78–81
  rectal, 162
Cones of retina, 254, 255
Conjunctiva, ocular, 252, 253
  palpebral, 248, 249
Connective tissue, 30–35
  adipose, 34, 35
  dense, 30–35
  embryonic, 34, 35
  loose (irregular), 28–31, 34, 35
Cornea, 250, 251
  limbus of, 252, 253
Corona radiata, of oocyte, 222, 223
Corpora cavernosa of penis, 218, 219
Corpus albicans, 220, 221, 224, 225
  cavernosum urethrae, 218, 219
  luteum, 220–227
  spongiosum, 218, 219
Corpuscles, Hassall's, 100, 101
  lamellar, 32, 33, 102, 103, 162, 163
  Meissner's, 104, 105
  Pacinian, 32, 33, 102, 103, 110, 111,
      162, 163
  renal, 188, 189
  splenic, 102, 103
  tactile, 104, 105
  thymic, 100, 101
Corti, organ of, 256, 257
  spiral ganglion of, 256, 257
Cortical labyrinth of kidney, 186, 187
Crypt, tonsillar, 98, 99
Crypts of Lieberkühn, 156–163
Cumulus oophorus, 222–225
Cuticle of hair, 108, 109

Dartos tunic, 218, 219
Decidual cells, 236, 237
Del Rio Hortega's stain, 70, 71, 168, 169
Demilunes, serous, 128, 129
Dendrite, 66, 67, 78–85
Dental alveolus, 122, 123
  pulp, 122, 123
  sac, 122, 123

Dentin, 120–123
  tubules, 120, 121
Dermal papillae, 104, 105, 108, 109
Dermis, 104, 105, 108, 109
Descemet's membrane, 250, 251
Desmosomes, 104
Duct, alveolar, of lung, 182–185
  bile, 164–167, 169
  cochlear, 256, 257
  intercalated, of pancreas, 172, 173
    of salivary glands, 124–127
  interlobular, of lacrimal gland, 250,
    251
    of mammary gland, 244, 245
    of pancreas, 172, 173
    of salivary glands, 172–179
  lactiferous, 244–247
  papillary, 190, 191
  striated, 124–127, 172, 173
Ductuli efferentes, 206, 207, 210, 211
Ductus deferens, 212, 213
  epididymis, 210, 211
Duodenum, 146–149
Dura mater, 80, 81

Ear, inner, 256, 257
Efferent ducts of testis, 206, 207, 210,
  211
Elastic fibers, 28–31
  in aorta, 88, 89
Eleiden, 104
Enamel, 120–123
  prisms, 120–123
  pulp, 120–123
  rods, 120–123
Endocardium, 90–93
Endocervix, 238, 239
Endometrium, 230–237
Endomysium 63, 64
Endoneurium, 74, 75
Endosteum, 42, 43
Endothelium of blood vessels, 86–89
Enteroendocrine cell, 150, 151
Eosinophil, 56–59
Epicardium, 90–93
Epidermis, 104, 105, 108, 109
Epididymis, duct of, 210, 211
Epiglottis, 176, 177
Epineurium, 74–77
Epithelium, 14–27
  ciliated, 20, 21
  germinal, of ovary, 220–223
  peritoneal, 14, 15
  pseudostratified, 20, 21
  simple columnar, 16, 17
  simple squamous, 14, 15
  stratified squamous, 18, 19
  striated columnar, 16, 17
  transitional, 20, 21
    of bladder, 194, 195

of ureter, 192, 193
Erythroblasts, 56–59
Erythrocytes, 52–59
Esophageal glands, 130–135
Esophageal-cardiac junction, 136, 137
Esophagus, 18, 19, 130–135
Eye, 252–255
Eyelid, 248, 249

Fallopian tube (uterine tube), 228, 229
Fasciculus cuneatus, 78–81
Fasciculus gracilis, 78–81
Fat cells, 28–31, 34–35
  droplets, 168–169
  tissue, 34, 35
Fibroblasts, 28–31
Fibrous connective tissue, 28–33
Filiform papillae, 114, 115
Follicle, hair, 104, 105, 108, 109
  ovarian, 220–225
  thyroid, 200, 201
Follicular cells, ovarian, 220, 221
  theca, 222–225
Fornix of cervix, 238, 239
Fovea centralis, 252
Foveolae, of stomach, 136–143
Fungiform papillae, 114, 115

Gallbladder, 170, 171
Ganglion, dorsal root, 76, 77
  parasympathetic, 128, 129, 148–151,
    156–161
  spiral, 256, 257
  sympathetic, 76, 77
Gastric glands, 136–143
Germinal center, of a lymph node,
  96–99
  of spleen, 102, 103
Germinal epithelium, of ovary, 220–223
Glands, accessory lacrimal, 248, 249
  adrenal, 204, 205
  anterior lingual, 114, 115
  Bowman's (olfactory), 174, 175
  Brunner's (duodenal), 146–149
  bulbourethral, 216, 217
  cardiac, 136, 137
  cervical, 238, 239
  compound alveolar, 26, 27
    tubuloalveolar, 24, 25
  duodenal, 146–149
  esophageal, 130–135
  gastric, 136–143
  intestinal, 146–163
  labial, 112, 113
  lacrimal, 250, 251
  Lieberkühn's (crypts of Lieberkühn),
    148–163
  mammary, 244–247
  Meibomian, 248, 249

Glands *(continued)*
   Moll's, 248, 249
   of vallate papilla, 116–117
   parathyroid, 202, 203
   parotid, 124, 125
   pituitary, 196–199
   posterior lingual, 118, 119
   prostate, 214, 215
   pyloric, 144, 145
   salivary, 124–129
   sebaceous, 104–108
   simple branched tubular, 22, 23
   sublingual, 128, 129
   submandibular, 126, 127
   sweat, 104–109
   thymus, 100, 101
   thyroid, 200–203
   tubular, 22, 23
   tubuloalveolar, 24, 25
   urethral, 218, 219
   uterine, 230–235
   von Ebner's, 116, 117
Glomerulus, of cerebellum, 82, 83
   of kidney, 186–189
Glomus, 110–111
Glycogen, liver, 168, 169
   vagina, 240, 241
Goblet cells, 16, 17, 20, 21
   of appendix, 158, 159
   of large intestine, 156, 157
   of rectum, 160, 161
   of small intestine, 148–153
Golgi stain of nerve cells, 68, 69
Granulocyte, 52–59
Granulosa lutein cell, 226, 227
Gray commissure, 78–81
   matter, 66–69, 78, 79, 82, 83

Hair, 104, 105, 108, 109
   bulb, 108, 109
   follicle, 108, 109
Hassall's corpuscle, 100, 101
Haversian canal, 40–43, 48, 49
   systems, 40–43, 48, 49
Heart: atrium, mitral valve, ventricle,
     90, 91
   pulmonary artery, valve, ventricle,
     92, 93
Helicotrema, 256, 257
Hemocytoblast, 56–59
Hemorrhoidal plexus, 162, 163
Henle's layer, 108, 109
   loop, 186
Hepatic artery, 164–167
   triad, 164, 165
Hepatic lamina (plate), 164–167
Hilus of a lymph node, 94, 95
Histiocytes, 28, 29
Holocrine secretion, 108
Howship's lacuna, 46–49

Huxley's layer, 104, 105
Hypophysis, 196–199

Ileum, 152, 153
Infundibular stalk of hypophysis, 196,
     197
Integument, 104–111
Intercalated disc, 62, 63
   duct, 124–129, 172, 173
Intercellular bridges of skin, 104, 105
Interglobular dentin, 120, 121
Interlobular duct, of lacrimal gland, 250,
     251
   of mammary gland, 246, 247
   of pancreas, 172, 173
   of salivary glands, 124–129
Interstitial cell of testis, 208, 209
Intestine, large, 154–158
   small, 148–153
   smooth muscle layers of, 62, 63
Involution of corpus luteum, 224, 225
Iris, 252, 253
Islets of Langerhans, 172, 173

Jejunum, 150, 151
Juxtaglomerular apparatus, 188, 189

Kidney, 186–191
Kupffer cells, 166, 167

Labial glands, 112, 113
Lacrimal gland, 250, 251
   accessory, 248, 249
Lacteal, central, 144, 152, 153
Lactiferous duct, 244–247
Lacunae, Howship's, 46–49
   of bone, 40–43, 46
   of cartilage, 36–39
   of Morgagni, 218, 219
Lamellae of bone, 40, 41
   circumferential, 40, 41
   inner circumferential, 40, 41
   interstitial, 40, 41
   outer circumferential, 40, 41
Lamina fusca (suprachoroid layer), of
     eye, 254, 255
Lamina propria, of appendix, 158, 159
   of bladder, 194, 195
   of cardia, 136, 137
   of cervix, 238, 239
   of ductus deferens, 212, 213
   of esophagus, 130–135
   of gallbladder, 170, 171
   of large intestine, 150–158
   of lip, 112, 113
   of nose, 174, 175
   of rectum, 160–163

Lamina propria (*continued*)
   of seminal vesicle, 216, 217
   of small intestine, 148–153
   of stomach, 138–145
   of tongue, 114–119
   of trachea, 180, 181
   of ureter, 192, 193
   of uterine tube, 228, 229
   of uterus, 230–235
   of vagina, 240, 241
Langerhans, islets of, 172, 173
Large intestine, 150–157, 160–163
Larynx, 176–179
Lens, 252, 253
  suspensory ligament of, 252, 253
Leukocytes, 52–55
Lieberkühn, crypts (glands) of, 148–163
Lip, 112, 113
Lissauer's tract, 78–81
Liver, Altmann's stain of, 168, 169
  Best's carmine stain of, 168, 169
  Del Rio Hortega's stain of, 168, 169
  glycogen in, 168, 169
  laminae (plates), 164–167
  lobules of, 164–169
  sinusoids of, 164–169
Lung, 182–185
Lutein cells, granulosa, 226, 227
    theca, 226, 227
Lymph nodes, 94–99
Lymphatic nodules, of appendix, 158, 159
  of ileum, 152, 153
  of lymph node, 94–97
  of spleen, 102, 103
  of tonsil, 98, 99, 118, 119
Lymphatic vessels, 86, 87
  afferent, of node, 94, 95
  efferent, of node, 94, 95
Lymphoblasts, 98, 99
Lymphocytes, 52–55, 93–103
  proliferation of, 98, 99

Macrophages, in bone marrow, 56, 57
  in connective tissue, 28, 29
  in liver (Kupffer cells), 166, 167
  in lymphatic tissue, 98, 99, 102, 103
  in placenta (Hofbauer cells), 236, 237
Macula lutea, 252, 253
Mallory-azan stain, of bone, 42, 43
  of esophagus, 134, 135
  of heart, 92, 93
  of nerve, 74, 75
Mammary glands, 26, 27, 244–247
Mast cells, 28, 29
May-Grünwald-Giemsa stain of blood, 52, 53, 58, 59
Medullary cord of a lymph node, 93–97
  ray of kidney, 186–191
  sinus of a lymph node, 93–97
Megakaryocytes, 46, 49, 58, 59

Meibomian glands, 248, 249
Meissner's corpuscle, 104, 105
Membrana granulosa, 221–223
Membrane, cell, 14, 15
Mesenchymal cell, undifferentiated, 30, 31
Mesentery, 154, 155
Mesothelium, of the peritoneum, 14, 15, 138, 139, 194, 195
  pleural, 182, 183
  uterine tube, 228, 229
Mesovarium, 220, 221
Metamyelocyte, 56, 57
Microglia, 66, 67, 70, 71
Mitochondria in liver cells, 168, 169
Modiolus, 256, 257
Moll, glands of, 248, 249
Monocyte, 52–55, 58, 59
Motor end plates, 64, 65
Mucosa, gastric, 138–143
  of bladder, 194, 195
  of cervix, 238, 239
  of ductus deferens, 212, 213
  of esophagus, 130–135
  of gallbladder, 170, 171
  of large intestine, 150–158
  of lip, 112, 113
  of rectum, 160–163
  of seminal vesicle, 216, 217
  of stomach, 138–145
  of trachea, 180, 181
  of uterine tube, 228, 229
  of vagina, 240, 241
  olfactory, 174, 175
Müller's cells, 254, 255
Muscle, cardiac, 62, 63
  ciliary, 252, 253
  muscle spindle, 64, 65
  orbicularis oculi, 248, 249
  orbicularis oris, 112, 113
  Riolan's, 248, 249
  skeletal, 60–65
  smooth, 60–63
  tarsal, 248, 249
  thyroarytenoid, 178, 179
  trachealis, 180, 181
  vocalis, 178, 179
Muscularis externa, of appendix, 158, 159
  of esophagus, 130, 131, 134, 135
  of large intestine, 154–157
  of small intestine, 148–153
  of stomach, 138, 139
Muscularis mucosae, of appendix, 158, 159
  of esophagus, 130–137
  of large intestine, 154–157
  of pylorus, 144, 145
  of rectum, 160, 161
  of small intestine, 148–153
  of stomach, 138–143

Myelinated nerve fibers, 72–75
  sheath, 72–75
Myelocyte, 58, 59
Myocardium, 90–93
  muscles of, 62, 63
Myoepithelial cell, 108, 109, 124–129
Myofibrils, 60, 61
Myometrium, 230–235

Nerve cell body, 66–69, 76–81
  fibers, 72–75
  terminations, transverse section of,
    72–75
Nervous tissue, 72–75
Neurofibrils, 64, 65, 72, 73
Neuroglia (neuroglial cells), 70, 71
  of the hypophysis, 198, 199
Neurolemma, 74, 75
Neurovascular bundle, 88, 89
Neutral red, blood cells, 54, 55
  connective tissue, 28, 29
Neutrophil, 52–59
Nissl bodies, 66, 67, 80, 81
Normoblast, 58, 59
Nose, 174, 175
Nucleus dorsalis, 80, 81
  lateral sympathetic, 80, 81

Odontoblast of teeth, 122, 123
Oligodendrocytes, 66, 67, 70, 71
Oocytes, 204–209
Optic papilla, 252, 253
Ora serrata, 252, 253
Organ of Corti, 256, 257
Orbicularis oculi muscle, 248, 249
  oris muscle, 112, 113
Os, cervical, 238, 239
Ossification, endochondral, 44–47
  intramembranous, 42–43
  secondary centers of, 50, 51
Osteoblasts, 42–49
Osteoclasts, 42, 43, 46–49
Osteocytes, 40, 42, 43, 46–49
Osteons, 40, 41
Ovarian follicles, 220–225
Ovary, 220–225
Oxyphilic cell (acidophilic cell) of
    parathyroids, 202, 203

Pacinian corpuscle, in dermis, 108–111
  in pancreas, 172, 173
  in tendon, 32, 33
Pancreas, 172, 173
  Gomori's stain of, 172, 173
Paneth cels, 150, 151
Papilla, circumvallate, 116–119
  filiform, 114, 115
  fungiform, 114, 115

of kidney, 186, 187, 190, 191
  of tongue, 114, 115
  optic, 252, 253
Papillary ducts, 190, 191
Parafollicular cells of the thyroid, 200,
    201
Parasympathetic ganglion, 138, 139,
    148–151, 156–161
Parathyroid glands, 202, 203
Parietal cells of stomach, 138–143
Parotid gland, 124, 125
Pars distalis of hypophysis, 196–199
Pars intermedia of hypophysis, 196, 197
Pars nervosa of hypophysis, 196, 197
Pars tuberalis of hypophysis, 196, 197
Penis, 218, 219
Perichondrium, 36–39, 44–47
Perimysium, 62, 63
Perineurium, 72–75
Periosteum, 42–47
Peritoneum, 138, 139, 148–159
Peroxidase reaction, 54, 55
Peyer's patch, 152, 153
Pia mater, 80, 81, 84, 85
Pituitary gland (hypophysis), 196–199
  azan stain of, 198, 199
Placenta, 236, 237
Plasma cell, 28, 29, 102, 103
Platelets, blood, 52–59
Pleura, 182, 183
Polymorphous cell of cerebral cortex, 84,
    85
Portal area of liver, 164, 165
Portal vein, 86, 87
  of liver, 164–167
Posterior chamber of eye, 252, 253
Predentin, 122, 123
Principal cell (chief cell) of parathyroids,
    202, 203
Prostate gland, 214, 215
Pulmonary trunk, heart, 92, 93
Pulmonary artery of lung, 182–185
Pulp cavity, tooth, 116, 117
Purkinje cells, of cerebellum, 82, 83
  fibers of heart, 92, 93
Pyloric glands of stomach, 144, 145
Pyloric sphincter, 146, 147
Pyloric-duodenal junction, 146, 147
Pyramid of kidney, 186, 187
Pyramidal cell of cerebral cortex, 84, 85

Ranvier, nodes of, 72–75
Rectal columns, 160
Rectum, 160–163
Red pulp of spleen, 102, 103
Reissner's (vestibular) membrane, 256,
    257
Renal corpuscle, 188, 189
  papilla, 186, 187, 190, 191
  pyramid, 186, 187

Reticular cell, of bone marrow, 56, 57
   of lymph node, 96, 97
Reticular fibers of liver, 168, 169
   of lymph node, 96, 97
Retina, 252–255
   blind, 252, 253
   ciliary, 252, 253
   iridial, 252
   optic, 252, 253
Retzius, lines of, 120, 121
Rods of retina, 254, 255
Root canal of tooth, 120, 121

Salivary glands, 124–127
Sarcolemma, 60, 62
Sarcoplasm, 60, 62, 63
Satellite cells, 76, 77
Scala tympani, 256, 257
   vestibuli, 256, 257
Scalp, 108, 109
Schmidt-Lantermann clefts, 72, 73
Schreger, bands of, 120, 121
Schwann sheath (neurolemma), 74, 75
Sclera, 252–255
Sebaceous gland, of eyelid, 248, 249
   of integument, 104, 105, 108, 109
   of lip, 112, 113
   of penis, 218, 219
Seminal vesicles, 216, 217
Seminiferous tubules, 206–209
Serosa, of gallbladder, 170, 171
   of large intestine, 154–157
   of small intestine, 148–153
   of stomach, 138, 139
Serous demilunes, 126, 127
Sertoli cell, 208, 209
Sinusoids, of bone marrow, 44, 45, 48,
      49, 56, 57
   of liver, 164–169
   of lymph node, 94–97
   of spleen, 102, 103
Skin, Cajal's trichromic stain of, 104, 105
   of palm, 104, 105
   of scalp, 108, 109
   thick, 104, 105, 110, 111
   thin, 104, 105
Small intestine, 148–153
Spermatid, 208, 209
Spermatocytes, primary, 208, 209
   secondary, 208, 209
Spermatogonium, 208, 209
Spermatozoa, 208, 209
Sphincter, anal, 162, 163
   pyloric, 146, 147
Spinal cord, 78–81
   anterior horn of, 66–69
   cervical region, 78, 79
   thoracic region, 80, 81
Spiral ganglion (of Corti), 256, 257
Spleen, 102, 103

Splenic cords (of Billroth), 102, 103
Spongiocytes, 204, 205
Stains (other than hematoxylin-eosin)
   Altmann's, mitochondria in liver cells,
      168, 169
   aniline blue, bone, 40, 41
      nerve, 74, 75
   azan, hypophysis, 198, 199
   Best's carmine, glycogen in liver, 168,
      169
   Cajal's silver, cerebellum, 82, 83
      cerebral cortex, 84, 85
      spinal cord, 78, 79
      trichromic, skin, 104, 105
   Celani's, 54, 55
   cresyl blue, reticulocytes, 54, 55
   Del Rio Hortega's, reticular fibers,
      168, 169
   Fontana's silver, enteroendocrine
      cells, 150, 151
   Gallego's, elastic fibers, 150, 151, 180,
      181
   Golgi's, nerve cells, 68, 69
   Gomori's chrome hematoxylin-
      phloxine, 172, 173
   hematoxylin-orcein, elastic cartilage,
      38, 39
   iodine, glycogen, in vaginal
      epithelium, 240, 241
   Janus green, mitochondria in
      leukocytes, 54, 55
   Mallory-azan, bone, 43
      esophagus, 134, 135
      nerve fibers, 74, 75
      Purkinje fibers, 92, 93
   May-Grünwald-Giemsa, bone marrow,
      58, 59
      peripheral blood, 52, 53
   neutral red, leukocytes, 54, 55
      loose connective tissue, 28, 29
   orcein, elastic fibers, aorta, 88, 89
      cartilage, 38, 39
   osmic acid, fat, 168, 169
      bile canaliculi, 166, 167
   Pappenheim's, 54, 55
   PAS hematoxylin, 110, 111
   Protargol, nerve fibers, 74, 75
   Shorr trichrome, 242, 243
   Van Gieson's, esophagus, 134, 135
   Verhoeff's, elastic fibers, 34, 35
Stellate cell, of cerebellum, 82, 83
   of cerebral cortex, 84, 85
   of liver (Kupffer cell), 166, 167
Stereocilia, 210, 211
Stomach, chief cells of, 136–143
   fundus or body of, 138–143
   gastric glands of, 136–143
   mucosa of fundus or body, 138–143
   parietal cells of, 136–143
   pyloric mucosa of, 144, 145
   zymogenic cells of, 136–143

Stratum corneum, 104–109
  basale, 104–109
  granulosum, of skin, 104, 105
  lucidum, 104, 105
  spinosum, 104–109
Striated border of epithelium, 16, 17,
     148–157
Striated duct, 124–127
Striations in muscle, 60–63
Stroma, corneal, 250, 251
  ovarian, 220–225
Subcapsular sinus (marginal sinus) of
     node, 94–99
Sublingual gland, 128, 129
Submandibular gland, 126, 127
Submucosa, of appendix, 158, 159
  of esophagus, 130–133
  of rectum, 160, 161
  of small intestine, 148–153
  of stomach, 138–143
Substantia propria of cornea, 250, 251
Sulcus, posterior median, of spinal cord,
     78–81
Suprachoroid layer of eye, 254, 255
Sweat glands, 104–109
Sympathetic ganglion, 76, 77, 88, 89
  cells, 76, 77
  lateral nucleus, of spinal cord, 80, 81
     cells, 80, 81

Tactile corpuscle (Meissner's), 104, 105
Tarsal gland, of eyelid, 248, 249
Tarsal muscle, 248, 249
Tarsus, 248, 249
Taste buds, 116, 117
Tectorial membrane, 256, 257
Teeth, 120–123
  development of, 122, 123
Tendon, 32, 33
Testis, 206–213
Theca externa, 222, 223
  follicular, 220–223
  interna, 222, 223
  lutein cell, 224, 225
Thymus gland, 100, 101
Thyroarytenoid muscle, 178, 179
Thyroid gand, 200, 201
Tissue, adipose, 34, 35
  bone, 40–43
  cardiac, 62, 63
  cartilage, 36–39
  connective, 28–35
     dense, 30–33, 34, 35
     embryonic, 34, 35
     loose, 28–31, 34, 35
  epithelial, 14–27
  fibrous connective, 28–33
  muscular, 60–63
  nervous, 72–75
  osteogenic connective, 48, 49

skeletal muscle, 60–63
  smooth muscle, 60–63
Tomes, fibers of, 122, 123
  granular layer of, 120, 121
  processes of, 122, 123
Tongue, 114–119
  longitudinal section of, 114, 115
  skeletal muscles of, 62, 63
  transverse section of, 116–119
Tonsil, laryngeal, 178, 179
  lingual, 118, 119
  palatine, 98, 99
Tooth, developing, 122, 123
Tooth, dried, 120, 121
Trabeculae, of bone, 42, 43
  of lymph node, 94–99
  of penis, 218, 219
  of spleen, 102, 103
Trachea, 180, 181
  cartilage of, 36, 37, 180, 181
  epithelium of, 20, 21
  glands of, 36, 37, 180, 181
Tracheal cartilage, 180, 181
  muscle, 180, 181
Tubules, collecting, of kidney, 188–191
  distal convoluted, 188, 189
  proximal convoluted, 188, 189
  seminiferous, 206–209
Tunica adventitia of an artery, 73, 86–89
  albuginea, of ovary, 220–223
     of penis, 218, 219
     of testis, 206, 207
  intima, 86–89, 92, 93
  media, 86–89, 92, 93

Ureter, 192, 193
Urethra, cavernous, 218, 219
  prostatic, 214, 215
Urinary bladder, 194, 195
Uterine glands, 230–235
Uterine tube, 228, 229
Uterus, follicular phase of, 230, 231
  menstrual phase of, 234, 235
  secretory phase of, 232, 233
Uvea, 252, 253

Vagina, 240, 241
  exfoliate cytology (smears), 242, 243
  glycogen in cells of, 240, 241
Vas deferens (ductus deferens), 212, 213
Vasa vasorum, 86–89
Veins, central, of liver, 164–169
  interlobular, of kidney, 186–189
  intralobular (central) of liver, 164–169
  portal, 86, 87
     of liver, 164–169
  renal, 186, 187
  transverse section of, 86, 87
  tunica adventitia of, 86, 87
     intima of, 86, 87
     media of, 86, 87

Ventral (anterior) median fissure, of
    spinal cord, 78–81
Ventricle, of heart, 90–93
  of larynx, 178, 179
Vermiform appendix (appendix), 158,
    159
Vestibular (Reissner's) membrane, 256,
    257
Villi, of intestine, 16, 17, 148–153
  of placenta, 236, 237
Visceral pleura of lung, 182, 183
Vitreous chamber of eye, 252, 253
    humor, 252, 253

Vocal cords (vocal ligaments), 178, 179
  folds, false, 178, 179
    true, 178, 179

White matter, of eye, 252, 253
  of spinal cord, 78–83
  pulp of spleen, 102, 103

Zona glomerulosa, of adrenals, 204, 205
Zona fasciculata, of adrenals, 204, 205
Zona pellucida, of oocyte, 222, 223
Zona reticularis, of adrenals, 204, 205
Zymogenic cells, of pancreas, 172, 173
  of stomach, 140–143